CARDIAC PACING
A PHYSIOLOGICAL APPROACH

Asit Das
MD (General Medicine) DNB (Cardiology)
Clinical Tutor
Department of Cardiology
Institute of Postgraduate Medical Education and Research (IPGMER)
and SSKM Hospital
Kolkata, West Bengal, India

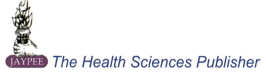

JAYPEE *The Health Sciences Publisher*
New Delhi | London | Philadelphia | Panama

Jaypee Brothers Medical Publishers (P) Ltd.

Headquarters
Jaypee Brothers Medical Publishers (P) Ltd
4838/24, Ansari Road, Daryaganj
New Delhi 110 002, India
Phone: +91-11-43574357
Fax: +91-11-43574314
E-mail: jaypee@jaypeebrothers.com

Overseas Offices

J.P. Medical Ltd
83, Victoria Street, London
SW1H 0HW (UK)
Phone: +44 20 3170 8910
Fax: +44 (0)20 3008 6180
E-mail: info@jpmedpub.com

Jaypee-Highlights Medical Publishers Inc.
City of Knowledge, Bld. 237, Clayton
Panama City, Panama
Phone: +1 507-301-0496
Fax: +1 507-301-0499
E-mail: cservice@jphmedical.com

Jaypee Medical Inc.
325, Chestnut Street
Suite 412, Philadelphia,
PA 19106, USA
Phone: +1 267-519-9789
E-mail: jpmed.us@gmail.com

Jaypee Brothers Medical Publishers (P) Ltd
17/1-B, Babar Road, Block-B, Shaymali
Mohammadpur, Dhaka-1207
Bangladesh
Mobile: +08801912003485
E-mail: jaypeedhaka@gmail.com

Jaypee Brothers Medical Publishers (P) Ltd
Bhotahity, Kathmandu, Nepal
Phone: +977-9741283608
E-mail: kathmandu@jaypeebrothers.com

Website: www.jaypeebrothers.com
Website: www.jaypeedigital.com

© 2016, Jaypee Brothers Medical Publishers

The views and opinions expressed in this book are solely those of the original contributor(s)/author(s) and do not necessarily represent those of editor(s) of the book.

All rights reserved. No part of this publication may be reproduced, stored or transmitted in any form or by any means, electronic, mechanical, photocopying, recording or otherwise, without the prior permission in writing of the publishers.

All brand names and product names used in this book are trade names, service marks, trademarks or registered trademarks of their respective owners. The publisher is not associated with any product or vendor mentioned in this book.

Medical knowledge and practice change constantly. This book is designed to provide accurate, authoritative information about the subject matter in question. However, readers are advised to check the most current information available on procedures included and check information from the manufacturer of each product to be administered, to verify the recommended dose, formula, method and duration of administration, adverse effects and contraindications. It is the responsibility of the practitioner to take all appropriate safety precautions. Neither the publisher nor the author(s)/editor(s) assume any liability for any injury and/or damage to persons or property arising from or related to use of material in this book.

This book is sold on the understanding that the publisher is not engaged in providing professional medical services. If such advice or services are required, the services of a competent medical professional should be sought.

Every effort has been made where necessary to contact holders of copyright to obtain permission to reproduce copyright material. If any have been inadvertently overlooked, the publisher will be pleased to make the necessary arrangements at the first opportunity.

Inquiries for bulk sales may be solicited at: jaypee@jaypeebrothers.com

Cardiac Pacing: A Physiological Approach

First Edition: **2016**
ISBN: 978-93-5250-182-3
Printed at Sanat Printers, Kundli.

Dedicated to

My parents Late Hrishikesh Dash and Smt Saraswati Dash for their unconditional love, great sacrifice and constant inspiration

My wife Arundhati and our daughter Anushka for their love, support and encouragement

All my teachers, Cardiologist friends, colleagues and Physicians, who will find the book useful.

Preface

Technological advancement has contributed to unprecedented developments in cardiac pacing in the last 50–60 years following the first implantable pacemaker in 1958. Cardiac pacing has evolved over the years. This revolution involves better engineering aspects of the device, more efficient batteries, functional designs and new materials. Latest technological innovation in the field of pacemaker is the development of leadless pacemaker. Contemporary pacemakers carry a number of functions that make them to provide more physiologic performance while avoiding the negative effects of unnecessary pacing. However, little work has been done to develop techniques to position the pacemaker leads into the sites which are more physiological. We have gathered knowledge and experience from the works of some pioneer investigators of this field. I have tried to assemble their works and find out easier way to physiological cardiac pacing in this book.

I hope with the book that readers should derive an improved understanding of the physiological cardiac pacing and know the strengths and weaknesses of various pacing strategies.

Asit Das

Acknowledgments

I am extremely grateful to my teachers who taught me about physiological cardiac pacing and insisted me to practice it. I am grateful to Dr Achyut Sarkar for his help. I sincerely thank all of the technical staff of the catheterization laboratory, whose efficiency made all the implant procedures safe for our patients. Finally, I acknowledge the cooperation of my patients on whom I have performed the implantations.

Contents

1. **History of Pacemaker** — 1

2. **Introduction to Physiological Pacing** — 16
   Adverse effects of RV Apical Pacing *16*
   Electrocardiographic Changes *16*
   Morphological Changes *22*
   Metabolic Changes *25*
   Mechanical *26*

3. **Managing Algorithm** — 41
   Strategies of reducing Pacing Burden *41*
   AV Search Hysteresis *42*
   Managed Ventricular Pacing (MVP) *43*
   Ventricular Intrinsic Preference (VIP) *47*
   AAIsafeR Mode *47*
   Reverse Mode Switch (RhythmiQ Mode) *50*
   Outcome Data *50*

4. **Selective Site: Right Ventricular Septal Pacing** — 60
   Anatomy *61*
   Radiology *66*
   Tools and Technique *68*
   Electrocardiographic Characteristics *72*
   Cardiomyopathy and RV Pacing *86*
   Evidence *86*

5. **Selective Site: His Bundle Pacing** — 90
   Anatomy *90*
   Electrocardiographic Characteristics *92*
   Indications *96*
   Implantation *98*

6. **Selective Site: Right Atrial Septal Pacing** — 106
   Anatomy *106*
   Electromechanics *108*
   Implantation *121*

7. **Case Discussion** — 138
   Case 1 *138*
   Case 2 *143*
   Case 3 *146*
   Case 4 *151*
   Case 5 *154*
   Case 6 *157*

8. **Introduction to Cardiac Resynchronization Therapy** — 163
   Indication *166*

9. Role of Pre-procedure ECG Analysis — 202
Role of Surface ECG *202*
Case 1 *210*
Case 2 *212*

10. Anatomy of Coronary Sinus — 215
Anatomy *215*
Venography *221*
Other Imaging Modalities *224*
Target Vein and Target Site *225*

11. Implantation Technique — 230
Approach *230*
Lead Implantation Order *231*
Placement of LV Lead *231*
Buddy Wire Technique *236*
Retrograde Buddy Wire Technique *237*
Venoplasty *238*
Anchor Balloon Technique *240*
Antegrade Snare Technique *242*
Retrograde Snare Technique *243*
Balloon-facilitated Delivery *243*
Placement of RV lead *245*
Anatomical Inter-lead Distance *247*
Electrical Inter-lead Distance *249*
Alternative Techniques *251*
Epicardial Pacing Techniques *253*
Endocardial Pacing Techniques *255*

12. Surface Electrocardiography: CRT Follow up — 259
ECG of Right Ventricular Pacing in CRT *259*
Case 1 *270*
Case 2 *273*
Case 3 *275*
Case 4 *281*
Case 5 *283*
Case 6 *288*
Fusion *290*

13. Optimizing Response — 295
Definition of Response *295*
Responders and Super-responders *296*
Cardiac Assist Devices *306*

14. Newer Advances — 309
Multisite and Multipoint LV Pacing *309*

Index *325*

CHAPTER 1

History of Pacemaker

The history of pacing is an exciting story of initiative and innovation, often in the face of criticism and opposition. It is a unique mix of medicine, technology and marketing which has developed into a major industry and has brought electrotherapy out of the labs and into the clinics. Electrotherapy has a simple core concept: the use of an outside source of electricity to stimulate human tissue in various ways to produce a beneficial therapeutic effect. Over the last sixty years or so, electrotherapy has shown an explosive development. This was the consequence of a remarkable co-operation among surgeons, physicians, engineers, chemists, businessmen and patients. Most of the scientists and physicians involved in electrotherapy faced significant criticism by the contemporary scientific community. Yet the speciality moved steadily on gaining medical respectability and now helps countless patients all over the world.

Since the era of Hippocrates (460–375BC) physicians were aware of syncope. Innovative works by different scientists at different times enriched the history of pacemakers gradually. In late 1800's an English doctor **John Mac William** collected and analyzed all the scattered data available at that time and laid down the basic concepts of modern pacing accurately identifying many of the treatment's problems. The first external cardiac pacemaker has been developed by two doctors working independently on the opposite sides of the world: the Australian anesthesiologist **Mark Lidwell** and the American physiologist **Albert Hyman**. Lidwell's device ran on alternating current and required a needle to be inserted into the patient's ventricle. In 1928, he used intermittent electrical stimulation of the heart to save the life of a child born in cardiac arrest. The child apparently recovered completely and survived but not much else is known of Lidwell's efforts. Hyman became interested in reviving the "stopped heart" by means of "intracardiac (his term) therapy". Initially this therapy consisted of the intracardiac injection of stimulant drugs such as epinephrine although he soon realized that it was not really the drug that restarted the heart but the needle that set up an action current of injury as it punctured the cardiac wall. Hyman's device, described in 1932 (Fig. 1.1) was powered by a spring-wound hand-cranked motor and called by Hyman himself an **"artificial pacemaker"**, a term still in current use.

In his device, the electrical impulses from a DC current generator were directed into the patient's right atrium through a bipolar needle electrode introduced via an intercostal space. Pacing could be delivered at rates of 30, 60 or 120 per minute. None of the models of this device build in the 1930's survives today. Hyman' work was frustrated and eventually derailed by technical problems and the attitude of the times. The medical and social community was not ready for accepting this electro stimulation. He faced considerable opposition, including that of the Journal of the American Medical Association and did not report his experiments. During the Second World War, Hyman unsuccessfully urged the US Navy to support his device for use in resuscitation of dying servicemen.

In the early 1950's mains-powered pacemakers were developed and were large bulky boxes filled with vacuum tubes that had to be wheeled around on carts and plugged into wall mains socket outlets to obtain their alternating current power. They were portable only in name since they could only go as far as the nearest electrical outlet. **John Hopps,** an electrical engineer, was recruited on a part-time basis by the National Research Council of Canada and designed what perhaps the first electronic device was specifically built as a cardiac pacemaker. The electrical impulses were transmitted via a bipolar catheter electrode to the atria using a transvenous approach. Atrial pacing was readily achieved and heart rate could be controlled with no uncomfortable chest wall contractions.

Paul Zoll from Boston had been given the credit for ushering in the modern era of clinical cardiac pacing. He had developed

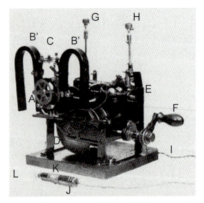

Fig. 1.1 Albert Hyman's "artificial pacemaker"

an external tabletop pacemaker that was successfully applied to the treatment of heart block. The electrodyne PM-65 pacemaker, designed by Zoll, comprised an electrocardiograph to monitor the cardiac rhythm and an electric pulse generator to pace the heart. The pulse generator was a modification of the electric stimulator used in physiology laboratories. It delivered periodic electric impulses at 2 ms pulse width and 50 to 150 volts alternating current pulse amplitude through a pair of 3 cm^2 metal electrodes strapped to the patient's chest directly over the heart. The electrodes irritated the skin and the patients of course found the repeated electric shocks painful. The mains-powered unit was bulky and heavy and was carried on a cart. It could only go as far as the extension cord would allow (Figs 1.2A and B).

In a garage in northeast Minneapolis **Earl E Bakken** and his brother-in-law **Palmer Hermundslie** had co-founded Medtronic on April 29th, 1949. The company had led a precarious existence as a repair service for hospital electrical equipment and regional distributor for other manufacturers. They would build new equipment on order or customize standard instruments for laboratory or clinical researchers. They would hang around hospital surgical suites setting up equipment, training personnel in its use and troubleshooting and repairing it as necessary. Meanwhile they forged working relationships with physicians and their staff.

The field of pediatric open heart surgery gave a major impetus to the development of pacemakers since heart block often accompanied impeccably performed intra-cardiac repairs of congenital defects. **C Walton Lillehei** was a leading cardiac surgeon at the University of Minnesota, Minneapolis and had attained international fame by the mid-50. Techniques had been developed to enter the heart and correct congenital defects while the circulation was supported. The rapidly

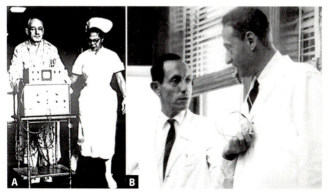

Figs 1.2A and B The PM-65: historic 1958 photo (patient was using the first catheter electrode), Paul Zoll and a colleague

evolving field of open heart surgery was to be a major driving force towards the development of cardiac pacing. Lillehei and his co-workers developed the myocardial wire: a multi-stranded, braided stainless steel wire in a Teflon sleeve. One end of this was implanted directly into the myocardium and the other end was exteriorized via a stab incision and connected to the physiology lab stimulator. An indifferent electrode was buried under the skin to complete the circuit. Effective pacing needed only 1.5 volts as there was direct contact with the myocardium. There was no rejection and no damage to the beating heart and the wire could be removed easily by tugging once normal conduction resumed. The first myocardial wire was implanted on the **30th January 1957** in a 3-year-old girl in whom heart block had complicated the repair of Fallot's tetralogy. Pacing was successful and the little girl soon regained sinus rhythm and survived. Myocardial wires started being implanted electively, ready for immediate use later should this become necessary. A technique for their implantation through a hollow needle was also developed for non-surgical patients who developed Stokes-Adams attacks. Problems soon became obvious: the stimulator was large and heavy, of limited portability and awe-inspiring especially for pediatric patients. Moreover, the system was fatally flawed since it depended totally on its external mains power supply and on the length and integrity of the extension power cord. If power supply failed, it was worthless.

On October 31st, 1957 a municipal power failure lasting three hours resulted in the tragic death of a baby. The hospital had emergency power generation in its surgical suites and recovery area but not in its patient rooms. The caregivers were once more reminded of the limitations of existing technology. The next day, Lillehei requested Bakken to come up with something better. Patient mobility needed improvement and concerns about power failure needed to be eliminated. Only after 4 weeks of experimentation and work, the first battery-powered, transistorized pacemaker was already in clinical use. The first production run of ten or so units were more. The dials had been recessed so that children would be less likely to adjust them and a little neon light blinked red with each stimulus.

In addition, two metal handles (borrowed from an old ECG machine) were been added such that a strap could secure the pacemaker to the body. The pacemaker was not only portable but wearable. This pacemaker became known as the 5800 (because it was made in 1958). Medical historians regard Bakken's pacemaker is one of the first successful applications of transistor technology to medical devices helping to launch the new field of "medical electronics" (Figs 1.3 and 1.4). In the

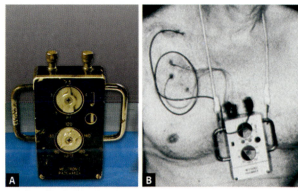

Figs 1.3A and B (A) One of the "first ten", (B) Wearable devices on patients (1958)

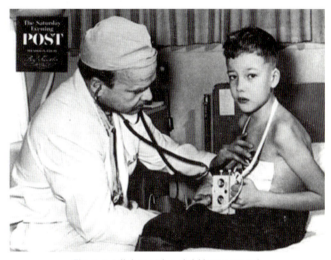

Fig. 1.4 Lillehei with a child being paced

entire history of medicine before 1957, there had never been a partly or completely implantable electrical device. It was however apparent that for long-term pacing a totally implanted device would have to be designed as ascending infection via the pacing electrodes occurred frequently.

Recurrent heart block in patients who had recovered from their postoperative heart block caused several deaths. It was apparent that these patients needed indefinite and not temporary pacing for them to survive. The myocardial wire developed exit block as scar tissue grew around the site of stimulation increasing electrical resistance and requiring a progressive increase in pacing stimulus voltage to maintain capture. The thoracic muscles began to twitch at these increased voltages. A totally implantable system with better designed electrodes needed to be designed. Meanwhile elsewhere, on the **16th July 1958** a transvenous catheter electrode was introduced fluoroscopically, via the basilic vein into the right ventricular outflow tract, in a patient with fixed complete heart block who required colon resection because of a malignancy. Pacing was continued for two hours, during the operative procedure, and ended with slowing of the stimulation rate until an unpaced idioventricular rhythm developed. The catheter was removed without complication and the patient resumed the idioventricular bradycardia.

On **October 8th, 1958** the first pacemaker implantation was performed in Sweden. The system had been developed by the surgeon **Ake Senning** and the physician inventor **Rune Elmqvist** and implanted on a 43-year-old engineer called **Arne Larsson.** This first experience with a fully implantable pacemaker system was reported at the Second International Conference on Medical electronics in 1959 and published as an abstract in 1960.

Ake Senning was the cardiac surgeon in charge of the Department of Thoracic Surgery at the Karolinska Hospital in Stockholm. He had observed Lillehei's work with temporary external pacing. Rune Elmqvist was a medical graduate who had not pursued a medical practice but became an engineer. He had designed a portable ECG machine in 1931. These two men began to collaborate closely in 1950 and developed fibrillators and defibrillators for open heart surgery. They realized that the main problem with external pacemakers was the open route for ascending infection along the lead and decided to design a fully implantable system.

Arne Larsson is the first human to receive an implanted pacemaker. He had been hospitalized with complete heart block and frequent Stokes-Adams attacks for 6 months. He was having 20 to 30 attacks daily and his prognosis was poor. Treatment was maximized with ephedrine, pentymal, atropine, isoprenaline, caffeine, digoxin and whisky. Else Marie was the patient's wife who pleaded with Elmqvist and Senning to help her seriously ill husband. She had read press reports about ongoing experiments with electrical stimulation of the heart and hounded down the two scientists for a solution that did not yet exist: **an implantable pacemaker**. To avoid publicity, the implantation was done in the evening when the operating rooms were empty. Via a left-sided thoracotomy two suture electrodes were implanted into the myocardium and tunnelled to the pacemaker box placed in the abdominal wall. The first pacemaker implanted functioned only a few hours but the second one implanted in the same patient had better longevity.

The pulse generator delivered impulses at an amplitude of 2 volts and a pulse width of 1.5 ms. The pulse rate was fixed at a constant rate of 70 to 80 beats per minute. The energy utilized was minimized since Elmqvist managed to obtain a few of the first silicon transistors imported into Sweden. These were more efficient than the older germanium transistors. With them Elmqvist designed a stable and efficient blocking oscillator with a small power consumption. The Ruben-Mallory cells with zinc as the anode and mercuric-oxide as the depolarizer were used. Although the cell potential remained constant, these cells had a short lifetime and released hydrogen gas at the zinc anode. The effect of this gas in a cell encapsulated in plastic was not known. For these reasons, nickel-cadmium rechargeable cells were then chosen. Two cells of 60 mA each were sealed, encapsulated and connected in series. Recharging was accomplished inductively. A coil antenna with a diameter of about 50 mm was connected to the cells via a silicon diode. This was inductively coupled across the patient's skin to a large external flexible coil 25 cm in diameter attached to the patient's abdomen with adhesive tape. Recharging was accomplished by a 150 kHz radio frequency current generated by an external mains-powered vacuum tube device connected to the external coil. The pacemaker required charging once a week. The entire unit was entirely hand-made and consisted of the nickel-cadmium batteries, the electronic circuit and the coil recharging antenna (Figs 1.5A and B). These were encapsulated in a new epoxy resin (Araldite) produced by Ciba-Geigy, which had excellent biocompatibility. The approximate diameter and thickness became 55 mm and 16 mm respectively, according to the dimensions of the ever so popular shoe polish can from Kiwi. Elmquist in fact produced two such units using these cans as moulds.

Rune Elmqvist soon ceased his involvement in pacing but remained active in other areas of medical technology. He died

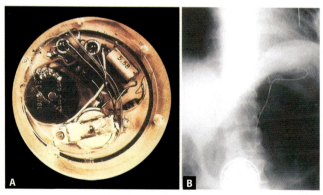

Figs 1.5A and B (A) First implanted pacemaker; (B) X-ray of Larsson showing pacemaker and leads

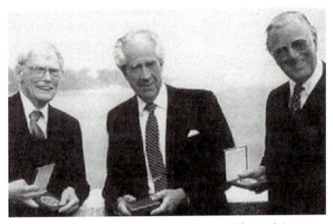

Fig. 1.6 Elmqvist, Senning and Larsson (left to right)

in 1997, aged 90. Ake Senning remained very active in the field of cardiac surgery. He died in 2000 at the age of 84. Arne Larsson survived both the engineer as well as the surgeon who had saved his life (Fig. 1.6). He required five lead systems and 22 pulse generators of 11 different models until his death on December 28th 2001 aged 86 of a malignancy totally unrelated to his conduction tissue disease or his pacemaker system.

Wilson Greatbatch was an electrical engineer teaching at the University of Buffalo where he was working on an oscillator to aid in the recording of tachycardias. He accidentally discovered the way to make an implantable pacemaker. **Dr William Chardack** was chief of surgery at Buffalo's Veteran's Hospital at the time. In Dr Chardack, Greatbatch had finally found a surgeon who believed in the viability of an implantable pacemaker.

On May 7, 1958, Greatbatch brought what would become the world's first implantable pacemaker to the animal lab at the hospital. There, Chardack and another surgeon, **Dr Andrew Gage,** exposed the heart of a dog to which they touched the two pacing wires. The heart proceeded to beat in synchrony with the device. The three looked at each other. Over the first two years experiments were made with animals. In 1959, Greatbatch patented the implantable pacemaker, and William Chardack reported the first success in a human with this unit in 1960. The procedure was completed in **June 1960** on a 77-year-old man in complete heart block. Chardack first implanted the lead and when threshold stabilized implanted the pulse generator. The patient survived uneventfully for 2 years before his death from natural causes. The three - Greatbatch and Drs Chardack and Gage - became known as the bow tie team (Fig. 1.7).

Faulty batteries, body fluids leaking into the encasement and broken leads caused numerous pacemaker failures that

History of Pacemaker

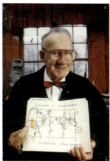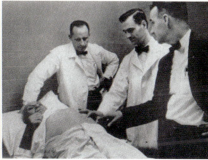

Fig. 1.7 Greatbatch and his "Bow Tie Team"

required emergency surgery. The main difficulty however was the lead. It was soon obvious that the myocardial wire was unsuitable as a long-term electrode. Stimulation threshold increased after a few weeks until exit block developed and no more capture was possible. Moreover, the wire could not resist the enormous repetitive mechanical stresses of bending. These technical problems contributed to the delay in the widespread use of implanted pacemakers for several years. Tight collaboration between engineers, physicians and patients was the fundamental driving force for the growth of a significant global industry. Well over 2 million pacemakers have been implanted worldwide since 1960.

- **Zoll** founded Electrodyne and continued developing pacemakers.
- **Earl Bakken** (co-founder of Medtronic Inc.) started producing the Chardack-Greatbatch pacemaker.
- **Wilson Greatbatch**, after a time with Medtronic, founded his company (Wilson Greatbatch Ltd.) and convinced the industry to change from mercury to lithium-iodine cells.
- The company ***Elema Schonander,*** for which Rune Elmqvist worked, became ***Siemens-Elema*** in 1974. Siemens then acquired Pacesetter Inc. in 1985 and combined them to form Siemens-Pacesetter which was then in turn acquired by St Jude Medical in 1994.

Other investigators followed a different line of approach in designing self-contained implantable pacemakers: inductive coupling. A pair of electrodes were sutured to the epicardium and connected to a coil antenna located subcutaneously. Minimal or no circuitry was implanted and no internal batteries were needed. This coil antenna was inductively coupled to an external coil taped to the patient's intact skin. This external coil was connected in turn to a transistorized pulse generator powered by an external battery. The electronic components, relatively unreliable at this time, were therefore located entirely outside the body. Glenn, Mauro, Longo, Lavietes and Mackay's technique utilized a radio-frequency oscillator. Later versions of this system included triple-helix; silicone insulated endocardial leads and rate-control via an external knob (which the patient himself could modify at will).

Atrial pacing with this device was used in 1969. Inductively-coupled pacemakers proved to be very successful with several hundreds of implants and survival rates of over 10 years. These devices were extensively used in the Birmingham (UK) region for a number of years, being produced by the Lucas factory, more commonly known for its automotive electrical products (until taken over by Bosch). One particular disadvantage of this device was that its removal (for example, for bathing) could result in bradycardia and syncope. They continued to be used until well into the 1970's and several patients with later generation pacemakers still have the implanted coils from their original devices.

On the 4th April 1959 **Samuel Hunter** (Professor of Surgery at St Paul) and **Norman Roth** (Chief Engineer at Medtronic) implanted a bipolar stainless steel electrode to pace a patient suffering from post-myocardial infarction complete heart block. The lead consisted of a pair of stainless steel wires secured in a silicone rubber base.

A new lead was developed in 1959 by Elema Schonander and the Telecom Company, Ericcson. This consisted of four thin bands of stainless steel wound around a core of polyester braid and insulated with soft polyethylene. It was estimated to resist over 184 million flex cycles, hence lasting for at least 6 years. The unipolar epicardial stimulation electrode was a platinum disc, 8 mm in diameter and insulated at the back. The Elema 135 (Fig. 1.8) rechargeable pacemaker was successfully implanted in Stockholm (1959), Uruguay (February 1960) and England (March 1960) but Elema Schonander never filed a patent application. The market prospects were perceived to be poor. Pacemakers were considered as an expensive service to prominent customers with little commercial value. The external charging system was too complicated especially for elderly patients.

Elmqvist constructed the Elema 137 pacemaker in 1960. Ruben-Mallory zinc-mercury oxide cells were used as the power source thus eliminating the need for periodic recharging of the previously utilized nickel-cadmium cells. The technique for inserting permanent transvenous bipolar pacing electrodes **without thoracotomy** was developed in 1962 by **Parsonnet**, et al. (in the US) and by **Ekstrom** et al. (in Sweden).

Pacemaker and lead technology continued to develop rapidly to make these devices reliable, automatic and flexible

History of Pacemaker 11

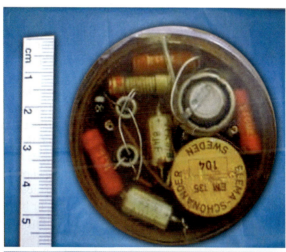

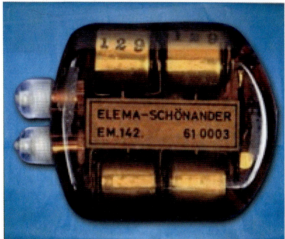

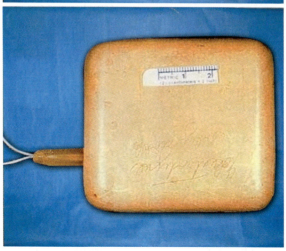

Fig. 1.8 The Elema 135, The Elema 142 (with non-rechargeable cells), Zoll device

in the therapy they provide. The therapeutic end-point shifted from saving life to enhancing its quality and simplifying follow-up. In mid 1960's transvenous leads replaced epicardial leads. Pacemakers and their leads could be implanted without a thoracotomy and without general anesthesia. "Demand" pacemakers were developed to sense the underlying cardiac activity and provide pacing only when needed. In 1970's lead design improved: "tined" for passive fixation and "screw-in" for active fixation. The lithium-iodine battery was developed to replace the mercury oxide-zinc battery that had been used till then. This resulted in greatly increased pacemaker longevity.

In 1972, an American-made radioisotope pacemaker was implanted by Parsonnet et al. These nuclear pacemakers had an expected life of 20 years but went out of fashion mainly due to the need for extensive regulatory paperwork. Titanium casing was developed to enclose the battery and circuitry. This replaced the epoxy resin and silicone rubber that was previously utilized to encase the internal components of the pacemaker. Pacemakers were made non-invasively programmable in the mid-1970. Using a radio-frequency telemetry link, most pacing parameters could be adjusted to follow the changing clinical needs of the patient. By the end of the 70's dual-chamber pacemakers were developed to pace and sense in both atria and ventricles. Synchronized timing made it possible to preserve the atrial contribution to ventricular filling as well as to track the intrinsic atrial rate. In the early 1980's steroid-eluting leads were developed. These eluted steroid from their tip and hence decreased the inflammatory response evoked by the presence of the lead tip (acting as a foreign body). Consequently, the early rise of capture threshold was blunted and safety was enhanced.

In 1981, Zoll patented and re-introduced a transcutaneous external pacemaker with a longer pulse width of 40 ms and a larger electrode surface area of 80 cm^2. This reduced the current necessary to capture the heart and thus improved patient comfort. This method of pacing could be applied very rapidly as a bridge to the establishment of pacing via the transvenous route. In the mid-1980's rate-responsive pacemakers were designed. A tiny sensor within the pacemaker box detected body movement and used this as a surrogate measure of activity. Signals from the sensor were filtered and applied to an algorithm to alter the pacing rate up or down. Thus, pacing rate would change according to the patient's activity level. Microprocessor-driven pacemakers appeared. These became very complex devices capable of detecting and storing events utilizing several algorithms. They delivered therapy and modified their internal pacing parameters according to the changing needs of the patient in an automatic manner. The rate-response pattern also adjusted itself automatically to the patient's activity level. Bi-ventricular pacing for heart failure was introduced with an additional specially-designed lead was introduced via the coronary sinus to the epicardial surface of the left ventricle (Fig. 1.9). The right ventricle (via the standard lead) and the left ventricle were paced simultaneously to attempt to resynchronize contraction of the left ventricular septum and left ventricular lateral walls. The improved contraction improved symptoms and survival. Automaticity progressively increased thus making follow-up visits easier and briefer. Pacemakers could also upload data telephonically to a central server via the internet. Latest addition to the list is MRI-compatible pacemaker. New pacing systems have recently been specifically designed by the major companies for safe use in the MRI environment (Fig. 1.10).

Permanently implantable pacing leads evolved from the temporary pacing wires that were first used to provide

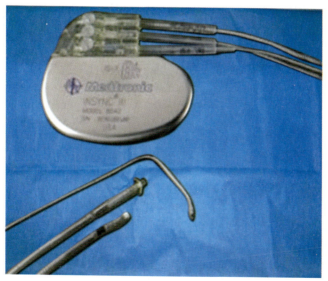

Fig. 1.9 Biventricular pacemaker

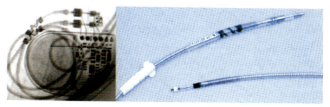

Fig. 1.10 MRI-compatible pacemaker and lead. System is identified by coil markers on the proximal lead and by device markings

bradycardia support. The initial permanent transvenous leads were unipolar and consisted of a basic conductor, an insulator, and a connector pin. The electrodes were large and polished with high-polarization properties, low electrode-tissue impedance, and excessive current drain. No lumen was present in these leads to allow for stylet insertion, so lead implantation was a long, difficult task. Also, no fixation mechanism was present, so lead displacement rates were high. The development of bipolar pacing leads minimized far-field over-sensing, requiring a major reconsideration of lead body design and structure, because two longitudinal conductors needed to coexist inside the lead, separated only by a thin layer of insulation. This and subsequent increases in complexity required advances in materials science so as not to compromise reliability.

The development of passive-fixation tines was a huge step forward and dramatically reduced the rate of re-operation for lead dislodgement compared with existing flange-tipped pacing leads. Active-fixation helices were introduced subsequently and further improved the stability of implanted leads. Modern electrodes were developed with small geometric surface area but large effective area as a result of porous surfaces, and these optimized the trade-off between high current density and low polarization. Chronic threshold rises and late exit block were still major problems in cardiac pacing at that stage, however, and remained so until the revolutionary incorporation of an elutable dexamethasone reservoir into a porous-tip electrode, essentially eliminating this complication. Although this likely resulted from the glucocorticoid and not the redesigned porous titanium-tip electrode, this remained unproved until a pioneering randomized double-blind trial compared two otherwise identical leads and electrodes, with and without steroid elution. This unequivocally demonstrated the benefit was the result of the dexamethasone. Subsequent advances have included the universal standardization of connector pins (and consequently device headers), improving lead longevity through the use of better component materials, and improving sensing through the use of narrower bipoles.

Latest technological innovation in the field of pacemaker is the development of leadless pacemaker. Leadless pacemaker is a very small (Fig. 1.11) device yet so powerful, a fully functional VVIR pacemaker which is implanted endocardially using 18F delivery system through femoral vein. Hence, exclude the chance of lead related problems (i.e. lead infection, fracture and exit block etc.). It can be implanted in a target site with a total procedural time of not more than 15 to 20 minutes. It can also be retrieved when required by catheter-based retrieval system.

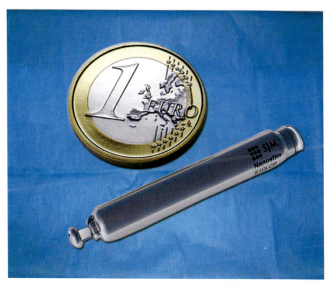

Fig. 1.11 Nanostim™ leadless pacemaker (Courtesy St Jude Medical)

BIBLIOGRAPHY

1. A Brief History of Cardiac Pacing by Glen Nelson.
2. Earl Bakken's Little White Box: The Complex Meanings of the First Transistorised Pacemaker by David Rhees and Kirk Jeffrey.
3. First Artificial Pacemaker: A Milestone in the History of Cardiac Electrostimulation.
4. History of Cardiac Rhythm Disorders by B Luderitz.
5. History of electrotherapy http://www.hrsonline.org/ep-history/.
6. Images Paediatric Cardiology. 2006;8(2):17-81.
7. Landmarks in Cardiac Surgery by Stephen Westaby.
8. One Man's Full Life by Earl Bakken.
9. The Bakken: A Library and Museum of Electricity in Life.
10. Wilson Greatbatch: Man of the Millennium by Joseph Radder.

CHAPTER 2

Introduction to Physiological Pacing

INTRODUCTION

From its first human implantation (October 8th, 1958 by Swidish Surgeon Ake Senning) the right ventricular apical pacing has saved millions of lives. But, within one decade it was proved to be nonphysiological as it causes several deleterious hemodynamic effects. Right ventricular apical pacing alters left ventricular electrical and mechanical activation. Chronic right ventricular apical pacing causes left ventricular dilatation and reduction in left ventricular ejection fraction by a process called 'remodeling'. It causes some cellular and subcellular changes which persist for long-time even in absence of continued pacing. These changes have been related to increased mortality and morbidity in patients with ventricular pacemakers.

ADVERSE EFFECTS OF RV APICAL PACING

In general, the negative effects of right ventricular (RV) apical pacing have been attributed to the abnormal electrical and mechanical activation pattern of the ventricles. During RV apical pacing, the conduction of the electrical wave front propagates through the myocardium, rather than through the His-Purkinje conduction system. As a result, the electrical wave front propagates more slowly and induces heterogeneity in electrical activation of the myocardium, comparable to left bundle branch block. This is characterized by a single breakthrough at the interventricular septum and the latest activation at the inferoposterior base of the left ventricular (LV). Various acute and long-term deleterious effects of right ventricular apical pacing are summarized in Table 2.1.

ELECTROCARDIOGRAPHIC CHANGES

Normal activation of the ventricles starts with conduction of the electrical impulse from the atrioventricular (AV) node to the His bundle. From the His bundle, at the superior margin of the muscular interventricular septum, the right bundle branch

Introduction to Physiological Pacing

Table 2.1 Short- and long-term effects of right ventricular (RV) apical pacing

Metabolic changes: • Changes in regional perfusion   • Changes in oxygen demand
Remodeling: • Asymmetric septal hypertrophy   • Left ventricular and left atrial dilatation   • Functional mitral regurgitation   • Histopathological changes
Hemodynamics: • Decreased cardiac output   • Increased left ventricular (LV) filling pressures
Mechanical function: • Changes in myocardial strain   • Interventricular mechanical dyssynchrony   • Intraventricular mechanical dyssynchrony
Miscellaneous: • Increased risk of atrial fibrillation   • Promotion of ventricular arrhythmia   • Activation of sympathetic nervous system

proceeds intramyocardially as a thin, unbranched extension of the His bundle along the right side of the interventricular septum and terminates in the Purkinje plexuses of the right ventricular (RV) apex, at the base of the anterior papillary muscle. The left bundle branch also has a short intramyocardial route in the interventricular septum before giving rise to its two branches: anterior and posterior fascicle. A third fascicle is also described recently, known as centroseptal fascicle, supplies the mid-septal area of the LV and arises either from the main left bundle branch or from its anterior or posterior subdivision, or from both. The anterior subdivision is longer and thinner than the posterior one. For this reason it is more vulnerable to damage, so that conduction disturbances along this fascicle are much more common than the ones involving the posterior fascicle. The three subdivisions continue in a network of Purkinje fibers, located subendocardially in the lower third of the septum and in the anterior free wall, and extending to the papillary muscles. The Purkinje fibers are long and large. The numbers of gap junctions in these fibers are very high resulting in their very fast conduction velocity. During normal antegrade excitation, fast propagation over these long fibers, together with the wide distribution of Purkinje—myocardial junctions, induces a high degree of electrical coordination between distant regions of the myocardium. His bundle as well as the right and the left bundle branches are electrically isolated from the adjacent working myocardium. The only sites where the Purkinje system and the normal working cells are electrically

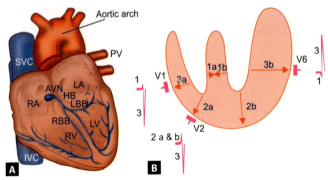

Figs 2.1A and B (A) Normal AV node and infranodal conduction system, (B) Diagram illustrating the mechanism of normal intraventricular conduction. With normal intraventricular conduction, activation of the ventricles begins in the left lower third of the interventricular septum and spreads transversely from left to right through the septum. This left-to-right vector, however, is opposed by the smaller right-to-left septal vector which originates from the right bundle branch, and which arises in the right side of the interventricular septum (vector 1). Paraseptal activation occurs next, spreading transversely from endocardial to epicardial surfaces (vector 2). This is followed by endocardial-epicardial activation of the free walls both in right and left side.
Abbreviations: SVC, superior vena cava; IVC, inferior vena cava; RA, right atrium; LA, left atrium; AVN, AV node; HB, common bundle of His; RBB, right bundle branch; LBB, left bundle branch; RV, right ventricle; LV, left ventricle.

coupled are the so-called Purkinje—myocardial junctions, located subendocardially both in the RV and in the LV. Impulse conduction in the Purkinje system is from base to apex and occurs quickly (3–4 m/s).[1] The activation of the myocardial muscular tissue in the septum occurs mainly from apex to base.[2] In the LV and RV free wall, impulse conduction also occurs from apex to base and from endocardium to epicardium. As a consequence of this impulse conduction, the posterobasal area is the last activated part of the ventricles. The electrical impulse is conducted approximately four times slower (0.3–1 m/s) in the normal myocardium than in the Purkinje system. In humans, total ventricular activation lasts 60–80 ms, corresponding with a QRS duration of 70–80 ms.[2]

Three-dimensional electroanatomical mapping data suggests that in the normal heart, the first site of endocardial ventricular activation (endocardial breakthrough site) is usually in the LV, at the interventricular septum or in the anterior region. Within approximately 10 ms the activation begins in the RV endocardium, near the insertion of the anterior papillary muscle, i.e. the exit of the right bundle branch.[7] After activation of these regions, depolarization wave fronts proceed simultaneously in the LV and RV, predominantly from apex to base and from septum to lateral wall in both ventricles (Figs 2.2A and B). The latest activated endocardial region of the RV is the basal area near the AV sulcus and the pulmonary conus. Overall, the posterolateral/basal area of the LV is the last part of the heart to be depolarized. Simultaneous depolarization wave front occurs centrifugally from the endocardium to the epicardium. However, the earliest ventricular epicardial activation site (epicardial breakthrough site) occurs usually at the pretrabecular area of the RV from where there is a radial spread towards the apex and the base, within the subepicardial layers.[7] In a normal heart, the duration of total ventricular electrical activation is 50–80 ms. The short ventricular activation time stresses the important role of the Purkinje fibers system in the synchronization of electrical myocardial activity. So, pacing in the right ventricular outflow tract (RVOT) septal region seems to produces a more physiological electrical activation sequence and endocardial-epicardial breakthrough pattern.

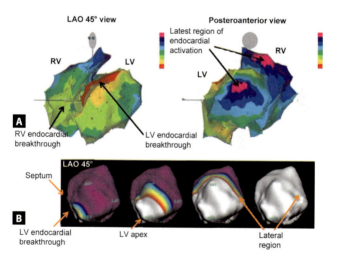

Figs 2.2A and B (A) Color-coded (red indicating the earliest and purple the latest activation site) 10 ms isochronal maps, obtained with contact electroanatomical mapping system, of biventricular activation in a normal heart. The earliest endocardial ventricular activation site (breakthrough site) is recorded in the LV anterior septal region (red spot). The latest activated regions are the posterolateral walls of both RV and LV; (B) Unipolar isopotential maps, recorded with noncontact mapping system of LV activation sequence in a normal heart. The LV endocardial breakthrough is recorded in the septum. The activation wave front (white spot) proceeds fast toward the anterior, then to the lateral region and finally to the posterior region.
(*Courtesy:* Cecilia Fantoni, Angelo Auricchio. Electrical activation sequence in 'Cardiac Resynchronization Therapy' 2nd edition, editor: Cheuk-Man Yu, David L. Hayes, Angelo Auricchio, pub. Blackwell Futura, 2008 with permission)
Abbreviation: LAO, left anterior oblique

Normally, the right ventricle (RV) contraction is a complicated peristaltic movement beginning in the inflow region and extending to the outflow tract.[3] The RV is largely silent during conventional electrocardiography because it generates weak electrical forces completed early in the QRS complex and mostly concealed by left ventricle (LV) depolarization. In patients with left bundle branch block (LBBB), surface electrocardiographic recordings demonstrated rapid initial myocardial activation (short rS duration) suggestive of intact right bundle branch (RBB) conduction despite the presence of LV conduction abnormalities.[4,5] The activation pattern likely reflects the course of the RBB, which passes down the septum to the base of the anterior papillary muscle and then fans out into multiple free-running false tendons terminating in the free wall as a profuse subendocardial Purkinje network. This generates nearly simultaneous activation of the free wall in a radial manner, likely responsible for initiation of RV contraction from the inflow tract to outflow tract.[6] In contrast, the LV free wall depolarizes from apex to base (Fig 2.3).

The electrical effects of RV pacing are similar to left bundle branch block (LBBB). The QRS configurations are similar. LV activation occurs transseptally after RV depolarization in both. The RV-paced wave-fronts propagated slowly from apex to base, in contrast to rapid and radial spread during intrinsic activation. The prolongation of the duration of global RV activation by RV pacing is driven by slow conduction areas generated locally around the stimulus site. Delay permits intrinsic right bundle branch-mediated conduction to contribute to RV free wall depolarization, resulting in varying degrees of wave-front fusion (Fig. 2.4). The pattern and duration of RV free wall activation are the outcome of the balance of intrinsic **(centrifugal)** and RV-paced **(centripetal)** wave-fronts. When RV-paced delays are less, global RV activation duration is not delayed (although direction of depolarization is different from intrinsic conduction). In contrast, when intrinsic AV conduction is absent or poor, the RV is committed to activation by the RV pacing and RV activation duration is longer. RV pacing also disturb septal depolarization.

Data from the literature indicate that the extent of synchrony and sequence of activation during ventricular pacing are determined by at least four myocardial properties: (1) the poor coupling of the ectopically generated impulse to the rapid conduction system. The impulses coming from the normal myocardium can enter the Purkinje system only at the apical part, the sites where during normal conduction the impulse exits this system. Therefore, in most cases the sequence of activation during ventricular pacing is governed

Introduction to Physiological Pacing

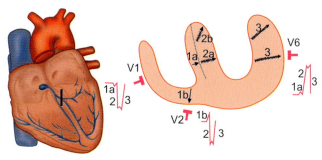

Fig. 2.3 *The mechanism of left bundle branch block:* Right septal activation—ventricular activation begins in the right side of the interventricular septum and proceeds from right to left through the septum. This results in a small right-to-left vector which is the normal right septal vector (vector 1a). Unlike normal intraventricular conduction, this is not opposed by a concomitant greater left-to-right force of the left septal mass. This unopposed vector will results in a small initial positive deflection in leads oriented to the left side of the interventricular septum (lead V6) and a small negative deflection in leads oriented to the right side of the interventricular septum (lead V1). This component is very small and needs sensitive ECG machine to record. *Delayed and anomalous left septal activation:* Following right septal activation, the activation process "jumps", the intraseptal physiological barrier (dotted line) and activates the left side of the septum in a delayed and anomalous fashion. This results in vectors of large magnitude which are directed to the left and posteriorly (vector 2). This results in a tall R wave in leads oriented to the left side of the septum (lead V6) and a deep S wave in the leads oriented to the right side of the septum (lead V1). Further delay in the activation of the superior region of the interventricular septum (vector 2b) may result in a slurred or notched plateau at the apex of the bizarre QRS complex recorded by left-oriented leads (lead V6), and a slurred or notched nadir in the right-oriented leads (lead V1). *Delayed and anomalous activation of the free left ventricular wall*: Septal activation is followed by delayed and anomalous activation of the free left ventricular wall. This results in a vector of large magnitude which is directed to the left and posteriorly as well as somewhat superiorly (vector 3) which is reflected by a tall R' deflection in left-oriented leads (lead V6) and a deep secondary S wave in right-oriented leads (lead V1)

by the slow conduction through the normal myocardium, away from the pacing site,[7] (2) because the conduction through the myocardium is up to four times slower than conduction through the Purkinje system, activation of the entire ventricular wall is more asynchronous than during normal sinus rhythm and atrial pacing, (3) the conduction velocity is approximately two times faster in the direction parallel to muscle fiber length (isotropic conduction) than in the direction perpendicular to them (anisotropic conduction).[8] Therefore, in a particular layer, the wave-front has an elliptic shape. Because fiber-orientation changes by more than 90° across the LV wall,

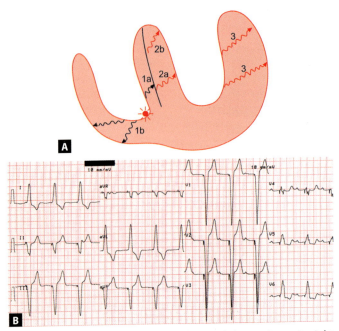

Figs 2.4A and B The mechanism of electrical dyssynchrony in right ventricular apical pacing: (A) Different vectors: blue arrow indicates the balanced vector of intrinsic (centrifugal) and RV-paced (centripetal) wave-fronts stimulating RV free wall and RV septum, red arrow indicates slow propagation of wave front though the myocardium activating LV septum and LV free wall, star indicates pacing site; (B) Resultant 12 lead surface ECG

and because impulses are also conducted in transmural direction, a complex three-dimensional helical wave-front is present in the LV wall during pacing,[9] (4) the most endocardial fibers, even though not part of the Purkinje system, conduct impulses faster than the fibers in the major part of the LV wall.[10]

To summarize, normal physiological activation of the ventricles is characterized by minimal asynchrony, monotonic activation, earlier LV than RV activation, and earlier apical than basal activation. During LBBB and RV apex pacing, the activation sequence deviates significantly from the physiological one.

MORPHOLOGICAL CHANGES

Normal cardiac contraction efficiently uses the geometric spiral arrangement of ventricular myocardial fibers. Activation of the specialized His-Purkinje system enables depolarization to occur in an established fashion with nearly simultaneous biventricular activation. However, cellular and molecular structures are not constant and are influenced and molded by electrical and hemodynamic forces. Therefore, alternative stimulus initiation can produce abnormal contraction patterns that affect ventricular synchrony changing regional myocardial blood flow with a redistribution of fiber strain.[11] This ultimately produces altered segmental wall shortening, abnormal metabolism, and inefficient work. The findings of more adverse cellular and subcellular alterations in patients with chronic RV apical pacing favors the concept that altered contractile stresses associated with chronic right ventricular apical pacing may adversely effect myocardial cellular growth.

Varying combination of the following various abnormal histopathological changes (Figs 2.5A and B) are noted in patients with prolonged right ventricular apical pacing:[12]
- Myofiber hypertrophy,
- Myofiber variation,
- Endocardial sclerosis,
- Fat infiltration,
- Interstitial fibrosis,
- Altered mitochondrial size, number, or histologies.

Studies have shown that these ultrastructural changes indicate that the site of origin of ventricular stimulation, *per se*, and not artificial electrical stimulation or loss of atrioventricular (AV) synchrony, appears to be responsible for the observed compensatory cellular remodeling as changes are not seen in patients with right ventricular septal pacing.[13]

Three important morphological alterations are noted in patients with chronic right ventricular apical pacing: **ventricular dilatation, asymmetric septal hypertrophy, and septal hypoperfusion**. These structural adaptations in the left ventricle are the results of asynchronous electrical activation from right ventricular apical pacing.

Left ventricular dilatation and dyssynchrony leading to deterioration of left ventricular function in chronic right ventricular apical pacing is secondary to a process also known as '**remodeling**'. Pacing at right ventricular apex disturbs the natural pattern of activation and contraction because conduction of the electrical wave front takes place slowly through ventricular myocardium rather than through the His-Purkinje system (electrical dyssynchrony). The mechanical effect of asynchronous electrical activation is dramatic because the various regions differ not only in the time of onset of contraction, but also in the pattern of contraction. Early contracting regions close to the pacing site stretch not-yet activated remote regions. This stretching further delays shortening of these late-activation regions and increases

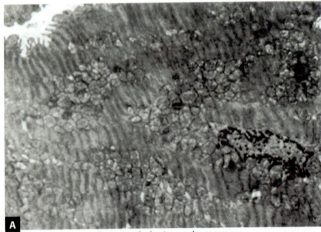
Prepaced electron microscopy

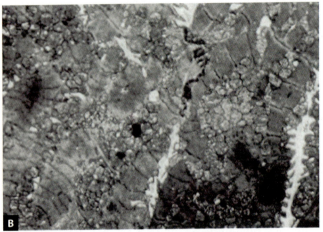
Postpaced electron microscopy

Figs 2.5A and B (A) Prepaced electron micrograph (EM) illustrating clumping of an increased number of relatively normal-appearing mitochondria but with preservation of the normal myofiber arrangement; (B) Postpaced EM compared with A, mitochondrial aggregates appear abnormal with variable sizes and shapes, distorting and thinning the surrounding myofibers. (Original magnification X12.500)
(*Courtesy:* Peter P Karpawich, Raja Rabah, and Joel E. Haas: Altered Cardiac Histology Following Apical Right Ventricular Pacing in Patients with Congenital Atrioventricular Block. PACE 1999; 22:1372-1377 with permission).

their force of local contraction by virtue of the (local) Frank-Starling mechanism. Because of their vigorous contraction, the late-activated regions impose loading on the earlier activated territories, which now undergo systolic paradoxical stretch. This reciprocated stretching of regions within the LV wall causes a less effective and energetically less efficient contraction.[14] The local differences in contraction pattern in the paced ventricle imply a redistribution of mechanical work, perfusion, and oxygen demand within the LV wall.[11] All these in long-term give rise to gradual dilatation of the left ventricle.

Asymmetrical hypertrophy in patients with RV apical pacing is most likely due to the redistribution of workload, as evidenced by the regional differences in circumferential shortening in systole (CSsys) and external work.[15] Regional differences in macroscopic hypertrophy are related to regional differences in myocyte diameter without differences in regional collagen content, indicating that the hypertrophy is due to a proportional increase of myocyte and collagen volume (discussed later).

Most interestingly, the mechanical dyssynchrony induced by RV apical pacing can persist even when the pacing is withdrawn (i.e. in absence of electrical asynchrony) probably because of cellular derangements, such as, myofibrillar cellular disarray, dystrophic calcification, disorganized mitochondria and down-regulation of proteins involved in calcium homeostasis and impulse conduction, in late-activated regions. Increased sympathetic stimulation, resulting in elevated myocardial catecholamine levels, also contributes to the development of asymmetric hypertrophy. The late-activated, most-hypertrophied regions show the most pronounced cellular derangements, such as down-regulation of proteins involved in calcium homeostasis and impulse conduction leading to dystrophic calcifications and disorganized mitochondria and myofibrillar cellular disarray.

METABOLIC CHANGES

Total myocardial work is reduced by 50% in early-activated regions and is increased by 50% in late-activated regions, as compared with the situation during normal electrical activation, as during atrial pacing.[16] Several studies report regional differences in myocardial blood flow, glucose uptake, and oxygen consumption during ventricular pacing, which are similar to the differences in mechanical workload. [17-19] As compared to sinus rhythm myocardial blood flow and oxygen consumption are approximately 30% lower in early-activated regions and approximately 30% higher in late-activated regions. Several observations support the idea that the regional differences in myocardial blood flow and oxygen consumption are caused by the regional differences in workload. Lactate extraction decreases and oxygen extraction increases when perfusion becomes insufficient. Regional perfusion adapts well to an altered mechanical load. Interestingly, the regional differences in blood flow during pacing disappear during total coronary vasodilatation by adenosine.[20] Therefore, it seems likely that regional differences in mechanical work increase regional oxygen requirements, which are met by local autoregulation of myocardial blood flow. Another explanation to this the regional differences in blood flow can be due to impediment of perfusion by the abnormal contraction and relaxation patterns at high heart rates (during rapid pacing) as it leaves less diastolic time for perfusion. However, considerable and/or frequent restriction of septal perfusion would have led to stunning or hibernation. Studies have shown that stunning is unlikely to occur, because systolic shortening does not deteriorate during longer lasting LBBB.[21] There are also no biochemical signs of hibernation. Hibernation, characterized by myocyte dedifferentiation due to longer lasting mild to moderate under perfusion, can increase myocardial glycogen three-fold. No signs of glycogen accumulation were observed in any study. The lack of hibernation is in agreement with a good balance between oxygen supply and demand in asynchronously activated ventricles which has previously been found during acute ventricular pacing. Throughout paced ventricles regional systolic shortening, mechanical work, and oxygen uptake are mutually related to each other. Moreover, under these conditions no lactate release occurs and complete vasodilatation attenuates the abnormal blood flow distribution, suggesting that coronary autoregulation is responsible for the effects. This is further supported by the immediate normalization of blood flow distribution upon resynchronization of the activation in chronic LBBB hearts. Therefore, the reduced septal contractility in the presence of reduced contractile performance, as frequently reported in patients, does not exclude adequate septal perfusion. Rather, the reduced septal perfusion during LBBB appears to be the result of autoregulation following a reduction in local oxygen demand in early activated myocardium (so, can be considered as 'functional'). The functional implication of reduced septal perfusion in LBBB hearts is under debate.

MECHANICAL

Impaired Pump Function

Normally synchronous mechanical activation and ventricular contraction is due to rapid and homogeneous electrical activation with minimal temporal dispersion throughout the left ventricular wall. Right ventricular apical pacing disturbs the natural pattern of activation and contraction as the evoked electrical wave front propagates slowly through ventricular myocardium rather than through the His-Purkinje system.

The dyssynchronous contraction patterns caused by abnormal ventricular activation during RV apex pacing induce a spectrum of systolic and diastolic hemodynamic abnormalities (Flow chart 2.1). An abnormality usually limited to ventricular pacing (not seen with indigenous LBBB) is uncoupling or improper timing of atrial and ventricular contraction, leading to impaired filling and mitral regurgitation.

Earliest ventricular depolarization occurs in the anterior right ventricle (RV) surface and latest at the posterior or posterolateral basal left ventricle (LV) surface (**Interventricular dyssynchrony**). As a result there is a considerable time delay between the opening of the pulmonic and aortic valves. This disruption to ventricular interdependence leads to paradoxical septal motion. However, this motion is not actually paradoxical, because it is really the net result of different forces. The motion is caused by dynamic alterations in transseptal pressure differences and presystolic shortening of septal muscle fibers as a result of the asynchrony between RV and LV. Abnormal septal motion results in a diminished contribution of the interventricular septum to LV ejection. However, delayed intraventricular activation is presumably the most important determinant of reduced pump function. The increased intraventricular asynchrony gives rise to prolonged isovolumic contraction and relaxation phases without an

Flow chart 2.1 Schematic relationship between the various consequences of asynchronous activation of the ventricles, resulting from ventricular pacing and the deterioration of pump function over time

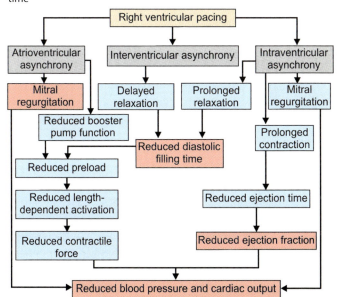

increase in the total duration of systole. As a result, the duration and the extent of ejection are reduced. Slow intramyocardial conduction during RV apical pacing prolongs QRS duration with left bundle branch block (**Electrical dyssynchrony**) and causes **intraventricular dyssynchrony** (electrical activation starts in the interventricular septum and ends with the posterior or posterolateral basal LV wall more than 100 msec later). Asynchronous electrical activation leads to asynchronous contraction. Region that are activated early also start to contract early. An additional cause of the reduction in pump function during asynchronous activation is mitral valve insufficiency. This diminishes LV pump function directly by reducing the volume ejected into the aorta and indirectly by reducing LV cavity volume.

During right ventricular apical pacing, local contraction patterns differ not only in the onset of contraction, but also, and more importantly, in the pattern of contraction (Figs 2.6A to E). These contraction patterns imply that opposing regions of the ventricular wall are out of phase and that energy generated by one region is dissipated in opposite regions. In patients with RV apical pacing, the early-contracting region is most often the lower septum. The earliest-contracting fibers can shorten rapidly by up to 10% just during the isovolumic contraction phase, because the remaining muscle fibers are still in a relaxed state. This rapid, early shortening is followed by an additional but modest systolic shortening, eventually followed by systolic stretch (from delayed mechanical contraction of other regions, in lateral wall), and premature relaxation. In late-activated regions, the fibers are stretched in the early systolic phase (up to 15%) from contraction of the early-activated region. Doubling of net systolic shortening and delayed relaxation occur in late-activated regions. This lack of coordination between early- and late-activated regions leads to lower output and reduced efficiency of the heart as a pump. This regional differences in contraction pattern most likely results from the local differences in myocardial fiber length during the early systolic phase. Furthermore, during ventricular pacing, regional systolic fiber shortening increases with greater isovolumic stretch. Similarly, a close correlation exists between the time of local electrical activation and the extent of systolic fiber shortening. Therefore, the regional differences in contraction pattern during ventricular pacing are most likely caused by regional differences in effective preload and local differences in the contraction force triggered by the Frank-Starling relation. Contraction of early-activated myocardium is energetically inefficient because LV pressure is low and ejection has not begun. Instead, stretching of remote regions not yet activated

Introduction to Physiological Pacing

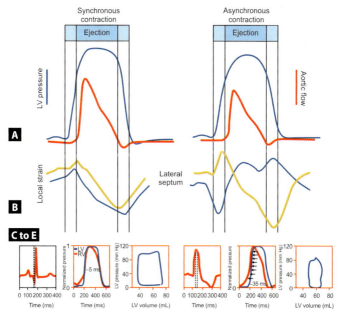

Figs 2.6A to E Effects of synchronous (left panel) and asynchronous (right panel) ventricular activation on LV and aortic pressure (A), regional strain (B), ventricular conduction (C), electrocardiographic tracings, RV and LV pressure signals (D), and pressure-volume loops (E). Asynchronous contraction causes reduction in ejection time and slows rates of rise and fall of LV pressure and aortic pressure and increases duration of isovolumetric contraction (IC) and relaxation (IR) (A). Onset of LV shortening (strain) is regionally delayed (negative deflection of curve) (B). Asynchronous electromechanical activation induces increased QRSd (C) and interventricular/intraventricular activation times (D), which instantaneously reduce stroke volume, stroke work, dP/dt_{max}, and dP/dt_{min}, indicating an acute reduction in pump function (E).
Courtesy: Sweeney MO, Prinzen FW: Ventricular pump function and pacing: physiological and clinical integration. Circ Arrhythmia Electrophysiol 1:127-139, 2008

absorbs the energy generated by the early-activated regions. This stretching further delays shortening of these late activation regions and increases their force of local contraction by virtue of the Frank-Starling mechanism (locally enhanced preload). Vigorous late systolic contraction at delayed sites occurs against high LV cavity pressures (locally enhanced after-load) and imposes loading on the earlier activated regions, which now undergo systolic paradoxical stretch. This reciprocated stretching of regions within the LV wall causes a less effective and energetically efficient contraction.

As a consequence of the slower contraction and relaxation, isovolumic contraction and relaxation phases last longer, thus leaving less time for ventricular filling and ejection. Therefore, it is not surprising that cardiac output and systolic arterial and LV pressures are also affected by dyssynchronous activation. In general, stroke volume is affected more than systolic LV pressure, presumably because baroreflex regulatory mechanisms partly compensate the decrease in blood pressure. In addition to reduced stroke volume at unchanged preload, ejection fraction is usually found to be depressed during ventricular pacing. Similarly, ventricular pacing can increase pulmonary wedge pressure. The negative inotropic effect of ventricular pacing under various loading conditions is clearly illustrated by a rightward shift of the LV function curve, that is, the relationship between cardiac output and mean atrial pressure.

The hemodynamic consequences of the asynchronous LV contraction are reductions in contractility and relaxation. These changes occur immediately on initiating RV apical pacing. The loss of pump function is indicated by decreases in stroke volume, stroke work, and slower rate of rise of LV pressure. Moreover, the left ventricle operates at a larger volume in order to recruit the Frank-Starling mechanism. Premature relaxation in early-activated regions, and delayed contraction in others also causes abnormal relaxation, as expressed as slower rate of fall of LV pressure, increase in the relaxation time, and decrease of E-wave velocity amplitude on Doppler echocardiograms. These changes also lead to prolongation of the isovolumetric contraction and relaxation times, which are characteristic for asynchronous hearts. The prolongation of the isovolumetric times occurs mainly at the expense of the diastolic filling time, leading to reduced preload.

Acute loss of pump function initiates compensatory responses (Fig. 2.7). Some of these responses, after a certain time and or degree of asynchrony, may result in further impairment of pump function and clinical heart failure. There are various triggers for these 'remodeling' processes. RVA apical pacing leads to stimulation of the sympathetic system, resulting in elevated myocardial catecholamine levels, and activation of the renin-angiotensin-aldosterone system. Regional differences in stretch and mechanical load heterogeneity are most likely important stimuli for remodeling processes. Chronic asynchronous LV activation results in regional and global structural changes indicated by asymmetric hypertrophy increased end-diastolic volume, and reduced ejection fraction, as well as locally different molecular abnormalities, including reductions in sarcoplasmic reticulum calcium-ATPase and phospholamban. Even stronger regional differences in gene expression are found in failing hearts with conduction abnormalities.

Introduction to Physiological Pacing

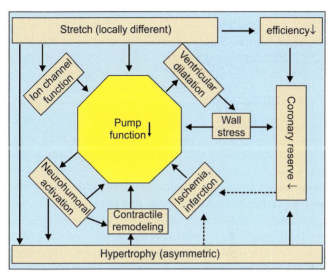

Fig. 2.7 Mechanisms of ventricular remodeling and progressive reduction in pump function during mechanical dyssynchrony induced by ventricular conduction delay (LBBB, RVA pacing). (From Sweeney MO, Prinzen FW: Ventricular pump function and pacing: physiological and clinical integration. Circ Arrhythmia Electrophysiol 1:127-139, 2008 with permission)

An adaptation of the heart to ventricular pacing occurs when the abnormal activation created by pacing is stopped but repolarization remains abnormal, a phenomenon called **cardiac memory**.[22,23] Several investigators found evidences that short-term cardiac memory (<1 hour) involves changes in ion channels and phosphorylation of target proteins, and that long-term cardiac memory (≈3 weeks of pacing) involves altered gene programming and protein expression.[24] Interestingly, in humans, cardiac memory appears to reach a steady state within 1 week. The repolarization abnormalities related to cardiac memory also have a mechanical counterpart. During sinus rhythm immediately after a period of ventricular pacing, relaxation is disturbed. Moreover, systolic function deteriorates between 2 hours and 1 week after ventricular pacing has been stopped. After ventricular pacing is stopped for 1 week, it takes 112 days for ejection fraction to return to its prepacing value. It seems likely that changes in the function of an ion channel, such as the L-type calcium channel, underlie the reduction in ejection fraction during the first week of ventricular pacing. Therefore, electrical and contractile remodeling appears to occur soon after the onset of asynchronous activation. In addition to the long-term effect on cardiac memory, longer-lasting (>1 month) ventricular pacing lead to major structural changes, such as ventricular dilatation and asymmetrical hypertrophy. The ventricular dilatation appears related to the LV operating at a larger volume. Global hypertrophy may be induced by this global dilatation, as well as by the greater sympathetic stimulation.

Mitral Regurgitation

Functional mitral regurgitation (MR) complicates and affects the prognosis of patients with coronary artery disease and congestive heart failure, and is usually associated with **incomplete mitral leaflet closure** (IMLC, defined as apically displaced coaptation with failure of the mitral leaflets to reach the level of the mitral annulus and without apparent intrinsic cusp abnormalities). It is usually accompanied by global left ventricular (LV) dysfunction and associated LV dilation which can potentially cause geometric changes in the mitral leaflet attachments. During systole mitral regurgitation is due to combined effect of reduced force to close the leaflets and geometric changes in the mitral leaflet attachments, causing augmented chordal tension and leaflet tethering. But, tethering is a potential mechanism of MR in terms of restricted leaflet opening during diastole, when the question of systolic dysfunction is no longer present.

Tethering

Tethering strongly depends on alterations in ventricular shape because the tethering forces that act on the mitral leaflets are higher in dilated, more spherical ventricles. Ventricular dilation and increased chamber sphericity increase the distance between the papillary muscles to the enlarged mitral annulus as well as to each other, restricting leaflet motion and increasing the force needed for effective mitral valve closure. In the larger ventricles, with increased separation between the mitral valve attachments, increased tethering and abnormally tensed chordae may interrupt further valve opening, aligning the anterior leaflet with the line connecting its anterior annular end and its posterior papillary muscle connection. It is also reasonable, then, that leaflet motion is limited in an anterior direction away from the papillary muscles (Fig. 2.8), whereas the increased side-to-side separation of those muscles actually allows for a wider orifice, preserving a normal total orifice area.[25] Measurably elevated chordal tension is noted when the leaflets reach their diastolic tether; it is, therefore ,reasonable that the leaflets can respond to altered tethering geometry by limited diastolic motion. This reduced excursion of the mitral leaflets is independent of transmitral flow.

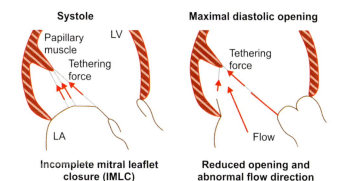

Fig. 2.8 Potential effects of augmented leaflet tethering on the mitral leaflets in a dilated left ventricle (LV) with systolic dysfunction: incomplete systolic leaflet closure because the leaflets are restricted from closing at the annular level (left), and reduced diastolic opening, redirecting inflow toward the papillary muscles (right). (Modified from Otsuji Y, et al: Restricted diastolic opening of the mitral leaflets in patients with left ventricular dysfunction: evidence for increased valve tethering. J Am Coll Cardiol 32:398-404, 1998)

Interpapillary Muscle Activation Delay

Sequence mapping with strain imaging revealed that the mechanical activation time delay between LV segments adjacent to the papillary muscles is associated with development of MR. A delay in peak strain at the mid lateral segment adjacent to the anterolateral papillary muscle, implying tethering of the mitral leaflet, which can be improved immediately after cardiac resynchronization (CRT) by coordinating the tethering forces on the papillary muscles and increasing the leaflet coaptational surface.[26]

Prolongation of Isovolumic Contraction Time

As a result of prolongation of isovolumic contraction time, there is development of a left ventricle-left atrial reverse pressure gradient when atrial contraction is not followed by an appropriately timed ventricular systole, diastolic MR is more likely with the incomplete mitral valve closure.[27] Normally, in early diastole left ventricular pressure rapidly decreased to a value lower than that of left atria pressure; this decrease results in a forward transmittal pressure gradient, opening of the mitral valve and early diastolic mitral flow. With ventricular filling the pressure at the apex increases faster than at the base or in the atrium, creating a mid-diastolic reverse transmitral gradient (Fig. 2.9). This results in rapid deceleration of early diastolic mitral flow and **near closure** of the mitral valve. Later in diastole, atrial contraction re-established a forward

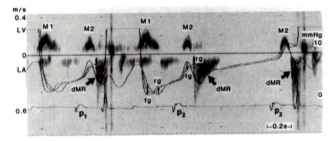

Fig. 2.9 Pulsed wave Doppler mitral flow velocity recording from the mitral valve annulus during first- and second-degree atrioventricular (AV) block (atria) pacing rate 75 beats/min. Left atrial (LA) pressure and left ventricular (LV) pressures from both the apex and the base of the ventricle are displayed. The beats of the paced P waves (p) are labeled: the first (p_1) and third (p_3) beats are conducted and the second (p_2) demonstrates AV block. Forward (left atrial to left ventricular) (fg) and reverse (left ventricle to left atrium) (rg) diastolic transmittal pressure gradients are indicated by the small arrows. Anterograde mitral flow in early diastole (M1) is associated with a forward transmitral pressure gradient (left aerial pressure > left ventricular pressure at base > left ventricular pressure at apex) and this flow slows and stops in association with a reverse pressure gradient (rg) (left ventricular pressure at apex > at base > in left atrium) of approximately the same magnitude. Similarly, mitral flow due to axial contraction (M2) is associates with a positive forward transmitral gradient. Diastolic mitral regurgitation (dMR) occurs during atrial relaxation, when a sudden decrease in atrial pressure results in a reverse transmittal pressure gradient that is larger in magnitude than either of the forward diastolic pressure gradients. The duration of diastolic regurgitation is longest with second-degree AV block (p_2), when there is no ventricular systole or increase in ventricular pressure to close the mitral valve. Diastolic mitral regurgitation is also seen on the first and third beats (p_1 and p_3), which have a PR interval of 195 and 205 ms, respectively. During these beats, the regurgitation terminates abruptly when left ventricular pressure increases and shuts the mitral valve. Large arrows indicate diastolic mitral regurgitation

pressure gradient, reopened the valve and again resulted in antegrade mitral flow. This flow is also slowed by a reverse transmitral gradient which is produced by either rapid increase in ventricular pressure or a rapid decrease in atrial pressure associated with atrial relaxation. Diastolic mitral regurgitation is seen after atrial contraction (during relaxation) during beats in which ventricular systole is absent or delayed. The peak velocity of regurgitation coincided closely in time to the peak reverse transmittal pressure gradient and the smallest mitral valve opening. Although the reverse transmittal gradients associated with rapid left ventricular filling and atrial relaxation cause near closure of the mitral valve leaflets on the M-mode echocardiogram, complete valve closure appears to occur only during the high pressures of ventricular contraction. Because the reverse transmittal pressure gradients nearly equal to or larger than the forward gradients, near closure of the valve after early ventricular filling and atrial contraction appears to be important to prevent severe diastolic regurgitation. As in single chamber RV apical pacing there is loss of atrioventricular synchrony atrial contraction is not properly timed to ventricular systole. So, there is development of mitral regurgitation.

Annular Dilatation

It is not a very important mechanism of mitral regurgitation in patients with right ventricular apical pacing.

Heart Failure

Multiple factors may contribute to heart failure associated with ventricular asynchrony. At least three candidate factors are readily identified: (1) reduced pump function caused by asynchronous contraction (dyssynchrony), (2) adverse remodeling caused by long-term dyssynchrony, (3) left-sided AV desynchronization, and (4) functional mitral regurgitation.

Atrial Fibrillation

Hemodynamic impairment of RV apical pacing may be caused by ventriculoatrial conduction and atrial contraction against a closed AV valve, which can result in elevated mean atrial pressure. Ventriculoatrial conduction can activate mechanical stretch receptors in the walls of the atria and pulmonary veins. Vagal afferents transmit these impulses centrally, and reflex peripheral vasodilatation results. In addition, various neurohormonal agents, such as atrial natriuretic peptide, are activated. These all result in vulnerability of atrial musculature for the development of different atrial arrhythmia (including atrial fibrillation).

To summarize, RV apical pacing causes abnormal electrical ventricular conduction, altered myocardial perfusion, histopathological alterations, ventricular dyssynchrony, left ventricular (LV) dilatation, and decreased LV function in an unpredictable way as a result of remodeling process consequent to abnormal ventricular activation and contraction, which ultimately results in an exacerbation of heart failure, atrial fibrillation, and an increased morbidity and mortality.

Definition of a Physiological Pacemaker

The criteria for a truly physiological pacemaker are:
- Maintenance of normal sequence and timing of atrial and ventricular activation over a wide range of heart rate (AV

synchrony) and maintenance the synchrony between right and left ventricles (Interventricular synchrony).
- Capability to vary the heart rate in response to the metabolic demand (Rate adaptability).
- Preservation of the normal rapid synchronous sequence of ventricular activation (Ventricular synchrony).

Trials of Dual Chamber Pacemaker as Physiological Pacemaker

Dual-chamber (DDD/R) pacing was developed to restore atrioventricular (AV) synchronization in patients with AV block and represented a significant technological advance. This led to an emphasis of AV synchronization in cardiac pacing, and DDD/R was quickly adopted as the 'physiologic' pacing mode. However, large randomized clinical trials in Sinus Node disease or AV block have reached a consensus that despite maintenance of AV synchrony, DDD/R pacing does not reduce death compared with single-chamber ventricular pacing (VVI/R) and has surprisingly modest or even negligible benefits for progression of heart failure (HF) and atrial fibrillation (AF) that emerge only after many years of follow-up.[28-30] The term **'physiological'** was used in Canadian Trial of Physiological Pacing (CTOPP) to reflect the terminology at the time of development of the trial.[28] Pacing the atrium and ventricle sequentially may solve the problem of unsynchronized contraction and prevention of atrial bradycardia, but the ventricular activation sequence is clearly not physiological. Studies using biventricular pacing have suggested improvement in patients with left bundle-branch block, and an extension of the theory behind this improvement suggests that right ventricular pacing might be deleterious. The Dual-chamber And VVI Implantable Defibrillator (DAVID) study randomized patients receiving implantable defibrillators (ICDs) either to backup pacing at 40 bpm or to DDD-R pacing at a rate of 70 bpm.[29] The composite end point of death or hospitalization with heart failure was greater in the group receiving DDD-R pacing than in the backup pacing group. This increased mortality and morbidity may be related to the increased heart rate or the right ventricular pacing or a combination of the two. The Mode Selection Trial in Sinus Node Dysfunction (MOST) implanted dual-chamber pacemakers in patients with sinus node disease.[30] The patients were then randomized to ventricular pacing versus dual-chamber pacing and followed up for a mean of 33.1 months. Congruent with the results of the CTOPP Extension, there was no difference in mortality, cardiovascular morbidity, or stroke. There was a very similar benefit with regard to reduction of atrial fibrillation and a significant but weak benefit with regard to hospitalization for heart failure. This mysterious inability to show an advantage of physiologic DDD/R versus nonphysiologic ventricular pacing may be explained by a factor common to all modes of ventricular pacing and also influencing short- and long-term cardiac pump function: **ventricular asynchrony.**

Two probable solutions to this problem are: **First** involves manipulation of pacing modes and timing cycle operation among patients with reliable atrioventricular (AV) conduction to minimize unnecessary ventricular pacing and preserve normal ventricular conduction (reduction of pacing burden (cumulative percent ventricular pacing [Cum%VP])) and the **second** involves pacing at alternate ventricular site(s) to attenuate the adverse effects imposed by ventricular desynchronization when ventricular pacing cannot be avoided and/or abnormal ventricular conduction is already present.

Strategies of Physiological Pacing

Before strategy formulation for a patient who needs a pacemaker, it is important to have an idea about the functional status of atrioventricular and ventricular conduction. Left ventricular pumping function should be assessed in all cases. Dyssynchrony assessment should be routinely done for patients in whom pacing burden is assumed to be high. Three possible situations are (Flow chart 2.2):

- *Both atrioventricular and ventricular conduction are normal:* Primary aim here is to protect ventricular synchrony. In presence of good LV pump function, the strategy is to implant a DDD/R pacemaker with **atrial-based pacing** algorithm. In patients with poor pump function, again the choice is atrial-based pacing and discontinue RV apical pacing if possible.
- *Ventricular conduction is normal with unreliable or absent atrioventricular conduction:* In this situation, the principle is prevent ventricular dyssynchrony by putting the lead in more physiological site as the increased pacing burden is inevitable. If the pump function is normal, choices are either RV septal or LV pacing or biventricular pacing. If the pump function is poor, options are His-bundle pacing or LV pacing or RV septal pacing. Biventricular pacing should be considered seriously if the patient is already on continuous RV pacing.
- *Abnormal ventricular conduction regardless of AV conduction status:* Here, the principle is restoration of ventricular synchrony. If the pump function is poor, the

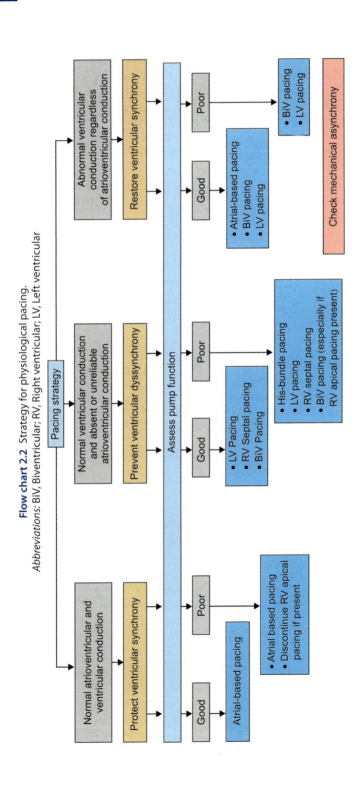

Flow chart 2.2 Strategy for physiological pacing.
Abbreviations: BiV, Biventricular; RV, Right ventricular; LV, Left ventricular

automatic choice is either viventricular pacing or LV pacing. In presence of normal pump function, the choice is atrial-based pacing if the AV conduction is normal and in presence abnormal AV conduction the strategy is to implant biventricular pacing or LV pacing.

REFERENCES

1. Myerburg RJ, Nilsson K, Gelband H. Physiology of canine intraventricular conduction and endocardial excitation. Circ Res. 1972;30:217-43.
2. Durrer D, van Dam RT, Freud GE, et al. Total excitation of the isolated human heart. Circulation. 1970;41:899-912.
3. March HW, Ross JK, Lower RR. Observations on the behavior of the right ventricular outflow tract, with reference to its developmental origins. Am J Med. 1962;32:835-45.
4. Kindwall KE, Brown J, Josephson ME. Electrocardiographic criteria for ventricular tachycardia in wide complex left bundle branch block morphology tachycardias. Am J Cardiol. 1988;61:1279-83.
5. Jia P, Ramanathan C, Ghanem RN, et al. Electrocardiographic imaging of cardiac resynchronization therapy in heart failure: observation of variable electrophysiologic responses. Heart Rhythm. 2006;3:296-310.
6. Lister JW, Klotz DH, Jomain SL, et al. Effect of pacemaker site on cardiac output and ventricular activation in dogs with complete heart block. Am J Cardiol. 1964;14:494-503.
7. Spach MS, Miller WT, Geselowitz DB, et al. The discontinuous nature of propagation in normal canine cardiac muscle. Evidence for recurrent discontinuities of intracellular resistance that affect the membrane currents. Circ Res. 1981;48:39-54.
8. Nagao K, Toyama J, Kodama I, Yamada K. Role of the conduction system in the endocardial excitation spread in the right ventricle. Am J Cardiol. 1981;48:864-70.
9. Frazier DW, Krassowska W, Chen P-S, et al. Transmural activations and stimulus potentials in three dimensional anisotropic canine myocardium. Circ Res. 1988;63:135-46.
10. Myerburg RJ, Gelband H, Nilsson K, et al. The role of canine superficial ventricular fibers in endocardial impulse conduction. Circ Res. 1978;42:27-35.
11. Prinzen FW. Augustijn CH, Arts T, et al. Redistribution of myocardial fiber strain and blood flow by asynchronous activation. Am J Physiol. 1990;259:H300-H308.
12. Aclomian CE, Boazoll J. Myofibrillar disarray produced in normal hearts by chronic electrical pacing. Am Heart J. 1986;112:79-83.
13. Lev M. The conduction system. In: SE Gould (Ed.). Pathology of the Heart and Blood Vessels, 3rd edn Springfield, IL, Charles C. Thomas Puh. 1968. pp.199-209.
14. Baller D, Wolpers H-G, Zipfers J, Bretschneider H-J. Comparison of the effects of right atrial, right ventricular apex, and atrioventricular sequential pacing on myocardial oxygen consumption and cardiac efficiency: a laboratory investigation. Pacing Clin Electrophysiol. 1988;11:394-403.

15. Van Oosterhout MF, Prinzen FW, Arts T et al. Asynchronous electrical activation induces asymmetrical hypertrophy of the left ventricular wall. Circulation. 1998;98:588-95.
16. Prinzen FW, Hunter WC, Wyman BT, et al. Mapping of regional myocardial strain and work during ventricular pacing: experimental study using magnetic resonance imaging tagging. J Am Coll Cardiol. 1999;33:1735-42.
17. Prinzen FW, Augustijn CH, Arts T, et al. Redistribution of myocardial fiber strain and blood flow by asynchronous activation. Am J Physiol. 1990;259:H300-H308.
18. Rosenbush SW, Ruggie N, Turner DA, et al. Sequence and timing of ventricular wall motion in patients with bundle branch block. Circulation. 1982;66:113-9.
19. Delhaas T, Arts T, Prinzen FW, et al. Regional fibre stress-fibre strain area as estimate of regional oxygen demand in the canine heart. J Physiol (London). 1994;477(3):481-96.
20. Amitzur G, Manor D, Pressman A, et al. Modulation of the arterial coronary blood flow by asynchronous activation with ventricular pacing. PACE. 1995;18:697-710.
21. Vernooy K, Verbeek XA, Peschar M, et al. Left bundle branch block induces ventricular remodeling and functional septal hypoperfusion. European Heart Journal. 2005;26:91-8.
22. Nahlawi M, Waligora M, Spies SM, et al. Left ventricular function during and after right ventricular pacing. J Am Coll Cardiol. 2004;44:1883-8.
23. Rosen MR. The heart remembers: clinical implications. Lancet. 2001;357:468-71.
24. Plotnikov AN, Yu H, Geller JC, et al. Role of L-type calcium channels in pacing-induced short-term and long-term cardiac memory in canine heart. Circulation. 2003;107:2844-9.
25. Otsuji Y, Handschumacher MD, Schwammenthal E, et al. Insights from three-dimensional echocardiography into the mechanism of functional mitral regurgitation: direct in vivo demonstration of altered leaflet tethering geometry. Circulation. 1997;96:1999-2008.
26. Hideaki K, Raveen B, David S. et al. A mechanism for immediate reduction in mitral regurgitation after cardiac resynchronization therapy insights from mechanical activation strain mapping. J Am Coll Cardiol. 2004;44:1619-25.
27. Appleton CP, Basnight MA, Gonzalez MS. Diastolic mitral regurgitation with atrioventricular conduction abnormalities: relation of mitral flow velocity to transmitral pressure gradients in conscious dogs. J Am Coll Cardiol. 1991;18:843-9.
28. Connolly SJ, Kerr CR, Gent M, et al. Effects of physiologic pacing versus ventricular pacing on the risk of stroke and death due to cardiovascular causes. N Engl J Med. 2000;342:1385-91.
29. The DAVID Trial Investigators. Dual-chamber pacing or ventricular backup pacing in patients with an implantable defibrillator. JAMA. 2002;288:3115-23.
30. Lamas GA, Lee KL, Sweeney MO, et al. Ventricular pacing or dual chamber pacing for sinus node dysfunction. N Engl J Med. 2002; 346:1854-62.

CHAPTER 3

Managing Algorithm

INTRODUCTION

Short- and long-term adverse hemodynamic effects of RV apical pacing are proven fact and lack of synchronized cardiac contraction was assumed to be the responsible mechanism. Contemporary thinking led to the assumption that pacing the atrium and ventricle sequentially may solve the problem of unsynchronized contraction and prevention of atrial bradycardia. So, dual chamber cardiac pacing (DDD/R) was introduced as the "physiologic" pacing mode. However, despite maintaining atrioventricular synchrony the dual chamber pacemakers (DDD/R) in different randomized controlled trials have failed to show its superiority over single chamber RV apical pacing in term of death, progression of heart failure and atrial fibrillation.[1-3] Retrospective analysis of the Mode Selection Trial (MOST) suggests that the risks of heart failure (HF) hospitalization and atrial fibrillation (AF) can be directly linked to right ventricular apex (RVA) pacing burden (cumulative percent ventricular pacing [Cum%VP]) regardless of pacing mode.[4] To minimize unnecessary ventricular pacing and preserve normal ventricular conduction manipulation of pacing modes and timing cycle operation among patients with reliable atrioventricular (AV) conduction can be done.

STRATEGIES OF REDUCING PACING BURDEN

The goals of optimized ventricular pacing when atrioventricular and ventricular conduction are normal are: (1) to prevent symptomatic bradycardia, (2) to provide chronotropic support if needed, (3) to maintain AV synchrony when necessary, and (4) to maintain normal ventricular activation sequence whenever possible.

The approaches have been proposed in pacemakers for providing atrial support while reducing ventricular pacing are (1) AAI pacing, (2) VVI/DDI pacing at low rate, (3) DDD with long AV delay, (4) Search AV hysteresis, (5) Advanced algorithms. By definition, AAI/R eliminates ventricular pacing and prevents bradycardia in patients with intact AV conduction. Problem with AAI pacing is the development of AV block requiring ventricular pacing and development of atrial fibrillation with bradycardia requiring ventricular pacing. Moreover, AAI pacing is not suitable for patients with moderate to severe AV nodal disease. An alternate approach to minimize ventricular pacing while precluding the possibility of syncope caused by AV block is to use DDD/R or DDI/R with long AV delays. Ideally dual-chamber pacemaker should provide atrial pacing, minimize ventricular pacing, and provide RV pacing if AV block or slow AF develops. This approach may yield functional AAI/R behavior in the context of a dual-chamber pacemaker. However, dual-chamber pacemakers impose limitations on maximum allowable AV delays to optimize upper-rate behavior and AF recognition and to prevent ventricular detection failures caused by cross-chamber blanking. The common consequence is high Cum%VP attributable to overlap with intrinsic AV conduction times, particularly during rate-responsive atrial pacing. Newer atrial-based dual-chamber minimal ventricular pacing modes have been developed to specifically overcome the inherent limitations of AAI/R, VVI/R, and DDD/R modes for reducing undesirable ventricular pacing. By selectively uncoupling atrial from ventricular pacing activity, these modes safely and effectively reduce mean Cum%VP to <5% in pacemaker patients. This reduction in Cum%VP is achieved without sacrificing atrial support, AV synchrony, and ventricular synchrony (unlike VVI/R), and without ventricular desynchronization because of RV apical pacing (unlike DDD/R or DDI/R).

AV SEARCH HYSTERESIS

AV search hysteresis is designed to reduce unnecessary RV pacing by allowing intrinsic AV conduction beyond the programmed AV delay during episodes of normal AV nodal function. Allowing intrinsic AV conduction via AV search hysteresis can improve hemodynamic performance and increase device longevity due to a reduced number of ventricular paces.[5] AV search hysteresis is an algorithm which is based on the programming of 2 AV delay—a short, physiologic delay and a longer AV delay. The device starts pacing with longer AV delay and continues at this setting if they find intrinsically conducted ventricular beats. If the device does not sense a QRS during the longer interval, pacing continues at the shorter physiologic programmed AV interval. It checks (or "search") for intrinsic conduction intermittently by switching to longer interval automatically after a specified number of cardiac cycles and able to program search frequency from 32–1024 cycles (Fig. 3.1). This is also known as **positive AV interval search hysteresis.** However, this algorithm is not absolutely protective as it may cause unsuccessful search (Fig. 3.2). On the contrary, the **negative AV interval search hysteresis** works in a reverse fashion. This algorithm attempts to maintain a paced QRS at all times instead of a non-paced QRS. The intention is to maintain the longest AV interval that results in a paced ventricular complex. By causing a LBBB pattern via early depolarization of the right ventricular apex, the high ventricular septum depolarizes in the later part of systole. This delayed contraction has the effect of reducing the outflow tract obstruction in patients with hypertrophic obstructive cardiomyopathy.

MANAGED VENTRICULAR PACING (MVP)

Managed ventricular pacing (MVP) is basically, functional AAIR pacing with backup dual chamber ventricular support in the presence of transient or persistent loss of conduction. Essentially, this algorithm operates in an AAI/R mode without AV restriction to minimize ventricular pacing. If ventricular sensing occurs prior to the following atrial beat, pacemaker remains in AAI/R mode.[6] If an A-A interval (either paced or sensed) occurs without an interpolated ventricular sensed beat, a ventricular paced beat (back up ventricular pacing) will be delivered 80 msec after the next programmed atrial beat. The maximum possible pause cannot, therefore exceeds twice the lower programmed cycle length plus 80 msec. If AV conduction doesn't occur over two of the last four A-A intervals (multiple heart blocks in a four beat window), the pacemaker perceives persistent loss of conduction and mode switches to DDD/R. MVP maintains the dual chamber DDD/R mode for 1 minute and then performs an "AV conduction check". The device monitors AV conduction by temporarily switching back to AAI/R timing during one A-A cycle. The AV conduction check is scheduled at 2 min, 4 min, 8 min and so on up to 16 hours after the transition to DDD/R has occurred. If spontaneous R-wave is sensed, the device reverts back to the AAI/R mode (Figs 3.3 and 3.4).

A "dynamic atrial refractory period" has been developed to avoid inappropriate switch to DDD/R mode caused by non-conducted premature atrial ectopic or far-field R-wave over-sensing. Dynamic ARP (atrial refractory period) is set to 600 ms if heart rate is slower than 75 bpm and 75% of R-R cycle length if heart rate is 75 bpm or faster. ARP cannot be longer than 600 ms. During atrial fibrillation, the device operates in DDI/R mode. With this approach the Cum%VP reduced from

44 Cardiac Pacing: A Physiological Approach

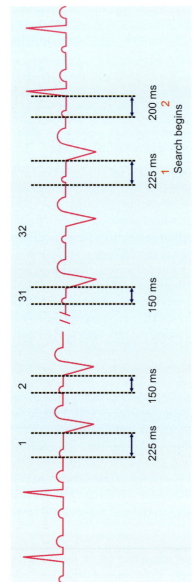

Fig. 3.1 Successful AV search hysteresis: During the search the AV Delay is extended to the long value. The intrinsic conduction occurs again so the long value is maintained (AV Delay is 150 ms. AV interval increase 50% during AV Search Interval is 32 cycles)

Managing Algorithm 45

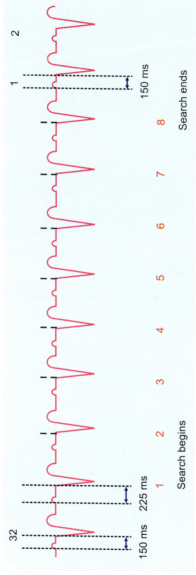

Fig. 3.2 Unsuccessful AV search hysteresis: In this case there is no intrinsic conduction during the search and AV delay returns to the normal AV delay after 8 beats and repeats sequence. The AV delay switches to the normal AV delay for a programmable number of cycles (nominal 32) followed by a search (AV Delay is 150 ms. AV interval increase 50% during AV Search Interval is 32 cycles)

46 Cardiac Pacing: A Physiological Approach

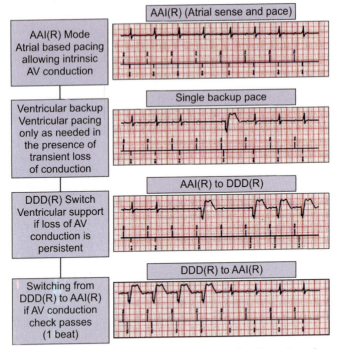

Fig. 3.3 Managed ventricular pacing (MVP): the algorithm allows for a single blocked beat before a back-up ventricular paced beat is delivered. Mode switch occurs only if two blocked beats occur. Two sequential blocked beats cannot occur because of back-up ventricular pacing

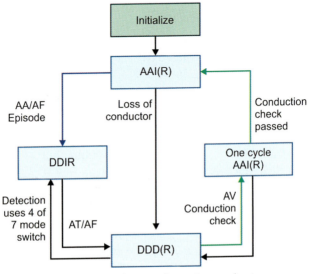

Fig. 3.4 Managed ventricular pacing: mechanism

a mean of 75% to 5%, with 80% of the patients being paced on the ventricle for < 1% of the time. This feature is most useful in patients with sinus node disease and intact AV conduction.

VENTRICULAR INTRINSIC PREFERENCE (VIP)

This algorithm is based on proven Auto-Intrinsic Conduction Search (AICS) algorithm by St. Jude Medical. VIP algorithm functions in DDD(R) mode with beat-by-beat ventricular support to maintain and restore AV synchrony (Fig. 3.5). By automatically adapting to changes in the patient's conduction patterns, this algorithm promotes intrinsic conduction and can limit unnecessary RV pacing to less than 10%.

When programmed optimally in appropriate patients it assures an appropriate AV delay if and when intermittent AV block occurs and permits normal upper rate pacing behavior. This algorithm extends the AV/PV interval every 30 sec to 30 min (programmable) to search for intrinsic conduction and extends the AV/PV interval whenever 3 consecutive R waves are sensed. This AV/PV extension is continued until consecutive V pacing occurs for 1, 2, or 3 beats (programmable). VIP is programmable from +50 to +150 ms in 25-ms steps, from +150 to +200 ms in 10-ms steps. It is recommended to use longest VIP to maximize intrinsic conduction. It allows for AV delay extension up to 450 msec. This promotes intrinsic activity and maintains physiologic heart rhythm. This mode also promotes optimal cardiac output, healthy conduction and improved hemodynamics.

AAIsafeR MODE

The AAIsafeR mode operates in the AAIR mode and switches to the DDDR mode when certain criteria are met (Fig. 3.6).[7] Mode switching from AAIR to DDDR occurs if:
- At least seven intervals between atrial paced or sensed events and ventricular sensed events exceed a predefined limit (programmable between 350 and 450 msec).
- If 3 of 12 sensed or paced atrial events are not followed by a ventricular sensed event, mode switching from AAIR to DDDR occurs.
- Two consecutive atrial events without consecutive ventricular sensed events results in mode switching.

To avoid prolonged pauses, DDDR pacing occurs if a programmable duration of ventricular asystole is detected (programmable between 2 and 4 seconds) independent of the relationship between atrial and ventricular events.

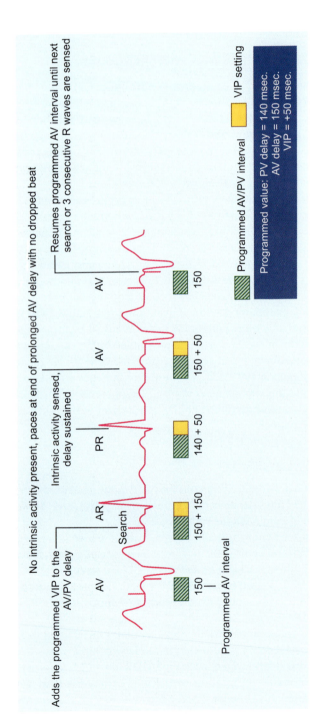

Fig. 3.5 Ventricular intrinsic preference (VIP): Beat-to-beat ventricular support

Managing Algorithm 49

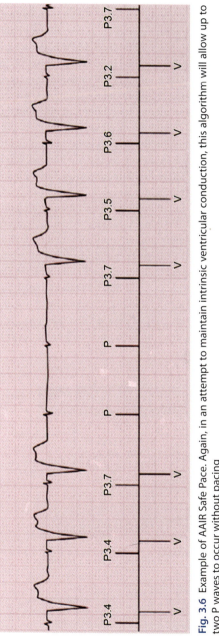

Fig. 3.6 Example of AAIR Safe Pace. Again, in an attempt to maintain intrinsic ventricular conduction, this algorithm will allow up to two P waves to occur without pacing

REVERSE MODE SWITCH (RHYTHMIQ MODE)

This algorithm provides AAI(R) at the lower rate limit (LRL) and/or sensor indicated rate according to the normal brady DDD(R) mode. The device provides back up VVI pacing at a rate of 15 pacing per minute (ppm) slower than the LRL. The back up VVI pacing rate is limited to no slower than 30 ppm and no faster than 60 ppm. When there is good conduction, ventricular pacing does not occur as the VVI backup mode runs in the background at a reduced LRL. The device monitors for loss of AV synchrony. If 3 slow ventricular beats are detected in a window of 11 beats, then the device automatically switches to DDD(R) mode (Fig. 3.7). A slow beat for this algorithm is defined as a ventricular pace or ventricular sensed event that is at least 150 msec slower than the AAI(R) pacing rate.[8] The 150 msec value is used to allow for normal variations between cardiac cycles.

OUTCOME DATA

SAVE PACe (The Search AV Extension and Managed Ventricular Pacing for Promoting Atrioventricular Conduction) trial has shown that the median percent ventricular pacing is lower in the minimal ventricular pacing group compared to the conventional DDDR group.[9] The percent atrial pacing was similar in both groups. A 40% reduction in the relative

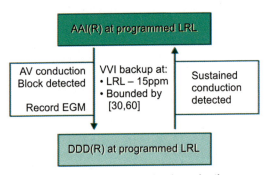

AV Conduction block:

- 3 Blocked ventricular events in a rolling window of 11 beats
  - Ventricular pacing
  - Ventricular sensing at least 150 ms slower than atrial pacing rate (LRL or SIR)

Sustained conduction

- Periodically engage AV search+:
  - 2 Ventricular pacing in a rolling window of 10 beats to fail
  - 25 Ventricular sensing to succeed

Fig. 3.7 RhythimiQ algorithm: mechanism

risk of developing persistent AF is seen with the strategy of minimizing ventricular pacing. But, no differences in mortality, hospitalization for heart failure, or cardioversion for AF were observed between the two groups. Although this study supports a strategy of minimizing ventricular pacing for prevention of AF, the magnitude of benefit has been overestimated by the study design.

Clinical studies report that MVP mode offers greater reduction in the percent ventricular pacing than search AV mode, except for patients with permanent AV block.[10] MVP is associated with a significant reduction in percent ventricular pacing for all categories of AV conduction except permanent AV block. However, whether such differences translate into improved clinical outcomes remains unknown. In MVP depending on device programming, prolonged AV delays of up to 600 msec may occur. These long AV delays cannot be considered physiologic and may result in pacemaker syndrome, with atrial contraction occurring early in diastole. This may be particularly decremental for patients with heart failure or mitral regurgitation. In the case of a ventricular premature beat, noncompetitive atrial pacing will extend the ventriculoatrial (VA) interval, resulting in an extension of the next atrial pacing interval. This results in atrial pacing rates below the programmed lower rate limit. Abrupt changes in ventricular cycle length (short-long-short) sequences have been reported to facilitate ventricular tachyarrhythmia onset in patients with implantable defibrillators. Such short-long-short sequences may be observed with the MVP mode and may constitute a form of ventricular proarrhythmia. Short-long-short sequences may also be observed with traditional DDDR programming preceding VT. Cases of torsade de pointes VT have been reported in pacemaker patients attributed to prolonged pauses secondary to programming in the MVP mode.[11] So, it is not suitable for patients with long QT syndrome or those with permanent complete heart block. VIP technology supposed to prevent potentially arrhythmogenic pauses by maintaining continuous AV synchrony. However, head-to-head comparison of efficacy of MVP, VIP, and Reverse mode switch algorithm in respect of reducing Cum%VP and prevention of atrial fibrillation is not available. Comparative analysis between VIP and MVP are given below:

Advantages of MVP

- Demonstrated reduction in ventricular pacing.
- Permits AAI functional pacing with ventricular backup.
- No pacing rate limitations.
- No specific DDD programming needed.

Disadvantages of MVP

- Permits non-conducted beats.
- Long V-V intervals of 2x Lower Rate +80 ms may occur.
- Search is triggered 1,2,4,8 . . . Minutes may result in more ventricular pacing with frequent block.
- Mode switch occurs with 2 of 4 blocked beats, frequent but intermittent block will stay AAIR.
- Extended V-V intervals may be proarrhythmic.
- Extremely long AV delays may exacerbate heart failure in certain patients.

Advantages of VIP

- Demonstrated reduction in ventricular pacing.
- Maximum AV delay up to 350 ms.
- Does not allow for dropped beats or extremely long A-V intervals.
- Permits programming of normal upper rate behavior.
- AV/PV extension can occur as frequently as every 30 sec and every time 3 consecutive R waves are sensed.
- 3 consecutive R waves will trigger AV/PV extension.
- Not affected by PVC's.
- May benefit patients with frequent intermittent block.

Disadvantages of VIP

- Not available above 110 ppm, programmed AV delay is restored.
- Does not allow true AAI type pacing.
- To optimize conduction, must program AV delay > 200 ms.
- Has not been demonstrated to reduce the % VP as dramatically as MVP.

Strategies of Reducing Atrial Fibrillation Burden

Atrial Pacing to Prevent Atrial Fibrillation

For atrial fibrillation (AF) to be established, it requires the appropriate triggers (premature atrial complex [PAC]) for initiation and appropriate atrial substrate (non-homogeneous refractoriness) for maintenance of re-entrant wavelets. Preventive pacing algorithms have been designed to suppress AF triggers, and new pacing lead designs may compensate for underlying atrial substrate by allowing pacing from multiple sites or alternative sites in the atria. The potential mechanisms of atrial pacing for prevention of AF are:

- Prevention of bradycardia-induced dispersion of atrial repolarization – a substrate for AF
- Suppression of frequent supra ventricular premature beats, which are triggers for AF, by atrial overdrive pacing, and
- Prevention of adverse atrial electrical remodeling that predisposes to AF by preservation of AV synchrony.

Suppression of Triggers

Premature atrial complex suppression can be achieved by permanently elevating the lower pacing rate or by dynamic overdrive pacing. Dynamic atrial overdrive pacing achieves a similar effect of ensuring constant atrial capture without having to program an elevated lower base rate. It allows for preservation of a normal circadian heart rate pattern. The pacing rate is increased incrementally upon detection of intrinsic atrial events until no further atrial sensed events occur. Pacing is maintained for a programmable duration before it is decreased again in steps until the intrinsic rate appears or lower pacing rate or sensor rate is reached. Again, sensing of atrial events will result in an increase of atrial pacing rate. **The Atrial Preference Pacing algorithm** (Medtronic, Minneapolis, Minnesota) monitors the P–P interval and paces 30 milliseconds shorter, while the **Dynamic Atrial Overdrive algorithm** (St Jude Medical, Sylmar, California) increases atrial paced rate for a programmable duration of time based on detection of intrinsic atrial activity (Fig. 3.8).

Effect on Atrial Substrate Suppression of Compensatory Pause

Premature atrial complexes also may initiate AF by altering the underlying atrial substrate to support re-entry. The short-long cycles caused by post extra systolic pauses following PACs may increase dispersion of atrial refractoriness making it conducive to the maintenance of re-entrant wavelets.[12]

Pacing algorithms, which respond to spontaneous PACs, have been designed to maintain homogeneous refractoriness. The pacing response to a PAC can be a single paced beat, a series of paced beats coupled with auto-adaptive decay, or pacing rate acceleration for a programmable duration.

The Atrial Therapy Efficacy and Safety Trial (ATTEST) evaluated the role of AT500 (Medtronic, Minneapolis, Minnesota) pacemakers that incorporated three different pacing algorithms (**Atrial Preference Pacing, Atrial Rate Stabilization and Post Mode Switching Overdrive**) in AF prevention.[13]

Reducing Dispersion of Refractoriness Multi-Site Pacing

Patients with paroxysmal AF can have profound intra- and inter- atrial conduction delay as evidenced by broader P waves on surface ECG. This conduction delay increases dispersion of atrial refractoriness, favoring induction of AF. Pacing may

Guidant
- Atrial pacing preference (APP)
    Increases atrial pacing rate when sensed atrial envents occur. Pacing rate is increased by shortening V-A interval by 10 ms. The V-A interval is lengthened (after a programmabel 2-128 cycles) by 10 ms increments till the next sensed atrial events. The APP is limited by the APP max pacing rate.

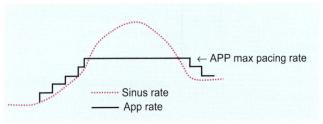

- ProACT
    Increase pacing rate in presence of PAC by pacing at 75% of the V-V interval prior to PAC.
    Pacing is gradually decreased back to lower rate limit.

Medtronic

Anti-Pace™ pacing algorithms
- Atrial preference pacing
    Pacing rate is increased (programmable decrement of 30–150 ms) when atrial event is sensed to ensure atrial pacing.
- Atrial rate stabilization (ARS)
    Paces after a PAC to avoid short-long cycles. The ARS interval is the last A-A interval plus a % of the last A-A interval.

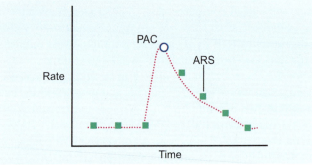

- Post-Mode switch overdrive pacing (PMOP)
    Paces DDIR at an elevated rate for a defined period of time, starting after a mode switch event.
    The overdrive rate is programmable from 34 bpm to 120 bpm and the overdrive duration is programmable from 0.5 to 120 minutes.

Contd...

Contd...

St Jude medical
- **Dynamic atrial overdrive**
  Increases atrial pacing rate when 2 P waves (need not be consecutive) in a 16 cycle window for a programmable number of cycles and then pacing rate is decreased (programmable cycle length extension) till atrial event is sensed again.

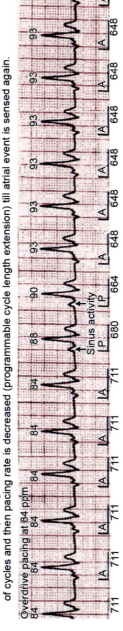

Fig. 3.8 Description of different dynamic atrial pacing algorithms

correct the conduction delay, and this can be achieved by simultaneous pacing from more than one site (multi-site or dual-site) to allow synchronization of left and right atrial activation. Dual-site pacing has been shown to be effective in preventing AF by reducing the conduction delay.[14]

Reducing Dispersion of Refractoriness: Alternative Site Atrial Pacing

Another method of shortening the total atrial activation time is by pacing the atrium from selected sites. Generally, it is accepted that routes of preferential interatrial conduction exist, and pacing at these sites will pre-excite the left atrium. **Bachmann's bundle** is the largest and most important anatomical interatrial communication and probably accounts for most interatrial conduction. The structure is a band of tissue that extends from the right of the superior vena cava transversally to the anterior wall of the left atrium up to the left atrial appendage. This alternative pacing site had been shown to be effective in AF prevention.[15]

Atrial Pacing for Atrial Fibrillation Termination

Anti-tachycardia pacing (ATP) has been used originally to treat VT episodes by the delivery of pacing impulses that are slightly faster than the detected arrhythmia. The aim is to "break" the tachycardia by forcing the myocardial circuit to conduct the faster impulses beyond its physiologic limits. Two types of ATP therapy are generally available: burst and ramp. Burst ATP consists of a sequence of paced beats delivered at a programmable rate that is faster (i.e., shorter cycle length) than the detected tachycardia. This sequence has a stable cycle length of variable but programmable duration (generally 8 cycles). Ramp pacing also consists of a sequence of paced beats, faster than the detected VT, but with a decremental cycle length; that is, each paced impulse in the sequence is faster (i.e., shorter cycle length) than the preceding cycle. The number of beats in each ramp is programmable, as is the rate by which each cycle shortens from the prior cycle. The ramp consisted of eight beats with 91% decrement between successive beats. Anti-tachycardia pacing (ATP) is a reliable mode of therapy in arrhythmias with a large excitable gap such as atrial flutter. On the other hand, AF with shorter excitable gap does not lend itself easily to pace termination. There are several potential advantages to incorporating ATP into devices for management of AF. Atrial flutter, atrial tachycardia (AT) and AF frequently can coexist in the same patient, and not uncommonly, atrial flutter can degenerate into AF. Delivery of ATP while the patient is in atrial flutter may prevent AF initiation. Alternatively, AF may be converted to atrial flutter with antiarrhythmic agents, and the availability of ATP would allow for termination of atrial flutter. The ATP algorithms for AT/AF termination in some study are **atrial burst + (atrial burst followed by two extra stimuli), atrial ramp (atrial auto-decremental ramp) and atrial 50 Hz burst pacing up to 3 seconds**.[16] The relatively lower success rate of pace termination is attributable to the shorter excitable gap present in AF as evidenced by the indirect relationship between successful outcome and underlying cycle length of the AT/AF. Prompt AF detection and delivery of ATP may prevent electrical remodeling after AF onset and promote sinus rhythm.

Newer Pacing and Therapeutic Algorithms

The irregularity of the ventricular depolarization during AF has been associated with poorer cardiac performance and increased sympathetic nervous system activation. Ventricular rate stabilization algorithms have been developed by various device manufacturers to regularize the R–R interval during AF in attempts to improve patients' symptoms. This can be achieved by increasing the ventricular pacing rate during AF, without causing a significant increase in mean heart rate and has been shown to suppress the R–R intervals at shorter cycle lengths and regularize the rate. Although a stand-alone atrial defibrillator has been shown to be effective, its role in AF management remains limited. Most current pacemakers are capable of storing intracardiac electrograms, sometimes allowing the clinician to distinguish between AF, AT, and atrial flutter.

OUTCOME DATA

Based on well-designed prospective clinical trials, only a few of these strategies can be recommended for routine clinical use in related subpopulations. From the available studies, several key considerations are apparent:
- The definition of physiologic pacing has evolved. It is no longer enough to maintain AV synchrony with a dual-chamber atrial-based pacemaker. When possible, intrinsic AV conduction should be promoted to minimize the deleterious effects of RV pacing. Therefore, mode selection is important (AAI)/DDD, DDI, or DDD with long AV delays). Unresolved questions include the maximum hemodynamically acceptable AV delay and the optimal site for RV pacing.[17]

- Pacing in chronic AF to promote ventricular rate regularization has limited clinical value, and careful attention should be paid to overall adequacy of rate control. An average ventricular rate greater than the upper pacing limit may lead to tachycardia-mediated cardiomyopathy and signals the need for more aggressive rate control or AVJ ablation.
- Pacing algorithms that attempt to prevent AF have limited value. As a sole indication, they are not widely accepted or recommended as a primary indication for pacemaker implantation in patients with paroxysmal or persistent AF.[18]
- Multisite and novel site pacing strategies do not have broad clinical applications at this time.

CONCLUSION

The risks of heart failure (HF) hospitalization and atrial fibrillation (AF) in patients with right ventricular apical pacing can be directly linked to pacing burden (cumulative percent ventricular pacing [Cum%VP]) regardless of pacing mode. Different advanced algorithms have been introduced to minimize ventricular pacing. Overall, these algorithms have been reported to be safe and well tolerated. Head-to-head comparison of the efficacy of all of these algorithms is not available. Available data indicates superiority of MVP over AV search hysteresis. However, MVP algorithm has been documented to cause long-short-long cycles, resulting in life-threatening arrhythmias. Algorithms for prevention of atrial fibrillation are effective. Pacing in chronic AF to promote ventricular rate regularization has limited clinical value. Multisite and high atrial septal pacing strategies do not have specific clinical applications at this time.

REFERENCES

1. Connolly SJ, Kerr CR, Gent M, et al., for the Canadian Trial of Physiological Pacing Investigators. Effects of physiological pacing versus ventricular pacing on the risk of stroke and death due to cardiovascular causes. N Engl J Med. 2000;342:1385-91.
2. Lamas GA, Lee KL, Sweeney MO, et al., for the MOST Investigators. Ventricular pacing or dual chamber pacing for sinus node dysfunction. N Engl J Med. 2002; 346:1854-62.
3. Toff WD, Camm AJ, Skehan JD, for the United Kingdom Pacing and Cardiovascular Events Trial (UKPACE) Investigators. Single chamber versus dual-chamber pacing for high-grade atrioventricular block. N Engl J Med. 2005;353:145-55.
4. Sweeney MO, Hellkamp AS, Ellenbogen KA, et al. Adverse effect of ventricular pacing on heart failure and atrial fibrillation among patients with normal baseline QRS duration in a clinical trial of

pacemaker therapy for sinus node dysfunction. Circulation. 2003; 23:2932-7.
5. Olshansky B, Day JD, Moore S, et al. Is dual-chamber programming inferior to single-chamber programming in an implantable cardioverter defibrillator? Results of the INTRINSIC RV (inhibition of unnecessary RV pacing with AVSH in ICDs) study. Circulation. 2007;115(1):9-16.
6. Sweeney MO, Bank AJ, Nsah E, et al. The search AV extension and managed ventricular pacing for promoting atrioventricular conduction (SAVE PACe) trial. Minimizing ventricular pacing to reduce atrial fibrillation in sinus-node disease. New England Journal of Medicine. 2007;356(10):1000-8.
7. Hanna G, Goodman J, Fahmy R, et al. Reduction of ventricular pacing in pacemaker patients using ventricular intrinsic preference: preliminary results from the VIP trial. Europace. 2008; (Suppl1):i1-i214.
8. Pioger G, Leny G, Nitzsché R, Ripart A. AAIsafeR limits ventricular pacing in unselected patients. Pacing Clin Electrophysiol 30 Suppl 1:S66-S70,2007.
9. Reference Guide, INCEPTA ICD, page 4-28, 358430-003 EN US01/11.
10. Sweeney MO, Bank AJ, Nsah E, et al. Search AV Extension and Managed Ventricular Pacing for Promoting Atrioventricular Conduction (SAVE PACe) Trial. Minimizing ventricular pacing to reduce atrial fibrillation in sinus node disease. N Engl J Med. 2007; 357:1000-8.
11. Pürerfellner H, Brandt J, Israel C, et al. Comparison of two strategies to reduce ventricular pacing in pacemaker patients. Pacing Clin Electrophysiol. 2008;31:167-76.
12. Vavasis C, Slotwiner DJ, Goldner BG, Cheung JW. Frequent recurrent polymorphic ventricular tachycardia during sleep due to managed ventricular pacing. Pacing Clin Electrophysiol. 2010; 33:641-4.
13. Murgatroyd FD, Nitzsche R, Slade AK, et al. A new pacing algorithm for overdrive suppression of atrial fibrillation. Pacing Clin Electrophysiol. 1994;17:1966-73.
14. Daubert C, Mabo PH, Berder V, et al. Atrial tachyarrhythmias associated with high degree interatrial conduction block: prevention by permanent atrial, resynchronisation. Eur J Cardiac Pacing Electrophysiol. 1994;1:35-44.
15. Daubert C, Leclercq C, Le Breton H, et al. Permanent left atrial pacing with a specifically designed coronary sinus lead. Pacing Clin Electrophysiol. 1997;20:2755-64.
16. Bailin SJ, Adler S, Giudici M. Prevention of chronic atrial fibrillation by pacing in the region of Bachmann's bundle: results of a multi-center randomized trial. J Cardiovasc Electrophysiol. 2001;12:912-7.
17. Andersen HR, Thuesen L, Bagger JP, et al. Prospective randomized trial of atrial versus ventricular pacing in sick-sinus syndrome. Lancet. 1994;344:1523-8.
18. Knight BP, Gersh BJ, Carlson MD, et al. Role of permanent pacing to prevent atrial fibrillation: science advisory from the American Heart Association Council on Clinical Cardiology (Subcommittee on Electrocardiography and Arrhythmias) and the Quality of Care and Outcomes Research Interdisciplinary Working Group, in collaboration with the Heart Rhythm Society. Circ. 2005; 111(2):240-3.

CHAPTER 4

Selective Site: Right Ventricular Septal Pacing

INTRODUCTION

The right ventricular (RV) apex has been used for decades as a safe and reliable pacing site because it is easily accessible and has a low dislodgement rate and an excellent pacing threshold and sensing characteristics. However, RV-apical pacing is non-physiological as it causes abnormal electrical ventricular conduction, altered myocardial perfusion, histopathological alterations, ventricular dyssynchrony, left ventricular (LV) dilatation, and decreased LV function in an unpredictable way as a result of remodeling process consequent to abnormal ventricular activation and contraction, which ultimately results in an exacerbation of heart failure, atrial fibrillation, and an increased morbidity and mortality.[1,2] But, so called "physiological" dual chamber DDD/R pacing failed to prove their superiority in different randomized control trials.[3] As a consequence, investigators searched for alternate pacing sites with a more physiological depolarization pattern which will result in better hemodynamics, less mitral valve regurgitation, less detrimental remodeling, and delaying, reducing, or eliminating long-term negative changes like perfusion defects and heart failure.[4-6] The idea of septal pacing is coined on the fact that the septal regions of the RVOT and mid RV are the first zones of the ventricle to depolarize, suggesting that pacing from these areas on the right side of the septum would achieve as normal a contraction pattern as possible. In contrast, the free wall of the RV is the last zone to be depolarized. In particular, RV septal pacing compared to apical pacing results in a shorter electrical activation delay and consequently less-mechanical dyssynchrony. But, RV septal pacing has not been widely accepted and utilized. One concern is that despite the perceived advantages of septal pacing, results of different trials to date are not confirmatory.

ANATOMY

The interior of right ventricle consists of two parts: rough inflow tract and smooth outflow tract or infundibulum. The inlet and outlet components of the ventricle, supporting and surrounding the cusps of the tricuspid and pulmonary valves respectively, are separated in the roof of the ventricle by the prominent thick, muscular supraventricular crest (crista supraventricularis). The posterolateral aspect of the crest provides a principal attachment for the anterosuperior cusp of the tricuspid valve. The septal limb of the crest may be continuous with, or embraced by, the septal limbs of the septomarginal trabecula. The septomarginal trabecula or septal band reinforces the septal surface where, at the base, it divides into limbs that embrace the supraventricular crest. Towards the apex, it supports the anterior papillary muscle of the tricuspid valve and, from this point, crosses to the parietal wall of the ventricle as the "moderator band". A further series of prominent trabeculae, the **septoparietal trabeculations**, extend from its anterior surface and run onto the parietal ventricular wall (Fig. 4.1). Below the level of the supraventricular crest (crista supraventricularis) lies the inferior portion of the septum,

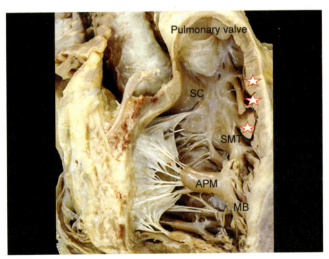

Fig. 4.1 Illustration of the heart highlighting the RV septal anatomy. The right ventricle has been opened from the front with the heart orientated anatomically. The RVOT is bordered by the pulmonary valve above and the superior aspect of the tricuspid apparatus below. The upper part of the septal wall is the conus arteriosus, bordered below by the supraventricular crest. To the anatomical left of the septomarginal trabeculation, this continues into the moderator band. The septoparietal trabeculations are shown with stars.
Abbreviations: SC, supraventricular crest; SMT, septomarginal trabeculation; APM, anterior papillary muscle of tricuspid valve; MB, moderator band

which, to the left of the septomarginal trabeculation, is a cul-de-sac filled with the septoparietal trabeculations and is ideal for pacing lead attachment as it is truly septal.

The lower border of the RVOT is defined as a horizontal line along the top of the tricuspid valve, whereas the pulmonary valve constitutes the upper border. Between these two, the interventricular septum on the one hand and the curved free wall on the other constitute the vertical borders. Three sites of lead placement within the RVOT are distinguishable, according to lead angulation. These sites are **anterior, septal, and free wall** (Fig. 4.2). The anterior 2/3 of the septal wall is the ideal site for lead attachment in septal pacing as it is the site for the septoparietal trabeculation. In a cross sectional view at the mid

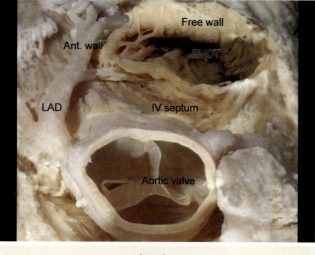

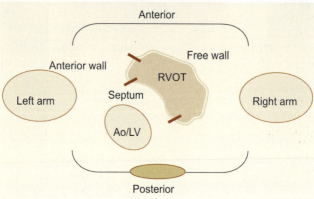

Fig. 4.2 Cross-section of the heart to demonstrate the relationship of the areas of the RVOT to surrounding structures. Depending on the level of the RVOT, behind the septum lies either the left ventricle or ascending aorta.
Abbreviations: LAD, left anterior descending artery; IV, interventricular; Ant, anterior; RVOT, right ventricular outflow tract; Ao, aorta; LA, left atrium

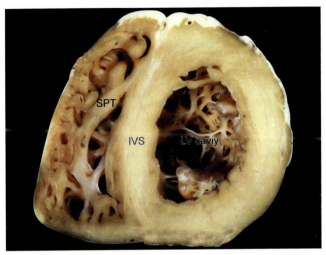

Fig. 4.3 A cross-section of the heart at mid-ventricular level to demonstrate the relationship of the septoparietal trabeculation and interventricular septum

Abbreviations: SPT, septoparietal trabeculation; IVS, interventricular septum; LV, left ventricle

ventricular level (at the papillary muscle level) anterior and middle third of the interventricular septum in its right side is also appropriate for septal lead attachment (Fig. 4.3).

Electrical Activation Sequence

With normal intraventricular conduction, activation of the ventricles begins in the left lower third of the interventricular septum and spreads transversely from left to right through the septum. This left-to-right vector, however, is opposed by the smaller right-to-left septal vector which originates from the right bundle branch, and which arises in the right side of the interventricular septum. Paraseptal activation occurs next, spreading transversely from endocardial to epicardial surfaces. This is followed by endocardial–epicardial activation of the free walls both in right and left side.

Three-dimensional electroanatomical mapping data suggests that in the normal heart, the first site of endocardial ventricular activation (endocardial breakthrough site) is usually in the LV, at the interventricular septum or in the anterior region. Within approximately 10 ms the activation begins in the RV endocardium, near the insertion of the anterior papillary muscle, i.e. the exit of the right bundle branch.[7] After activation of these regions, depolarization wave fronts proceed simultaneously in the LV and RV, predominantly from apex to base and from septum to lateral wall in both ventricles. The latest activated endocardial region of the RV is the basal area near the AV sulcus and the pulmonary conus. Overall, the posterolateral/basal area of the LV is the last part of the heart to be depolarized. Simultaneous depolarization wave front occurs centrifugally from the endocardium to the epicardium. However, the earliest ventricular epicardial activation site (epicardial breakthrough site) occurs usually at the pretrabecular area of the RV from where there is a radial spread towards the apex and the base, within the subepicardial layers.[7] In a normal heart, the duration of total ventricular electrical activation is 50–80 ms. The short ventricular activation time stresses the important role of the Purkinje fibers system in the synchronization of electrical myocardial activity. So, pacing in the RVOT septal region seems to produces a more physiological electrical activation sequence and endocardial-epicardial breakthrough pattern.

RV Apical vs RV Septal Pacing

It is now widely recognized that prolonged RV apical pacing is associated with progressive LV dysfunction which leads to exacerbation of heart failure, atrial fibrillation, and increased morbidity and mortality. This effect is due to the process known as remodeling. **Remodeling** of left ventricle because of chronic RV pacing is due to modified regional blood flow patterns, increased oxygen consumption without increase in blood flow (60% change in blood flow between early and later activated regions) and abnormal thickening of LV wall. RV apical pacing also leads to an altered left ventricular electrical and mechanical activation. Altered ventricular function in chronic RV apical pacing is due to less work produced for given LV end diastolic volume and delayed papillary muscle activation (**valvular insufficiency**). Ultrastructurally, it causes a change in the myocardium known as **cellular disarray** which includes fibrosis (away from pacing lead location), fat deposition, calcification and mitochondrial abnormalities. RV septal pacing differs from conventional RV apical pacing in various ways:

- Histologically, in comparison to apical pacing, RV septal pacing patients do not show calcification, degenerative changes, or altered mitochondrial morphology in follow up (Fig. 4.4).
- RVOT septal pacing produces narrower QRS complex in comparison to RV apical pacing probably by stimulating part of normal conduction system. RVOT septal pacing normalizes the axis of depolarization. Cardiac output is higher with RVOT vs RV apical pacing in patients with narrow

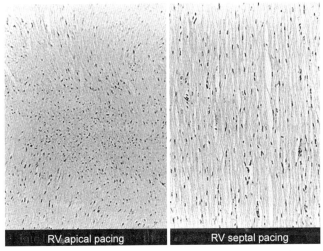

Fig. 4.4 4 months follow up of RV apical pacing versus RV septal pacing

baseline QRS. QRS duration do not always reflect activation front. **However, in cases of wide native QRS complex it fails to normalize QRS duration. The wider the native QRS, the wider is the RVOT paced QRS probably due to involvement of the His-Purkinje system and they are also associated with late transition in precordial leads.** Multiple studies have shown that narrow QRS complex do not always lead to better hemodynamic outcome. In contrast, some study has shown improved function without shortening QRS duration in biventricular pacing.

- Maintenance of AV contraction sequence is just as important as electrical activation. Improvement of LV function with RV pacing site varies with different AV delays. Studies have shown that trend toward more improvement with shorter AV delays with septal versus apical pacing. Rather than individual optimization, set to near normal value of 100 ms shows no differences between RVOT and apical pacing. So, individual optimization may be the best alternative.

- In a healthy heart, as the helically arranged myocardial fibers contract, the walls of the LV **shorten longitudinally, thicken radially, and rotate around the long axis.** Although this coordinated motion is complicated, it can be simplified using two-dimensional echocardiographic projections. The magnitude of motion and timing between different wall segments can be measured with tissue Doppler imaging (TDI) and speckle tracking echocardiography (STE) so that longitudinal, radial and rotational motion can be assessed. Since RV pacing artificially stimulates the ventricles at a location other than the His-Purkinje system, the action potential is propagated more slowly through myocytes rather than through the specialized conduction system. Electrical activation then becomes heterogeneous, with early activation near the pacing site, and delayed activation at distant locations. The resultant LV mechanical contraction becomes dyssynchronous. RV apical pacing reduces longitudinal LV systolic function and increases dyssynchrony. The peak radial strain and the time to reach peak radial strain in 6 short-axis segments become heterogeneous after long-term RV pacing. The radial strain is **most reduced and peaked earliest** in septal and anteroseptal regions, and **increased in magnitude and delayed** in lateral and posterior regions. In chronically paced humans, it has been found that both basal and apical peak rotation and peak systolic torsion are lower than in age-matched non-paced controls. In addition, apical rotation is found to be in the reverse direction from normal in about 1/3 of paced patients. RVOT pacing results in superior radial synchrony using STE, as well as better coronary blood flow dynamics. Some investigators showed that longitudinal LV function is better in RVOT pacing than in apical pacing. Tse, et al., measured regional wall motion abnormalities in a long-term study of 24 patients with complete atrioventricular block paced from either the RV apex or RVOT for a period of 18 months (Tse et al. 2002). Changes in perfusion and dyssynchrony were not different between pacing sites after 6 months, but RVOT pacing resulted in significant reductions in perfusion defects and dyssynchrony after 18 months.[8]

RADIOLOGY

For RVOT lead placement, four fluoroscopic views are essential:
1. ***Posteroanterior (PA) view:*** It is the initial view to work with and best for guiding the lead into the RVOT and mid-RV. The view, however, gives little help as to which RVOT segment the lead is actually attached to. When two leads lie in the RVOT, one septal and one free wall, the latter is usually pointing upward or superior, although this finding is not consistent.
2. ***40° Right anterior oblique (RAO):*** It is used to exclude inadvertent positioning of the lead in the coronary sinus and great cardiac vein. A lead in the coronary sinus/great cardiac vein mimics the RVOT in the PA view. The RAO view confirms the posterior aspect of the lead in the cardiac venous system. The same principle can be applied to RV apical pacing and inadvertent positioning of the lead in the middle or lateral cardiac vein.

3. **40° Left anterior oblique (LAO):** Differentiation between the septal, anterior, and free wall aspects of the RV are best defined by the 40° left anterior oblique (LAO) view. Interventricular septum is an oblique structure and is situated posteriorly. So, in left anterior oblique (LAO) view the septal lead points towards the spine. **The septal position is characterized by a posterior orientation of the lead tip** (Fig. 4.5), whilst **the free wall positioning is seen with the lead tip facing anterior. With anterior wall placement, the tip faces upwards** (Fig. 4.6).
4. **Left lateral (LL):** A fourth view, the 90° left lateral (LL), is also very valuable, but almost impossible to achieve during an implant using single plane fluoroscopy, because of sterile drapes, lead shields, arm boards, and monitoring equipment. A posterior projection of the lead tip indicates septal placement and is **100% specific** (Fig. 4.7). In comparison, a lead on the free wall passes anteriorly toward the sternum. The anterior segment of the RVOT, particularly the junction with the septum, where the anterior descending

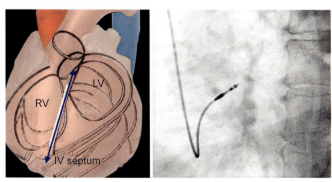

Fig. 4.5 Forty-degree left anterior oblique. Left anterior oblique (LAO) views of the heart. Left, anatomic diagram showing position of right ventricle (RV) and interventricular septum (IV septum); LV, left ventricle. Right, fluoroscopic image showing pacing lead in the septum

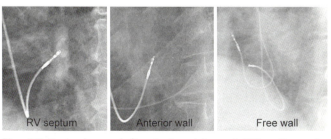

Fig. 4.6 Forty-degree left anterior oblique (LAO) radiographs demonstrating lead position on the septum (pointing posteriorly towards the spine), anterior wall (pointing upwards) and free wall

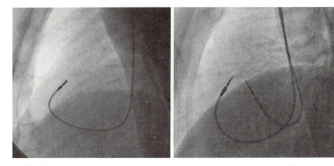

Fig. 4.7 Left lateral radiograph displaying leads with septal location pointing posteriorly towards the spine

coronary artery lies, is a transition zone. Not surprisingly the appearances lie between the other two described lead tip positions. In both LAO and LL projections, the lead tip points superiorly in anterior segment location of the lead.

TOOLS AND TECHNIQUE

1st step is to achieve the venous access to subclavian vein either by cephalic cut down or by direct puncture (preferably extrathoracic than intrathoracic) in either side (preferably in left side because of natural curve from left). **2nd step** is to position the lead onto the septum in the outflow tract or mid cavity. The main challenge in septal pacing is to shape a stylet that consistently places the lead on the RV septum, whether it is the RVOT or mid-RV. Innovative works by Prof Hary Mond resulted in the development of Mond's stylet. Firstly, a generous curve is created using the distal 5–6 cm of wire. Then the terminal 2 cm is bent to create a swan neck deformity. However, to reliably position leads on the RV septum, a posterior angulation is essential (Fig. 4.8). Such a shaped stylet is now commercially available (Mond's stylet; St Jude Medical, USA). They are available in two curves—a medium curve and a broad curve. In general, the medium curve is used first and the broad curve is reserved for the grossly enlarged right ventricle. Two stylets with differing stiffness are provided with each model: a soft with a green handle (diameter 0.35 mm) and a firm with a yellow handle (diameter 0.38 mm). The choice of stylet stiffness is physician preference although lead manipulation is easier with the firm stylet.

The stylet for septal lead placement can be hand prepared at the time of implant. To prevent damage to the lead, stylet shaping is preferred to shaping a stylet-loaded lead. Holding the curved end of the stylet with the summit superior, the terminal straight bend is shaped toward the operator or forwards. It

Selective Site: Right Ventricular Septal Pacing

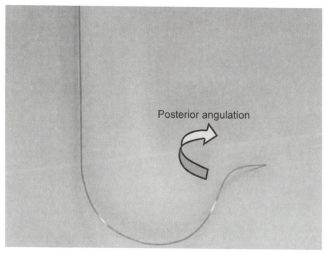

Fig. 4.8 The hand-fashioned stylet demonstrating the curve, bent distal portion, and posterior angulation (arrow)

is also advisable to gently shape the curve forwards as well. The same procedure is performed if the stylet-loaded lead is manually shaped. The concern is damage to the anode ring. Therefore, this portion must lie within the terminal straight bend some distance from the curve.

There are a number of advantages using the commercially prepared stylet. (1) The commercially prepared shape is consistent. With hand shaping, there is a surprisingly long and occasionally difficult learning curve with a bizarre array of shapes obtained. (2) Because the stylet is shaped upside down to the way it is inserted, the angulation during preparation is the reverse with the lead being shaped forwards. Inadvertent shaping the opposite way will consistently position the lead on the free wall.[9] (3) Loading the commercially prepared stylet is easy and smooth. Because the hand-fashioned stylet has a number of acute bends, loading can be difficult and frequently leads to stylet distortion. (4) The commercially prepared stylet is manufactured from tempered steel, which alters the internal stresses by heat treatment. This results in the shaped stylet having flexible memory and thus retains its shape as the lead is manipulated in the heart. The hand-fashioned stylet has poor memory and distorts easily. (5) The commercially prepared stylet is available with two curves and stylet wire stiffness.

The question is whether the commercially prepared stylet places the lead onto a better septal position. Studies are currently underway to determine this. Irrespective of which type of stylet is used, there have been no instances of lead dislodgement, excellent long-term stimulation thresholds and no perforation, pericarditis, or pericardial tamponade. Clinical experience with the hand-fashioned stylet suggests that it is very successful at RVOT septal and mid-RV septal placement in over 90% of cases.[10]

After obtaining the venous access, the lead is advanced into the pulmonary artery through the right atrium right ventricle. Because the lead must be directed from the right atrium into the RV and then the pulmonary artery, it should be at least 58 cm in length, particularly when implanted from the left side. Any commercially available 6 or 7-French active-fixation lead can be used. Prior to lead insertion, the septal stylet should be loaded into the lead. Some operators prefer to use a slightly curved hand-prepared stylet to position the lead in the right atrium or even pulmonary artery and later insert the septal stylet. There are a number of methods to insert the lead tip into the pulmonary artery. The PA or approximately 10° RAO projection is recommended **(1)** On occasion; the lead tip can be passed directly across the tricuspid valve into the body of the RV and from there into the pulmonary artery. However, this is generally difficult to perform. **(2)** The most common technique is to advance the lead loaded fully with the septal stylet across the tricuspid valve and directed toward the RV apex. With the stylet slightly withdrawn, the body of the lead is arched into the RVOT and then the tip is prolapsed into the pulmonary artery. **(3)** Another method is to cross the tricuspid valve with the body of the lead. Once the loop of lead is close to the pulmonary artery, the stylet can be partially withdrawn and the tip is maneuvered into the pulmonary artery. **(4)** In difficult cases and, in particular, patients with significant tricuspid regurgitation and enlarged right-sided chambers, a stylet with a generous simple curve can be used to place the lead into the pulmonary artery. The stylet can then be exchanged with the septal stylet. It is important to confirm that the lead tip is in the pulmonary artery. Once in the pulmonary artery, the lead, with septal stylet fully inserted, is retracted into the RVOT or mid-RV and contact is made with the septal wall. This is best achieved using the PA projection. This can be confirmed by gently inserting more lead and the tip is seen to arch against the wall. If after a number of attempts contact is not achieved, then the procedure is repeated with the stylet partially withdrawn to allow the angle of the tip to change in order to make contact with the septum. In very large RV chambers, it is not surprising that contact may not be possible. In this situation, a wider stylet can be used. Once the lead tip makes contact with the septal wall, the screw should be immediately deployed. The standard technique uses an "inverted V" clip-on tool. Once the screw is deployed, the stylet should be gently withdrawn to the right atrium to confirm wall attachment. The 40° LAO projection should now be performed to confirm septal positioning.

Last step is RV lead testing about 5 minutes following screw deployment (allow the stimulation threshold to fall and plateau following the initial trauma to the endomyocardium) include R-wave size and stimulation threshold. Following satisfactory lead testing, a generous loop of lead is left in the right atrium and RV to prevent lead dislodgement. This can usually be determined by inserting more lead without stylet, until it bends across the tricuspid annulus. The amount of lead in the heart obviously depends on the cardiac size and whether the lead tip lies in the RVOT or mid-RV, but the final loop and angle of lead attachment are remarkably consistent in appearance.

The benefits of septal lead attachment are obvious. The lead cannot perforate the septal wall and the highest stimulation detected in 100 cases at 1 year was 1.5 V with 94% of cases <1 V.[11] In contrast, free wall pacing may perforate the RV with high threshold exit block, pericarditis, pericardial effusion, or tamponade. Pacing of the anterior wall may damage the left anterior descending coronary artery.

The techniques described also apply to the implantation of cardioverter-defibrillator (ICD) leads. Because of their complicated and stiff terminal portion, it seems intuitive that all ICD leads have the potential to perforate the RV apex. In contrast, ICD leads secured to the more muscular RVOT septal or mid-RV septal walls will not perforate.[12] The septal positions also have the potential of physiologic and hemodynamic benefits if ventricular pacing is also required. Furthermore, current evidence suggests that defibrillation thresholds are not adversely affected by septal positioning.[13]

But the Mond's stylet is not always available at our center. With hand shaping, there is bizarre array of shapes obtained making it difficult for use. So, **alternatively,** the RVOT septal position can be achieved with a different method. At first, the lead is advanced into the RVOT using a 'modified U-curve'. Then the stylet is withdrawn for few centimeters and slowly pulled back to the desired segment. Now, the lead stylet assembly is gentle rotation clock-wise or anti-clockwise for different patients along with the help of differently shaped styled will send the lead to the desired position (Fig. 4.9). A posteriorly facing lead in LAO view suggests septal location of the lead and left lateral view confirms its position in the septum. Now, the lead is screwed up in RAO caudal projection and the parameters are checked.

Dr Srivatsa has suggested another alternative technique for septal lead attachment.[14] Their stylet is basically a kind of modified Mond's stylet with more acute primary curve and less

Cardiac Pacing: A Physiological Approach

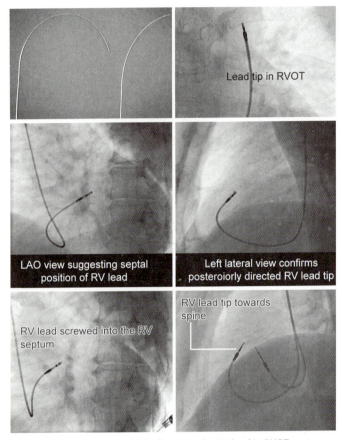

Fig. 4.9 Alternative method of putting the RV lead in RVOT septum

acute secondary curve. He has advised right ventriculogram with Swan-Ganz catheter during dragging the lead from RVOT to the target area in RAO projection (Fig. 4.10).

ELECTROCARDIOGRAPHIC CHARACTERISTICS

The 12-lead ECG of RVOT septal and mid-RV septal pacing is associated with a shorter QRS duration than elsewhere in the RV and in particular the RVOT free wall. This suggests that pacing from the RV septal areas, although not as good as intrinsic conduction or direct His bundle pacing, may be more desirable for chronic RV pacing compared to the RV apex as a narrow QRS is associated with improved LV dynamics.[15] The ECG can be specifically analyzed for **(1)** QRS amplitude and duration in all limb leads; **(2)** presence of "notching" of R in inferior leads II, III, and/or aVF; **(3)** QRS transition pattern in the precordial leads with a change at or beyond lead V4

Selective Site: Right Ventricular Septal Pacing

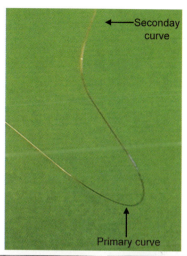

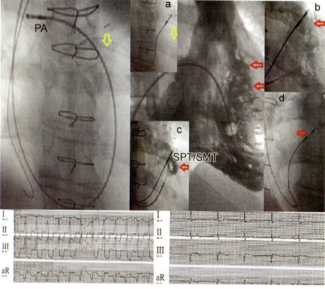

Fig. 4.10 Another alternative technique: A: Initial position of the RV lead in the right main PA achieved by using a simple shallow curved stylet to advance from RA to RVOT and then to PA. B: Comparison RV ventriculogram showing the angiographic location (open arrows) of the septoparietal trabeculations. Inset a RVOT septal lead being dragged inferiorly with modified Mond stylet in place from PA to septum. Inset b Lead screwed into place into SPT zone identified during pull back contrast injection. Inset c confirmation of lead location by a small bolus of contrast injection clearly delineating the septo-marginal trabeculation and septo-parietal trabeculation. Inset d steep (left anterior technique) LAO view showing lead in position against high septal location. C and D: Paced and unpaced ECG leads showing the isoelectric/slight positive lead I vector and inferior axis of the paced ECG (Courtesy Sanjoy S. Srivatsa. Finding the sweet spot for non-apical RV pacing. Journal of Invasive Cardiology 2014;26(3):140-7)

defined as a late transition; and **(4)** QRS morphology in limb lead I. Dixit and his colleagues have described different ECG morphology during pace mapping from different quadrants of RVOT[16] (Fig. 4.11). As discussed earlier in this chapter the target site in septal pacing is site 2 and 3 in septal wall, the ECG morphology during pace mapping from these sites need careful observation (Fig. 4.12).

Salient findings on 12-lead ECG that can help to distinguish RVOT or mid-RV septal from free wall sites of origin include:
- *Inferior leads (Lead II, III, and aVF):* Monophasic R waves indicate RVOT location of the lead. Taller and narrower QRS indicate septal location and smaller amplitude and increased width of the QRS points to a free-wall site of origin. Presences of notching of the R wave indicate free wall location and absence of notching in the R wave indicates septal location.
- *QRS duration:* QRS duration tends to be slightly shorter with septal and anterior RVOT pacing than with free wall RVTO pacing.
- *QRS vector and morphology:* Septal pacing is significantly more frequently associated with a negative complex in

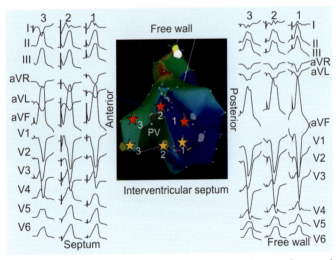

Fig. 4.11 Twelve-lead ECG pace maps from anterior, intermediate, and posterior sites (3, 2, and 1, respectively) of the RVOT septum and free wall. All pace maps show an LBBB morphology and inferior frontal plane axis. Lead I is negative in the anterior sites (site 3) and positive in the posterior sites (site 1). R waves in the inferior leads are broader, shorter, and notched in free wall pace map sites (Courtesy Dixit S, Gerstenfeld EP, Callans DJ, Marchlinski FE. Electrocardiographic patterns of superior right ventricular outflow tract tachycardias: distinguishing septal and free-wall sites of origin. J Cardiovasc Electrophysiol 2003; 14:1–7)

Selective Site: Right Ventricular Septal Pacing

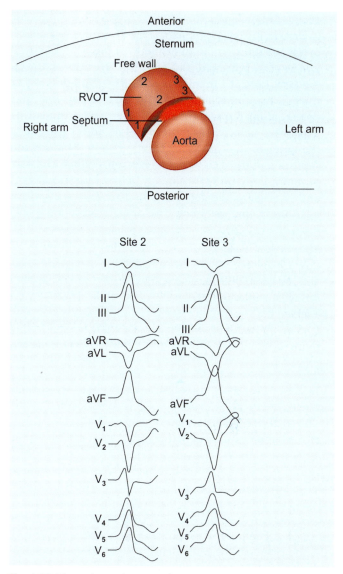

Fig. 4.12 The unique electrocardiogram (ECG) morphologies from septal sites 2, and 3. (Courtesy Dixit S, Gerstenfeld EP, Callans DJ, Marchlinski FE. Electrocardiographic patterns of superior right ventricular outflow tract tachycardias: distinguishing septal and free-wall sites of origin. J Cardiovasc Electrophysiol 2003; 14:1–7)

lead I than anterior and free wall RVOT pacing. However, a negative QRS complex is not specific for septal pacing. Limb lead I is useful in discriminating left anterior from right posterior locations along the free wall and the septum of the superior RVOT. The QRS morphologic appearance in lead I changes from a monomorphic R-wave to a monomorphic Q-wave as the pacing catheter is moved from the posterior to the anterior septum. **In general, for both the free-wall and septal rightward and posterior location (site 1), the QRS in lead I manifests a positive QRS polarity (r waves). In comparison, the leftward and anterior sites (site 3) along the septum and the free wall demonstrate a negative polarity (qs pattern). Sites midway between the anterior and posterior locations (site 2) along the septum and the free wall demonstrates either biphasic or multiphasic QRS morphology in lead I (qr/rs pattern) or an isoelectric segment preceding the q or r wave with a net polarity that was isoelectric.** Septal stimulation results more often in a negative deflection in lead aVL also.

- *Precordial QRS transition:* This event is earliest (towards V1) at the septal sites of pacing and later at the anterior sites, and latest (towards V6) at free wall RV outflow pacing sites. Similarly, the horizontal plane axis shows progressively more clockwise rotation in septal, anterior, and free wall RV outflow pacing sites. Precordial transition in ECGs using the transition zone index (TZI), adapted from the pace-mapping study by Shima for arrhythmogenic focus can be used (Figs 4.13 and 4.14).[17]

Figures 4.15 and 4.16 show 12-lead surface ECG of 2 patients with satisfactory radiological as well as electrocardiographic features of RVOT septal pacing.

However, all cases of septal pacing do not exhibit all the criteria in electrocardiography. Particularly, in presence of infra-nodal disease in form of either of the bundle branch block or interventricular conduction delay, the ECG features of a typical septal pacing do not match. Figures 4.17 and 4.18 are two examples of this kind. About 35% of the patients with RVOT septal pacing may have precordial transition at or beyond V4 and about 15% of the radiological confirmed septal pacing patients have R wave notching in inferior leads.[18]

Mid-septum versus RVOT Septum

The septal stylet can successfully position active-fixation leads in either the RVOT or mid-RV.[19] The determination of where the lead lies, however, is subjective. The boundary between the two sites can be represented by a His-bundle catheter passed adjacent to the roof of the tricuspid valve toward the lateral wall. In practice, in the vast majority of cases, this is not difficult to judge during fluoroscopy (Figs 4.19 and 4.20).

The pacing parameters of R-wave sensing, stimulation threshold and impedance are similar for the RVOT septum

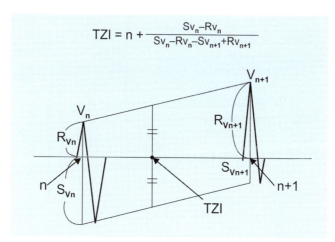

Fig. 4.13 Transitional zone index: In the precordial leads, the QRS complex changes from predominantly negative to predominantly positive. R-wave transition takes place between Vn and Vn+1. The transitional zone index is defined as the abscissa of the point at which the R-wave amplitude and S-wave amplitude are equal. Transitional zone index can be calculated by measuring the amplitude of the R-wave and S-wave at Vn and Vn+1

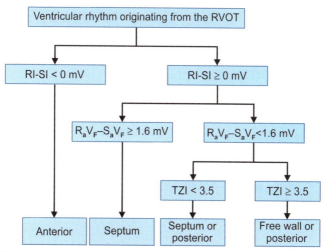

Fig. 4.14 Transitional zone index: A flow chart for differentiating the origin of the ventricular arrhythmia in the RVOT based on the surface 12-lead ECG

and mid-RV septum. The QRS width is slightly higher with RVOT septal pacing compared to mid-RV septal pacing without reaching statistical significance. RVOT septal pacing is associated with a predominant S wave in lead I in 46% of

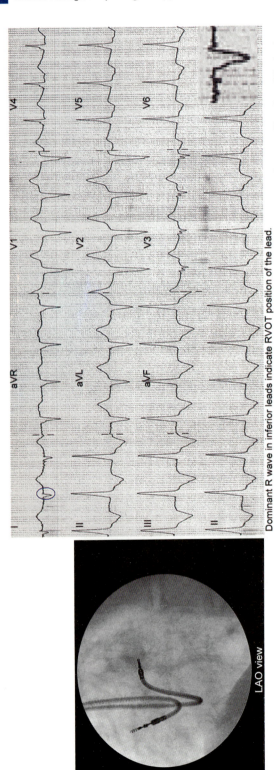

Fig. 4.15 Left anterior oblique fluoroscopic view of a typically positioned RV septal lead with its electrocardiographic features. Lead is positioned in the anterior part of interventricular septum (Site 3)

Dominant R wave in inferior leads indicate RVOT position of the lead.
Early precordial transition and lack of notching on R wave in the inferior leads confirm septal location of the lead.
Morphology in lead I suggest location of the RV lead in the anterior part of the interventricular septum.

Selective Site: Right Ventricular Septal Pacing

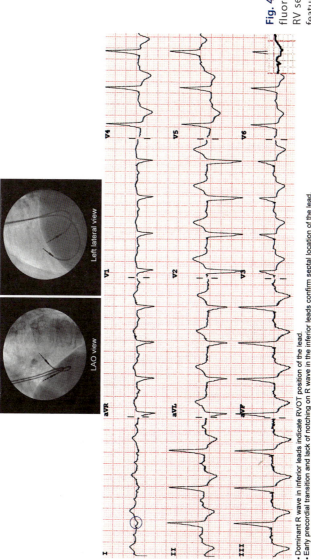

Fig. 4.16 Left Anterior oblique and left lateral fluoroscopic view of a typically positioned RV septal lead with its electrocardiographic features. Lead is positioned in the anterior part of interventricular septum (Site 3)

- Dominant R wave in inferior leads indicate RVOT position of the lead.
- Early precordial transition and lack of notching on R wave in the inferior leads confirm septal location of the lead.
- Morphology in lead I suggest location of the RV lead in the anterior part of the interventricular septum.

Cardiac Pacing: A Physiological Approach

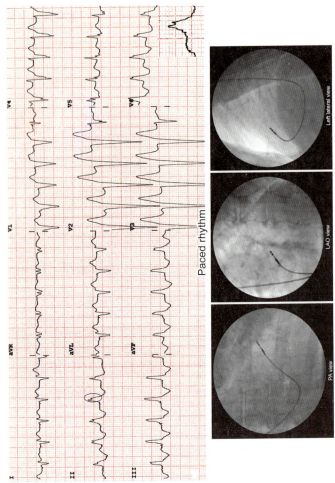

Paced rhythm

Contd...

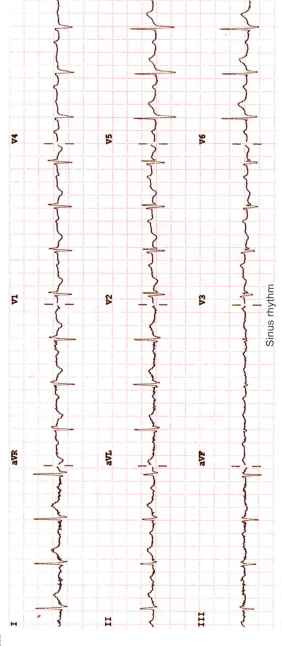

Fig. 4.17 Fluoroscopic PA view, left anterior oblique view (40 degree), and left lateral view confirm the RVOT septal position of the lead (middle row). But, the paced rhythm shows notched R wave in inferior leads and late precordial transition. Notably, the patient has right bundle branch block in sinus rhythm

Sinus rhythm

Contd...

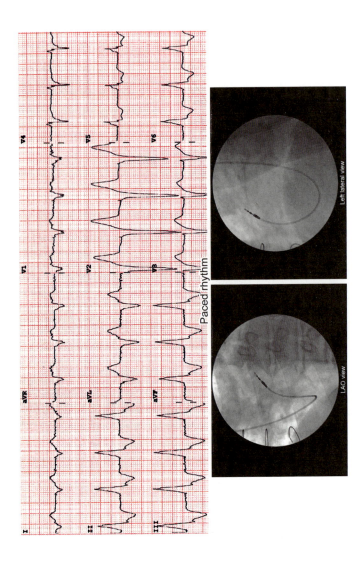

Contd...

Selective Site: Right Ventricular Septal Pacing

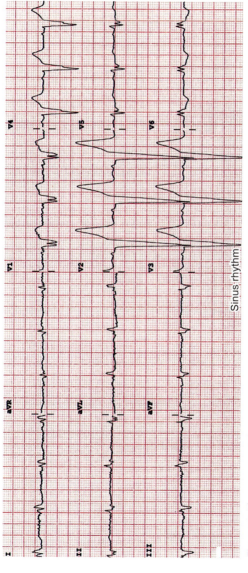

Fig. 4.18 Fluoroscopic left anterior oblique view (40 degree), and left lateral view confirm RVOT septal position of the lead (middle row). But, the paced rhythm shows notched R wave in inferior leads and late precordial transition. Note, there is marginal improvement in QRS duration. Also, note the patient has complete left bundle branch block in sinus rhythm

Contd...

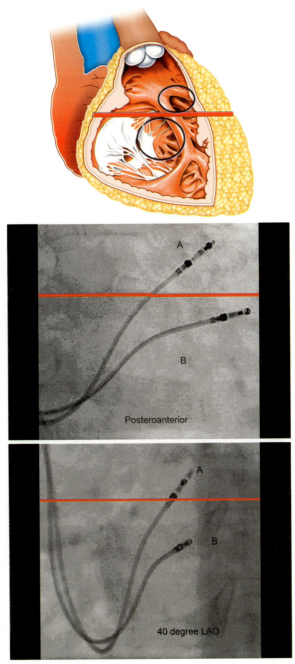

Fig. 4.19 Left: Illustration of the right ventricle (RV) septum. The red heavy line is the boundary between the RV outflow tract (RVOT) above and the mid-RV below (black circles). This line represents a His-bundle catheter passed across the roof of the tricuspid valve. Right: Radiographic views; posterior-anterior (PA) and 40 degree left anterior oblique (LAO) of the leads on the RV septum. The superior lead is in the RVOT (A) and the inferior lead in the mid-RV (B). The LAO view confirms the positioning of the leads on the septum

Selective Site: Right Ventricular Septal Pacing

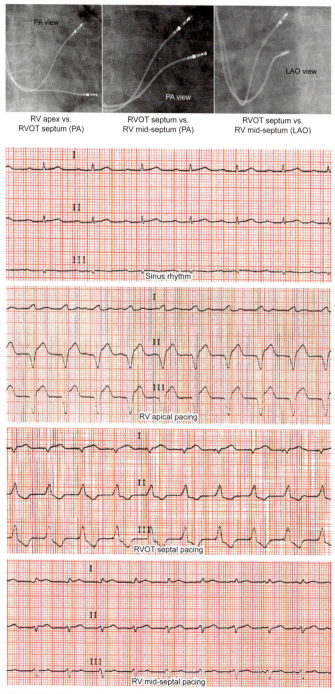

Fig. 4.20 RV apical pacing vs RVOT septal pacing vs RV mid-septal pacing in same patient: RVOT septal pacing produces narrower QRS duration (130 ms) than RV apical pacing (150 ms). Mid-septal pacing shows even narrower QRS (125 ms) complex.

patients, an R wave in 26%, and an isoelectric wave in 28%.[19,20] Why these differences occur is not well understood.

CARDIOMYOPATHY AND RV PACING

RV apical pacing improves cardiac output in hypertrophic obstructive cardiomyopathy whereas RV septal pacing worsens (Gadler, 1996). In dilated cardiomyopathy with symptomatic congestive heart failure cardiac output is higher in RV septal pacing relative to RV apical pacing with shorter AV delays (Cowell, 1994). However, other studies failed to demonstrate the benefit.

EVIDENCE

Study results of different trials comparing RV apical versus RV septal pacing are heterogeneous. Moreno and colleagues in a double-blind prospective randomized study have shown that after 1-year follow-up in persistently pacemaker-dependent patients, with no clinical evidence of severe CHF, midseptal ventricular lead placement is superior to the apical location. They observed significant improvements in both clinical (6-minute walk) and functional (LVEF) parameters.[21]

Using echocardiography as the "gold standard" to directly visualize and define the exact pacing sites and to examine the long-term impact of RV septal versus apical pacing on LV synchrony and function, Leung and colleagues have shown that long-term heterogeneous RV septal pacing may have more deleterious effects on LV function compared with apical pacing despite achieving a narrower QRS complex.[22] Heterogeneous RV septal pacing was associated with lower LVEF, higher LV end-systolic volume index, higher LV mass index, lower circumferential strain, and higher circumferential dyssynchrony. Further analysis comparing apical pacing with "true" septal pacing at the septoparietal trabeculations were not performed due to the small number of patients. Furthermore, patients were not properly randomized to receive RV septal or apical pacing. Echocardiographic determinations of LV function were also not available at the time of insertion of permanent pacemakers. Therefore, patients with possible pre-existing cardiomyopathy cannot be completely excluded and comparable clinical and echocardiographic parameters between the 2 groups of patients with pacing could not be ensured.

Several other studies also failed to prove the superiority of the RV septal pacing over the apical pacing. These clinical studies are flawed in that the leads were positioned in the

RVOT and not necessarily septal.[23-27] When attempting to prove the physiologic and hemodynamic benefits of septal pacing, it seems illogical to choose the RVOT with a mix of both septal and free wall pacing. The potential benefits of septal pacing would possibly be negated by free-wall pacing and thus it is not surprising that there has been no consistent benefit over RV apical pacing demonstrated. Indeed, if one examines RVOT pacing studies, where a septal RVOT pacing site was specified, improved outcomes both acutely and in the medium-term has been consistently demonstrated in the RVOT group compared to apical pacing groups. This is in contrast to the heterogeneous results of studies which did not specify RVOT pacing site. Therefore, the true septal aspect of the RVOT is the ideal target for placing a ventricular lead. Combined RV apex and RVOT pacing in patients resulted in shorter QRS duration than RVOT pacing alone but did not lead to further improvement of cardiac output.[28]

CONCLUSION

Long-term adverse electromechanical and hemodynamics of RV apical pacing is a proven fact. Reliable access and placement of the RV leads in the RVOT septum or mid septum are feasible using conventional active-fixation leads. Little is known about difference in outcomes between RVOT septal and RV mid septal pacing. But, placement of the leads in these sites need careful and better confirmation in posteroanterior, left anterior oblique and left lateral projection in fluoroscopy. Patients with normal ventricular conduction distal to the AV node (or Infra-Hisian conduction) may show the most benefits. Role of paced QRS duration in hemodynamic function needs clarity. More chronic studies with more selective patient criteria are needed. Even then, the detrimental effects of long-term RV apical are significant enough to suggest that it is high time to leave the RV apex.

REFERENCES

1. Tse HF, Lau CP. Long-term effect of right ventricular pacing on myocardial perfusion and function. J Am Coll Cardiol. 1997;29: 744-9.
2. Thambo JB, Bordachar P, Garrigue S, et al. Detrimental ventricular remodeling in patients with congenital complete heart block and chronic right ventricular apical pacing. Circulation. 2004;110: 3766-72.
3. Stuart J Connollly, Charles R Ker, et al. Effects of physiologic pacing versus ventricular pacing on the risk of stroke and death due to cardiovascular cause. NEJM. 2000;342:1385-91

4. De Cock CC, Giudici MC, Twisk JW. Comparison of the hemodynamic effects of right ventricular outflow-tract pacing with right ventricular apex pacing: A quantitative review. Europace. 2003;5:275-8.
5. Harris ZI, Gammage MD. Alternative right ventricular pacing sites—where are we going? Europace. 2000;2:93-8.
6. Karpawich PP, Justice CD, Chang CH, et al. Septal ventricular pacing in the immature canine heart: A new perspective. Am Heart J. 1991;12:827-33.
7. Durrer D, Dam v. RT, Freud GE, et al. Total excitation of the isolated human heart. Circulation. 1970;41:899-912.
8. Tse HF, C Yu, KK Wong, V Tsang, YL Leung, WY Ho, CP Lau. "Functional abnormalities in patients with permanent right ventricular pacing: the effect of sites of electrical stimulation. Journal of the American College of Cardiology. 2002;40(8):1451-8.
9. McGavigan AD, Roberts-Thompson KC, Hillock RJ Stevenson IH, Mond HG. Right ventricular outflow tract pacing: Radiographic and electrocardiographic correlates of lead position. Pacing Clin Electrophysiol. 2006;29:1063-8.
10. Mond HG, Hillock RJ, Stevenson IH, McGavigan AD. The right ventricular outflow tract: The road to septal pacing. Pacing Clin Electrophysiol. 2007;30:482-91.
11. Rosso R, Teh AW, Medi C, Thuy TH, Balasubraman R, Mond HG. Right ventricular septal pacing: The success of stylet-driven active fixation leads. Pacing Clin Electrophysiol. 2010;33:49-53.
12. Medi C, Mond HG. Right ventricular outflow tract pacing: Long-term follow-up of ventricular lead performance. Pacing Clin Electrophysiol. 2009;32:172-6.
13. Corbisiero R, Armbruster R. Does size really matter? A comparison of the Riata lead family based on size and its relation to performance. Pacing Clin Electrophysiol. 2008;31:722-6.
14. Sanjoy S. Srivatsa. Finding the sweet spot for non-apical RV pacing. Journal of Invasive Cardiology. 2014;26 (3):140-7.
15. Crossley GH, Boyce K, Roelke M, Evans J Yousuf D, Syed Z Vicari R. A prospective randomized trial of defibrillation thresholds from the right ventricular outflow tract and the right ventricular apex. Pacing Clin Electrophysiol. 2009;32:166-71.
16. Schwaab B, Frohlig G, Alexander C, Kindermann M, Hellwig N, Schwerdt H, Kirsch CM, et al. Influence of right ventricular stimulation site on left ventricular function in atrial synchronous ventricular pacing. J Am Coll Cardiol. 1999;33:317-23.
17. Dixit S, Gerstenfeld EP, Callans DJ, Marchlinski FE. Electrocardiographic patterns of superior right ventricular outflow tract tachycardias: distinguishing septal and free-wall sites of origin. J Cardiovasc Electrophysiol. 2003;14:1-7.
18. Shima T, Ohnishi Y, Inoue T et al. The relation between the pacing sites in the right ventricular outflow tract and QRS morphology in the 12-lead ECG. Jpn Circ J. 1998;62:399-404.
19. Jippe C Balt, Norbert M van Hemel, Hein JJ Wellens, Willem G de Voogt. Radiological and electrocardiographic characterization of right ventricular outflow tract pacing;Europace. 2010;12: 1739-44.
20. Rosso R, Medi C, Teh AW, Thuy TH, Feldman A, Lee G, Mond HG. Right ventricular septal pacing:A comparative study of outflow

tract and mid ventricular sites. Pacing Clin Electrophysiol. 2010;33:1169-73.
21. Luis Molina, Richard Sutton, William Gandoy, Nicola´ S Reyes, Susano Lara, Froyla´ N Limo, et al. Medium-term effects of septal and apical pacing in pacemaker-dependent patients: A double-blind prospective randomized study. PACE. 2014;37: 207-14.
22. Arnold CT Ng, Christine Allman, Jane Vidaic, Grad D Health, Hui Tie, Andrew P Hopkins, Dominic Y Leung. Long-term impact of right ventricular septal versus apical pacing on left ventricular synchrony and function in patients with second- or third-degree heart block. Am J Cardiol. 2009;103:1096 -101.
23. Mera F, DeeLurgio DB, Patterson RE, Merlino JD, Wade ME, Le´on AR. A comparison of ventricular function during high right ventricular septal and apical pacing after His-bundle ablation for refractory atrial fibrillation. Pacing Clin Electrophysiol. 1999;22:1234-9.
24. Victor F, Mabo P, Mansour H, Pavin D, Kabalu G, DePlace C, et al. A randomized comparison of permanent septal versus apical right ventricular pacing: Short-term results. J Cardiovasc Electrophysiol. 2006;17:238-42.
25. Stambler BS, Ellenbogen KA, Zhang X, Porter TR, Xie F, Malik R, et al. Right ventricular outflow versus apical pacing in paced patients with congestive heart failure and atrial fibrillation. J Cardiovasc Electrophysiol. 2003;14:1180-6.
26. Gong X, Su Y, Pan W, Cui J, Liu S, Shu X. Is right ventricular outflow tract pacing superior to right ventricular apex pacing in patients with normal cardiac function? Clin Cardiol. 2009;32:695-9.
27. Yoon HJ, Jin SW, Her SH, Lee JM, Shin WS, Kim JH, et al. Acute changes in cardiac synchrony and output according to RV pacing sites in Koreans with normal cardiac function. Echocardiography. 2009;26:665-74.
28. Rosso R, Medi C, Teh AW, Thuy TH, Feldman A, Lee G, Mond HG. Right ventricular septal pacing: A comparative study of outflow tract and mid ventricular sites. Pacing Clin Electrophysiol. 2010;33:1169-73.

CHAPTER 5

Selective Site: His Bundle Pacing

INTRODUCTION

Prolonged right ventricular apical pacing has the potential for ventricular function deterioration, mitral valve dysfunction, proarrhythmic effects, and a higher mortality in certain patient groups.[1,2] The outflow tract has been used as the alternative to the apex; however, the results have been not so encouraging.[3] The QRS morphology during direct His bundle pacing is identical to the baseline QRS as it utilizes the native His–Purkinje conduction system. Direct His-bundle pacing (HBP) does not induce interventricular or intraventricular asynchrony or trigger the myocardial perfusion disorders described with right ventricular apical pacing as it produces ventricular contraction via the specific conduction system.[4] His-bundle pacing is sufficiently well-documented in cases of supra-Hisian blocks.[5] Surprisingly, HBP can also correct many conduction disturbances usually considered to be infra-Hisian and, therefore, can be used in selected cases under such circumstances.[6]

ANATOMY

Anatomy of the atrioventricular (AV) junctional area is complex. The most important structure in it is atrioventricular (AV) node. The atrioventricular (AV) node consists of three different regions: the compact portion or AV node itself, the transitional cells zone also called nodal approach, and the penetrating part or His bundle.[7] The compact portion of the AV node is divided from and becomes the penetrating portion of the His bundle at the point where it enters the central fibrous body (Fig. 5.1). The AV node is divided on the basis of electrophysiological characteristics into **AN, N,** and **NH regions.** The AV nodal tissue conducts the electrical impulses very slowly; indeed, it takes approximately 80 ms to travel from the atrial to the ventricular side of the node. This delay between atrial and ventricular activation has functional importance, because it allows optimal ventricular filling. Cells of the lower part of

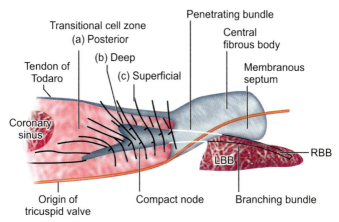

Fig. 5.1 Diagram of a cross-section through the AV junction perpendicular to the endocardial atrial surface. The compact node is covered with a superficial layer of transitional cells, providing a connection between the atrial tissue and the compact node. The compact node, in turn, connects to the bundle of His

the AV node may exhibit spontaneous depolarization and consequent firing activity at an intrinsic lower rate compared with the sinus node. The AV node has its posterior and left atrial extensions that are engaged by transitional tissue. Its posterior extension and transitional tissue in the posterior triangle of Koch are longitudinally arranged parallel to the tricuspid annulus with scant side-to-side connections. The AV node is richly innervated by both adrenergic and cholinergic fibers.

From the AV node, the electrical impulse reaches the His bundle that continues to the distal part of the AV node, perforates the central fibrous body and penetrates the membranous septum (Fig. 5.2). The central fibrous body (annulus fibrosus) electrically isolates the atrial and ventricular myocardium, so that the AV node is the only physiologic electrical connection between atria and ventricles. The proximal cells of the His bundle are very similar to the AV nodal cells, while the distal cells resemble those of the ventricular proximal branches (Purkinje cells). Within this distal system, the electrical impulse is conducted approximately four times faster (3–4 m/s) than in the working myocardium (0.3–1 m/s).[8] This difference is due to the fact that Purkinje cells are longer and have a higher content of gap junctions. Interestingly, neither sympathetic nor vagal stimulation affects normal conduction in the His bundle. The ventricular conduction system is trifascicular; a right bundle branch, and an anterior and posterior branch of the left bundle. These structures originate from the His bundle, at the superior margin of the muscular interventricular septum, immediately beneath the membranous septum.

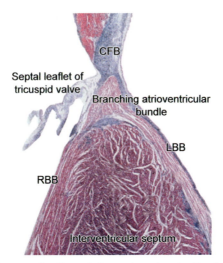

Fig. 5.2 Cross-section through the septum showing the descending right bundle branch and left bundle branches.
Abbreviations: CFB, central fibrous body; RBB, right bundle branch; LBB, left bundle branch

The right bundle branch proceeds intramyocardially as a thin, unbranched extension of the His bundle along the right side of the interventricular septum until it terminates in the Purkinje plexuses of the right ventricular (RV) apex, at the base of the anterior papillary muscle. Similarly, the left bundle branch also has a short intramyocardial route in the interventricular septum before giving rise to its two branches.

ELECTROCARDIOGRAPHIC CHARACTERISTICS

When the His bundle (HB) is correctly captured, activation of the ventricles is mediated by the His-Purkinje system, thus preserving synchronous contraction.[9] Although a QRS identical to the intrinsic one has always been taken as the hallmark of His bundle pacing, simultaneous activation of the His bundle and the ventricle may result in a QRS that is slightly different from the intrinsic one, without likely impairing synchronous activation of the heart. The term para-Hisian pacing (PHP) has been used to define this latter form of stimulation. However, the type of His bundle stimulation is dependent on pacing stimulus amplitude and overlapping may occur between selective HB pacing (SHBP), PHP.[10]

Selective His bundle pacing (SHBP) is defined according to the following criteria:
- His-Purkinje-mediated cardiac activation and repolarization, as evidenced by ECG narrow paced QRS complex with concordance of QRS and T-wave complexes with native QRS;

- The pace-ventricular interval (Vp-V) is isoelectric and almost identical to the His-ventricular interval (H-V) reflecting His-Purkinje conduction time;
- *Output criteria:* At low output, the HB is captured, while on increasing the output both the HB and ventricular fibers are captured (widening of QRS at high output).

Para-Hisian pacing (PHP) is defined according to the following criteria:
- The distal pole of the lead (screw-in) must be positioned as much as possible next to the mapping dipole of the electrophysiological catheter of reference (within 1 cm in the right and left oblique projections).
- The duration of the paced QRS can be larger than the spontaneous QRS, but the duration must be at least 50 ms shorter than the QRS obtained with RV apical pacing and, in any case, not more than 120–130 ms with the electrical axis of the paced QRS must be concordant with the electrical axis of the spontaneous QRS.
- Pace-ventricular interval (the interval between the spike and start of the paced QRS) significantly shorter than His-ventricular interval of the original rhythm, with value close to zero.
- *Output criteria:* On increasing the output step by step, at low output only myocardial fibers are captured, resulting in a wide QRS (i.e. interventricular septal stimulation), while at high output both myocardial fibers and the HB are captured, with a shortening of QRS (shortening of QRS at high output).

Para-Hisian pacing (PHP), which is simpler and more reliable, seems to guarantee physiological ventricular activation of the high muscular part of the intraventricular septum, and also early invasion of the His-Purkinje conduction system, very similar to the activation that can be achieved by direct His bundle pacing. It is difficult to prove that narrowing of the QRS during PHP is due to capture of latent His-Purkinje tissue. Coincident septal ventricular and His-bundle capture makes it difficult to distinguish the components of ventricular activation from local ventricular capture and subsequent ventricular activation via the His-Purkinje system.

Septal ventricular pacing (SVP) stimulation that captured only myocardial fibers is manifested with a large paced QRS at each output level and a discordant QRS and T-wave complexes with native QRS.

So, if the QRS shortens as the output level is decreased, direct or selective His bundle pacing (SHBP) is obtained; if, on the contrary, the QRS widens as the output level is decreased, PHP is obtained. From a **speculative point** of view, this behavior is explained by the distance of the lead helix from the HB, and may be predicted from the signal recorded by the lead. When high amplitude (near-field) His signal is recorded, the distal helix is very close to the HB and SHBP is obtained because less energy is needed to capture the His than to capture the ventricle. When a far-field signal is recorded, the lead helix is away from the His bundle and PHP is obtained because more energy is needed to capture the His bundle than to capture the ventricle. From an **anatomical point** of view, the node becomes the penetrating bundle of His when the conduction axis becomes engulfed within the insulating tissues of the central fibrous body.

It is likely that in SHBP patients the helix reaches the HB at a level where it is not surrounded by ventricular myocytes (approach from the apex of Koch triangle). After its course in the central fibrous body, the penetrating part of the bundle turns slightly leftward and emerges from the fibrous tissue on the crest of the muscular ventricular septum. In PHP patients, the helix probably reaches the bundle at this ventricular level. If this is the case, it is difficult to pace selectively the His, i.e. to avoid activation of ventricular septum even at low output since the helix crosses muscular septum to reach the HB.

The exact site of block or conduction delay producing bundle branch block patterns is not certain in all cases. According to the theory of the longitudinal dissociation of the His bundle, the fibers ascribed to the right and left branches are histologically differentiated and isolated inside the trunk.[11] Injury to the trunk may damage these fibers, showing up in the ECG as a bundle-branch block or complete block. Stimulation of the portion distal to the injury normalizes the QRS complex. Similarly, disease in the purkinje network of either ventricle can give rise to bundle-branch block. Hence, complete branch blocks can be classified according to the site as either central (His bundle) or peripheral (branches or Purkinje system), depending on whether or not they disappear with HBP. Three patterns of pacing are possible:

Pattern 1

- *Presence of latency and disappearance of bundle branch and complete AV block with normalization of QRS complex:* It occurs in the presence of a central block, when the His-bundle capture is 'pure' and distal to the blocked region; ventricular depolarization occurs via the Purkinje system, explaining the QRS normalization with latency.

Pattern 2

- *Absence of latency with the disappearance of bundle-branch and complete AV block without normalization of QRS complex:* It is caused by a 'fusion' caused by capture of the His bundle and the adjacent myocardium (PHP). Right ventricular pre-excitation would be present and induce loss of latency and disappearance of right bundle-branch block independently of its central or peripheral site due to the right ventricular pre-excitation. In the presence of left bundle-branch block (LBBB), this pattern is found solely at its central site because the QRS complexes here is the result of a fusion between His-bundle and myocardial capture. The left ventricular activation via Purkinje, explains the disappearance of LBBB. The activation via para-Hisian myocardial fibers pre-excites the right ventricle, which explains the loss of latency and absence of QRS normalization.

Pattern 3

- *Presence of latency and persistent bundle branch or complete infra-Hisian AV block:* This pattern is seen in the presence of a peripheral block with 'pure' HBP, explaining the persistent blocks with latency. This pattern can also be found in central blocks, if His-bundle capture is pure and prior to the blocked region. His bundle pacing is considered **unsuitable** for patients with this pattern.

In case of an AV block with a narrow QRS complex, pure His-bundle capture induces a QRS complex with a morphology and repolarization identical to native, because the impulse is conducted to the ventricles via a specific conduction system. The latency is equivalent to the conduction time from the His bundle capture region to the start of ventricular depolarization and is also equivalent to the HV interval. Latency is defined as the interval from the pacemaker stimulus to the onset of the earliest paced QRS complex. Fused capture (PHP) may be explained as capture of both the His bundle and the adjacent myocardium, giving rise to two activation fronts: one via a specific conduction system and the other via right anteroseptal myocardium. The QRS complexes are the result of the fusion of both fronts, which explains the absence of latency and the pre-excited aspect of the QRS complex. Pure and fused captures can often be observed in the same electrocardiogram tracing, depending on output energy and lead contact with the His-bundle area. In the case of blocks with a wide QRS complex, His bundle pacing (HBP) is known to be capable of correcting bundle-branch blocks, and obtain a normal QRS complex in the presence of complete AV block considered 'infra-Hisian'.[12]

INDICATIONS

At present, there is no strong recommendation for His bundle pacing for any special patient subset in any guideline. However, the His-bundle can be considered as an ideal pacing site to prevent dysynchrony of the ventricles and maintain normal activation pattern as it causes normal His-Purkinje system mediated activation of the myocardium leadings to rapid sequential synchronous multi-site depolarization of myocardial cells and efficient ventricular contraction. So, in my opinion it should be considered in all **patients with the indication of permanent pacing for AV conduction disturbance.**

Cardiac resynchronization therapy is an established therapy for patients with LV dysfunction with wide QRS (LBBB). It is done by pacing the left and the right ventricle with two separate leads. The benefit of biventricular pacing (BiV) for cardiac resynchronization therapy is not seen in 30–40% of patients, as measured by symptom improvement, left ventricular (LV) remodeling, and/or reduced mortality.[13] Deshmukh and his colleagues have shown improvement in these patients with His bundle pacing in term of increase in LVEF, decrease in LVEDD and LVESD, reducing cardiac size in chest X-ray during follow-up.[14] Echocardiographic studies performed in these patients indicated that during His pacing, the heart contracts in a normal fashion. Paradoxical septal excursion, which was previously described by others during RV apical pacing, and in left bundle-branch block, is not observed with His bundle pacing.[15,16] Dilated cardiomyopathy with ventricular dysfunction is a known consequence of chronic cardiac supraventricular tachyarrhythmia that can often be reversed by restoring a normal rhythm using cardioversion or ablative techniques. These patients can be benefited with AV node ablation followed by His bundle pacing for recurrent and resistant arrhythmia with tachycardiomyopathy.

In contrasts to non-physiologic biventricular pacing (BiV) in which ventricular activation occurs in response to RV endocardial and LV epicardial pacing, "physiologic" ventricular activation by previously latent His-Purkinje tissue during direct His bundle pacing as evidenced by narrowing of the QRS in response to His bundle pacing shows better promise as an alternative to LV lead. At least, it can be **an alternative option to LV lead for patients in whom cardiac resynchronization therapy is indicated but the LV lead implantation is not possible via coronary sinus due to anatomical reason.**

It has been seen that His bundle pacing has the potential for elimination of AV block or bundle-branch block, leading to a narrow QRS complex (≤120 ms) in about half of the patients with complete bundle branch block (particularly LBBB) (central type).[9] So, it should be considered strongly in **patients with complete LBBB who is otherwise going for pacemaker implantation and having normalization of QRS complex with temporary pacing by mapping catheter positioned in His bundle.**

Problems

There are certain problems unique for the His bundle pacing and for these problems we prefer para-Hisian pacing in all cases rather than direct His bundle pacing:

- *Threshold:* The His-bundle penetrates deep into the membranous septum, and, owing to the fibrous structure (less myocardium) of this area, the pacing thresholds are higher than those observed in other RV pacing sites (i.e. RV apex or septal). Almost all available series shows final permanent lead threshold for pacing close to 2 V. The series from Spain shows highest threshold (as high as 2.5 V at 1 msec pulse width).[17] It can be overcome with para-hisian pacing. His-bundle pacing entails greater energy consumption due to the higher stimulation threshold. A higher degree of fibrosis that causes a thicker layer of unexcitable tissue between lead and excitable myocardium, and calcification of this region, could explain this phenomenon.
- *Lead stability:* As the His-bundle is a deeper structure, the conventional 1.5-mm helix of the screw-in lead may be proved inadequate in its ability to sufficiently penetrate the membranous septum leading to repeated dislodgment of the lead tip. It can be overcome with lead having extralong helix (1.8 mm). To overcome this problem, some operators push the lead tip into the membranous septum as much as possible before extracting the helix. Of course, this maneuver can be dangerous sometimes as it can injure the His bundle itself.
- *Success rate:* Low success rate is another challenge for His bundle pacing. With the best effort and available equipment in skilled hands, the success rate is close to 65–70%.[17]
- Because the His-region block can become enlarged and encompass the lead site, an additional safety lead should be considered at the apex or right outflow tract to prevent asystole, especially in patients with pure His-bundle capture. This lengthens the surgical procedure time and results in a higher cost. In the case of para-Hisian pacing, it may be possible to avoid the safety lead because ventricular contraction is assured via myocardial capture.

IMPLANTATION

1st Step (Figs 5.3 and 5.4)

A quadripolar catheter with 2 mm inter-electrode spacing is inserted via femoral vein puncture and advanced to right ventricular (RV) apex. Pacing through the catheter is performed and QRS duration as well as configuration is noted. Then the catheter is withdrawn to a point near the AV septum superior to the tricuspid valve. Subsequent mapping and localization of the His bundle is done in the right anterior oblique fluoroscopic projection to best visualize the tricuspid annulus. To ascertain the optimal position of the catheter, the largest bipolar His

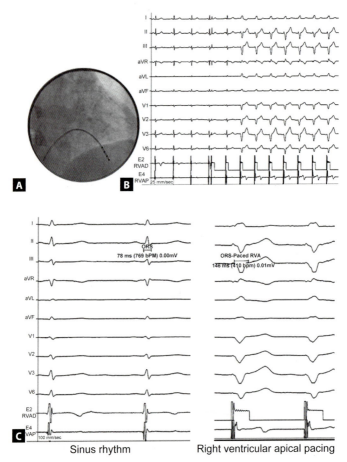

Figs 5.3A to C (A) Quadripolar EP catheter is placed in the RV apex (Right anterior oblique view); (B) Transition from sinus to paced rhythm; (C) Measurement of QRS duration. Left panel in sinus rhythm and right panel shows paced rhythm from RV apex. Note the sinus QRS duration is 78 msec and paced QRS duration is 146 msec

Selective Site: His Bundle Pacing

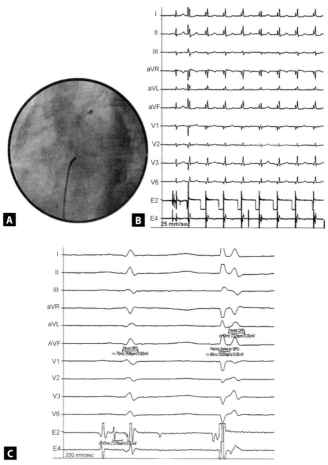

Figs 5.4A to C (A) Quadripolar EP catheter is placed in the His bundle (Left anterior oblique view); (B) Transition from sinus to paced rhythm (1st beat is sinus and subsequent beats are paced); (C) Measurement of QRS duration. Note the sinus QRS duration is 78 msec and paced QRS duration is 84 msec. Also note, the pacing spike to beginning of QRS complex is 48 msec (which is equal to sinus rhythm HV interval) indicates true His bundle capture

bundle potential is recorded and pacing is performed to verify His bundle capture.

2nd Step

Subsequently, a steerable catheter (Selectsite) is inserted into the right atrium via the subclavian vein, and anatomical mapping of the triangle of Koch is performed (Figs 5.5A and B). In particular, the os of the coronary sinus and the tendon of Todaro are located. To locate the tendon, the catheter is advanced into the ventricle at the level of the HB and then

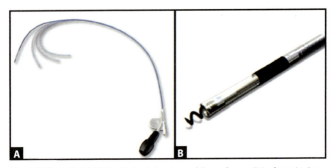

Figs 5.5A and B (A) The Selectsite steerable catheter (Medtronic, Inc., Minneapolis, Minn.); (B) The Selectsite catheter with the lead inside

pulled back in left anterior oblique (LAO) projection until a leftward deviation indicated the site of the tendon. Through the catheter, a bipolar, lumen less screw in, steroid-eluting, 4.1-Fr lead (Select Sure Model 3830–69, Medtronic) is advanced and unipolar mapping of the triangle of Koch is performed until the best near-field His bundle signal is recorded. This electrophysiologic mapping is guided by the quadripolar catheter previously positioned with the distal bipole on the His. Once the His signal has been recorded by means of the pacing lead, a clockwise turn is applied in order to fix the lead to the heart. Subsequently, the steerable catheter is retracted by 3 or 4 cm in order to allow electrical measurements by the lead.

In most of our labs the steerable catheter is not available. So, we take a regular screw-in lead through a 7F PLI sheath into the RV through the left subclavian vein and advanced in anteroposterior (AP) projection close to the distal dipole of the quadripolar diagnostic EP catheter. A modified J-shaped stylet with a secondary distal curve orthogonal to the J plane allows the lead to be properly oriented when rotated medially toward the AV septum. Iterative adjustments to the stylet shape are required because of individual patient anatomy. Then, in left anterior oblique (LAO) projection, it is gently rotated counterclockwise toward the His-bundle and positioned exactly on the distal dipole of the quadripolar diagnostic catheter. Using the exposed screw as a temporary anchor point, the lead is positioned near the mapping catheter and adjusted to obtain the largest His potential. Slight movements of the quadripolar His bundle catheter and permanent pacing lead are frequently required to achieve optimal positioning. The correct position is confirmed in right anterior oblique (RAO) projection and the lead is then screwed in by means of 4 or 5 clockwise rotations. Occasionally, a slight advancement of the helix by a half-turn at a time is required to achieve consistent capture. The

Selective Site: His Bundle Pacing

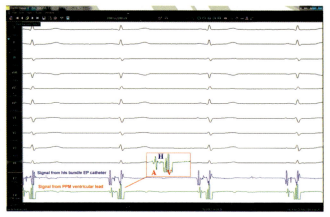

Figs 5.6 Simultaneous signal from the EP catheter positioned in the His bundle and permanent pacemaker ventricular lead (Same patient as in Figs 5.3 and 5.4).

bipolar signal through this lead should show an atrial potential followed by His deflection and ventricular signal (Fig. 5.6).

Lead placement in the His-bundle region can be difficult with the conventional lead because it must be anchored parallel to the plane of contact with the AV septum, something for which it is not designed. The close proximity of the tricuspid valve and its movements contribute to the greater instability of the lead. At present, the technique may be tedious and time-consuming in some patients, because multiple attempts are necessary. This can increase the rate of complications (particularly, infection of the system). So, we limit the time dedicated to the His-bundle lead implantation to not more than 25 min of fluoroscopy time.

Owing to the fibrous structure of the membranous septum where the His-bundle penetrates deep into, the pacing thresholds are higher than those observed in other RV pacing sites. Moreover, the EGM recorded in the His region can be regarded as a ventricular far-field signal; this could explain the lower amplitude of the recorded ventricular EGM.

3rd Step

At this point, temporary pacing is started from the lead at different output levels in order to evaluate the types of the stimulations obtained[12] (discussed earlier). The most significant challenge encountered during His bundle pacing is the inability to precisely direct the stylet-controlled lead tip to the small (≤2 mm in diameter) target, especially during cardiac contraction and relaxation. Moreover, difficulty is frequently encountered when attempting to engage the screw into the membranous septum. Gross dislodgment of the lead tip requiring multiple reattempts is a common occurrence. The observation that a slight advancement of the pacing helix into the septum often yield significantly lower pacing thresholds suggests that the conventional 1.5 mm helix is inadequate in its ability to sufficiently penetrate the membranous septum. Lead parameters are tested few minutes later. QRS width is measured (Figs 5.7A to D).

After satisfactory results on testing, the position of the lead is accepted. Fluoroscopic appearances of the permanent His bundle or Para-Hisian ventricular lead are not well characterized in any of the literature.

Outcome

At present, there is no long-term follow-up study or randomized control trial report is available to suggest that His bundle is the most effective pacing site to maintain long-term hemodynamic beneficial effect in patient undergoing permanent pacemaker implantation. However, few anecdotal reports indicating superiority of His bundle pacing over other sites of right ventricular pacing are available. Barold and his colleagues have shown that only His bundle pacing, guided by fluoroscopy and electrophysiology ensures homogeneous values of electromechanical activation during stimulation whereas both septal and apical RV pacing induces variable effect.[18] Deshmukh and his colleagues have demonstrated that permanent, direct His bundle pacing is attainable in many patients and that this type of pacing provides sustained hemodynamic improvement in a subset of patients with chronic atrial fibrillation and LV dysfunction.[5]

CONCLUSION

His bundle pacing undoubtedly is the most physiological in all respect. At present, the technique of His bundle pacing is tedious and time-consuming in some patients, because multiple attempts are necessary. This can increase the rate of complications and increased procedure time as well as high fluoroscopy time. So, we have to limit the time dedicated to the His-bundle lead implantation. Availability of the steerable lead delivery system with dedicated lead will increase the success rate. With the current advent of thinner MRI-friendly lead design should improve the success rate further. New types of batteries that are able to withstand higher energy consumption

Selective Site: His Bundle Pacing

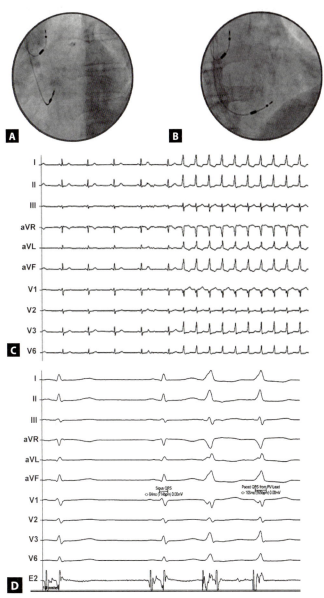

Figs 5.7A to D (A) Fluoroscopic left anterior oblique view; (B) Fluoroscopic right anterior oblique view; (C) Transition from sinus to paced rhythm; (D) Measurement of QRS duration. Note the sinus QRS duration is 84 msec and paced QRS duration is 108 msec (Same patient as in Figs 5.3, 5.4 and 5.6)

without significant reduction of their lifespan are now available and are supposed to be useful.

REFERENCES

1. Nahlawi M, Waligora M, Spies SM, Bonow RO, Kadish AH, Goldberger JJ. Left ventricular function during and after right ventricular pacing. J Am Coll Cardiol. 2004;44:1883-8.
2. Barold SS, Ovsyshcher EI. Pacemaker-induced mitral regurgitation. Pacing Clin Electrophysiol. 2005;28:357-60.
3. De Cock CC, Giudici MC, Twisk JW. Comparison of the haemodynamic effects of right ventricular outflow-tract pacing with right ventricular apex pacing: a quantitative review. Europace. 2003;5:275-8.
4. Catanzariti D, Maines M, Cemin C, Broso G, Marotta T, Vergara G. Permanent direct His bundle pacing does not induce ventricular dyssynchrony unlike conventional right ventricular apical pacing: an intrapatient acute comparison study. J Interv Card Electrophysiol. 2006;16:81-92.
5. Deshmukh P, Casavant DA, Romanyshyn M, Anderson K. Permanent, direct His bundle pacing: a novel approach to cardiac pacing in patients with normal His-Purkinje activation. Circulation. 2000;101:869-77.
6. Morin͂a-Vazquez P, Barba-Pichardo R, Venegas-Gamero J, Herrera Carranza M. Cardiac resynchronization through selective His bundle pacing in a patient with the so-called infra His atrioventricular block. Pacing Clin Electrophysiol 2005;28:726-9.
7. Scher AM, Young AC, Malmgreen AL et al. Activation of the interventricular septum. Circ Res. 1955;3:56-64.
8. James TN, Sherf L. Fine structure of the His bundle. Circulation 1971;44:9-28.
9. Amitani S, Miyahara K, Sohara H, Kakura H, Koga M, Moriyama Y, Taira A, Nagano S, Miura N, Misumi K, Sakamoto H. Experimental His-Bundle pacing: Histopathological and electrophysiological examination. Pacing Clin Electrophysiol. 1999;22:562-6.
10. Cantu` F, De filippo P, Cardano P, De luca A, Gvazzi A. Validation of Criteria for Selective His Bundle and Para-Hisian permanent pacing. Pacing Clin Electrophysiol. 2006;29:1326-33.
11. El-Sherif N, Amay YLF, Schonfield C, et al. Normalization of bundle-branch block patterns by distal His bundle pacing. Clinical and experimental evidence of longitudinal dissociation in the pathologic his bundle. Circulation. 1978;57:473-83.
12. Barba-Pichardo R, Morin͂a-Va´zquez P, Venegas-Gamero J, Frutos-Lo´pez M, Moreno-Lozano V, Herrera-Carranza M. Posibilidades y realidades de la estimulacio ´n permanente del haz de His. Rev Esp Cardiol. 2008;61:1096-9.
13. Young JB, Abraham WT, Smith AL, et al. Combined cardiac resynchronization and implantable cardioversion defibrillation in advanced chronic heart failure: the MIRACLE ICD Trial. JAMA. 2003;289:2685-94.
14. Pramod Deshmukh, David A Casavant, Mary Romanyshyn, Kathleen Anderson. Permanent, Direct His-Bundle Pacing: a Novel Approach to Cardiac Pacing in Patients with Normal His-Purkinje Activation. Circulation. 2000;101:869-77.
15. Leclercq C, Gras D, Helloco A, Nicol L, Mabo P, Daubert C. Hemodynamic importance of preserving left ventricular activation in permanent cardiac pacing. Am Heart J. 1995;129:1133-41.

16. Grines CL, Boshore TM, Boudoulas H, Olson S, Shafer P, Wooley CF. Functional abnormalities in isolated left bundle branch block: the effect of interventricular asynchrony. Circulation. 1989;79:845-53.
17. Rafael Barba-Pichardo, Pablo Moriña-Vázquez, Juan M José Venegas-Gamero, Manuel Herrera-Carranza. Permanent His-bundle pacing: seeking physiological ventricular pacing. Europace. 2010;12:527-33.
18. Gianni Pastore, Francesco Zanon, Franco Noventa, Enrico Baracca, Silvio Aggio, Giorgio Corbucci, Roberto Cazzin, Loris Roncon, Serge S. Barold. Variability of Left Ventricular Electromechanical Activation during Right Ventricular Pacing: implications for the Selection of the Optimal Pacing Site. Pacing Clin Electrophysiol. 2010;33:566-74.

CHAPTER 6

Selective Site: Right Atrial Septal Pacing

INTRODUCTION

The conventional site for placement of right atrial lead has been challenged as inadequate and non-physiologic as it has been shown to result in a higher incidence of atrial fibrillation.[1] It is believed that the prolonged times of signal conduction from high to low atrium that can occur with pacing from the right atrial appendage may play an important role in the induction of atrial fibrillation. In selective site atrial pacing, the atrial septum is chosen to improve intra-atrial and interatrial conduction and minimize dispersion of refractoriness. This in turn may improve atrial hemodynamics and reduce the incidence of paroxysmal atrial tachyarrhythmias like atrial fibrillation. Low atrial septal selective and multi-site atrial pacings have been shown to reduce the incidence of atrial fibrillation.[2] Upper atrial septal pacing is known to pace both the atria simultaneously.

ANATOMY

The interior of the right atrium consists of posterior smooth part known as *sinus venarum* which receives the termination of large veins (superior vena cava, inferior vena cava and coronary sinus) and anterior rough part known as *atrium proper*. These two parts are separated by a smooth muscle ridge, the **crista terminalis.** The interatrial septum is oblique in transverse plane, so the right atrium is both anterior and to the right of the left atrium. The left atrium (LA) is located to the left and mainly posterior to the interatrial septum. The RA is somewhat larger than the left, but its wall is thinner. The openings of the superior vena cava is situated in the upper and posterior part of the right atrium, directed downwards and forwards and have no valve. The opening of the inferior vena cava is situated in the lower and posterior part of the right atrium, close to the atrial septum and guarded by a rudimentary semilunar valve, **eustachian valve,** which is formed by duplication of endocardium containing a few muscle fibres. It is attached by its convex margin to the anterior wall of the opening; it's concave free margin projects into the atrium, and presents right and left horn. Right horn is continuous with the lower end of crista terminalis, and the left horn with the anterior limb of limbus fossa ovalis. The opening of the coronary sinus is situated between the opening of inferior vena cava and right atrioventricular orifice, in the lower part of interatrial septum. The opening is guarded at its lower margin by an incomplete semicircular valve, known as the *thebesian valve.*

Crista terminalis consists of muscle that is more prominent superiorly, tapering toward its inferolateral end. It extends from the upper part of the interatrial septum, passes laterally in front of the opening of the superior vena cava and skirts round the right side of the opening. The ridge runs downwards along the right wall of the atrium and ends below by joining with the right horn of the valve of inferior vena cava. Externally, the crista terminalis corresponds to a seam known as the sulcus terminalis, the pectinate muscles travel laterally in a parallel fashion from the crista terminalis along the RA free wall. The atrial wall between the pectinate muscle bundles is almost paper thin and translucent. An extensive muscular pouch, the auricle, projects anteriorly to overlap the right side of the ascending aorta. The auricle is a broad, triangular structure and has a wide junction with the true atrial component. It is filled with pectinate muscles. The pectinate muscles spread throughout the entire wall of the atrial appendage, extending to the lateral and inferior walls of the atrium. The pectinate muscles never reach the orifice of the tricuspid valve. The **vestibule** is a smooth muscular rim that surrounds the tricuspid valve orifice.

The interatrial septum forms the posterior or medial wall of the RA. The central ovoid portion, which is thin and fibrous, forms a shallow depression known as the **fossa ovalis.** The remainder of the septum is muscular, forming a ridge known as the limbus fossa ovalis. A triangular zone, the **Koch's triangle,** is a landmark indicating the site of the atrioventricular node and its atrial connections. The **anterior border** is marked by a hinge of the septal leaflet of the tricuspid valve. The coronary sinus (CS) terminates in the inferoposterior aspect of the RA and forms the **inferior border** of Koch's triangle. The **posterolateral border** is formed by the round, palpable, collagenous, subendocardial tendon of Todaro which extends dorsally from the central fibrous body to the left horn of the valve of inferior vena cava (Fig. 6.1). Epicardially, the sinus node is located in the groove adjacent to the SVC-RA junction. The RA musculature extends from the SVC externally and terminates at the entrance of the inferior vena cava.

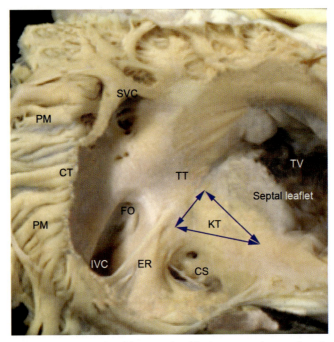

Fig. 6.1 The landmarks of the triangle of Koch are superimposed on the exposed right atrial cavity. The relationship of the structural landmarks to the coronary sinus (CS) is seen. ICV, inferior vena cava; SCV, superior caval vein; CT, crista terminalis; PM, pectinate muscle, FO, fossa ovalis; ER, eustachian ridge; TT, tendon of Todaro; TV, tricuspid valve; KT, Koch's triangle

ELECTROMECHANICS

The right atrium and left atrium are activated nearly simultaneously (within 50–80 msec) during sinus rhythm. The spread of activation within each atrium and from one atrium to the other follow preferential pathways for impulse propagation. These preferential pathways consist of circumferential and longitudinal muscle bundles, but they are generally not considered to be part of the specialized conduction system. In a study, it has been suggested that four distinct sites serve as electrical connections between the right and the left atrium: (1) the high septal right atrium or **Bachmann's bundle**, a circumferential muscle bundle at the anterior wall of the left atrium. In 1907, Bachmann described a distinct band of muscle tissue extending from the base of the LA appendage, called the anterior interatrial band. Bachmann's bundle was later defined as a band of fibers traversing the LA, curving posteriorly within the interatrial septum, and reaching the crest of the atrioventricular node.[3] BB diverges into fibers in the anterior and posterior left atrium. One bundle of fibers advances anteriorly toward the left atrial appendage and the other advances posteriorly between the pulmonary veins. BB serves to conduct cardiac impulses from right to left atrium, (2) the region of Koch's triangle, with left posterior extension of the AV node, (3) the fossa ovalis, and (4) the coronary sinus level with connections limbus between the coronary sinus muscle cover and the left atrium.[4] In the right atrium, the crista terminalis and its medial extension has been suggested to favor the spread of activation in a longitudinal direction, whereas transverse conduction has been found to be limited even in normal hearts. In the left atrium, circumferential muscle fibers along the mitral annulus have been described by some investigators.

Permanent atrial pacing has been proposed as one of the nonpharmacological alternative approaches in selected patient groups with presumed bradycardia-dependent atrial fibrillation (AF).[5] On the other hand, the development of novel atrial pacing techniques such as biatrial, bifocal right atrial and single site inter-atrial septum pacing has extended the indications for pacemaker therapy to symptomatic drug refractory AF by prevention of paroxysmal AF (PAF). The rationale for these new approaches is modification of the electrophysiological properties of the atria in order to influence the presumed mechanisms related to the pathogenesis of atrial tachyarrhythmia.[6]

Assessment of atrial conduction delay can be done in two ways:
1. *Electrocardiographically:* P wave duration is traditionally measured in lead II and a value of **more than 120 ms** is abnormal. The ECG often shows a wide and notched P wave in lead II together with a wide terminal negativity in V1 commonly described as *left atrial enlargement*. Such a configuration probably reflects atrial conduction disorder rather than biatrial or left atrial hypertrophy/ dilatation. But the typical aspect of the so-called "interatrial conduction block" is characterized by a left-axis deviation of the P wave terminal vector beyond – 30 degrees in the frontal plane and divergence (> 90 degrees) between the initial P wave vector (linked to early activation of right atrium) and the terminal vector. These ECG abnormalities are frequently associated with echocardiographic left atrial dilatation, and there is a statistically significant relationship between the size of the left atrium and interatrial conduction.[7]
2. *Electrophysiologically:* Typically, the right **intra-atrial conduction time** is measured from the beginning of the P wave, or the intracardiac signal recorded in the upper part of the right atrium, to the onset of atrial depolarization in the para-Hisian bundle region. Its normal value is generally between 30 and 60 ms (Fig. 6.2). **Interatrial conduction**

time is measured from the beginning of the P wave or upper right atrium depolarization to the onset of left atrial depolarization recorded at the level of the distal coronary sinus. It is normally between 60 and 85 ms (Fig. 6.3).

Two potential mechanisms produce atrial conduction disorders: **(1)** spatial dispersion of refractory periods or anisotropy resulting from scarce side-to-side electrical coupling, and **(2)** generally discrete fibrosis disrupting the arrangement of atrial muscle fiber bundles or to major ultrastructural abnormalities.[8]

The left atrium acts as both conduit and pump. So, its ability to transfer blood to the ventricle essentially defines

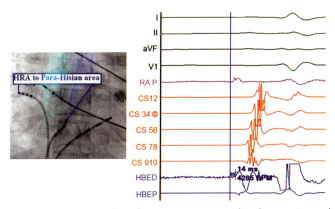

Fig. 6.2 Right intraatrial conduction time measured as the time interval of atrial depolarization between high right atrium (RAP) and His bundle (HBED). In this case it is 14 ms. A decapolar EP catheter placed in coronary sinus and 2 quadripolar catheter placed in high right atrium and His bundle respectively

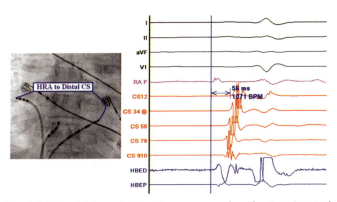

Fig. 6.3 Interatrial conduction time measured as the time interval of atrial depolarization between high right atrium (RAP) and distal coronary sinus (CS 1,2). In this case it is 58 ms. A decapolar EP catheter placed in coronary sinus and 2 quadripolar catheter placed in high right atrium and His bundle respectively

left ventricular filling. As a result the left atrial volume can be considered as an useful indicator of the presence, chronicity, and severity of left ventricular diastolic dysfunction. Left ventricular diastole begins when the aortic valve closes and includes isovolumic relaxation, rapid early ventricular filling, diastasis, and left atrial contraction (Fig. 6.4). The initial phase, prior to mitral valve opening, involves the rapid, energy-dependent relaxation of the left ventricular myocardium to its resting unstressed length. This process is associated with a brisk decline in left ventricular pressure. Once ventricular pressure falls below left atrial pressure (which is rising), the mitral valve opens. The interval between aortic valve closure and mitral opening is referred to as isovolumic relaxation. The next step involves filling the left ventricle as rapidly as possible without resulting in a significant increase in pressure. After the mitral valve opens, ventricular pressure continues to fall; creating a pressure gradient between the left atrium and the left ventricle and blood is pulled through the mitral valve. This event is reflected by the large E wave on mitral valve Doppler recordings in healthy individuals. As the left ventricle begins to fill, the pressure within the chamber rises and the rate of inflow slows. Continued filling in mid-diastole occurs only if left ventricular compliance is sufficiently low, or if left atrial pressure is sufficiently high, to allow the forward flow of blood. The final phase of left ventricular filling results from atrial contraction and ends with mitral valve closure. Atrial contraction, after the P wave on the ECG, produces a surge of blood into the ventricle at the end of diastole, causing the final and optimal filling of the ventricle. This "atrial kick" adds about 20% to the volume of the ventricles and reflected by the A wave on mitral valve Doppler. If diastolic pressure rises too quickly, left ventricular filling will be reduced and prematurely terminated. If a compensatory increase in left atrial pressure is required to maintain left ventricular filling, pulmonary venous pressure will rise as a result, leading to symptoms. In atrial fibrillation there is loss of atrial systole, which results in decrease in effective LV stroke volume by 25% at low heart rates and by almost 50% at higher heart rates.

Atrial conduction delay either spontaneous or induced by right atrial pacing, delays left atrial systole and modifies, or even in extreme cases cancels, its contribution to ventricular filling with the resultant risk of left heart AV asynchrony (Figs 6.5 and 6.6). As a result, this increases risk of diastolic mitral regurgitation and atrial fibrillation. During intrinsic conduction, significant delay of left atrial contraction can occur in patients with sinus rhythm and atrial conduction disorders (which can be demonstrated by analyzing mitral

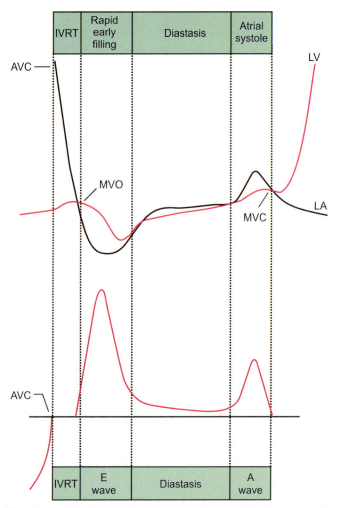

Fig. 6.4 The four stages of diastole are illustrated in this schematic. The upper tracing illustrates the left ventricular and left atrial pressure curves, whereas the lower tracing demonstrates the associated transmitral filling pattern, recorded with Doppler. Isovolumic relaxation begins with aortic valve closure (AVC) and ends with mitral valve opening (MVO), at which point, left ventricular filling begins. This is the result of a pressure gradient between the left atrium and the left ventricle and is coincident with the mitral E wave. A period of diastasis, during mid-diastole, is characterized by relatively little additional filling. In late diastole, atrial systole once again creates a transmitral pressure gradient and results in the Doppler A wave, terminating with mitral valve closure (MVC). IVRT, isovolumic relaxation time

flow). Investigators have shown that the beginning of active ventricular filling is delayed by an average of 50 msec in patients with significant intraatrial conduction delay than patients without any significant abnormality.[9] However,

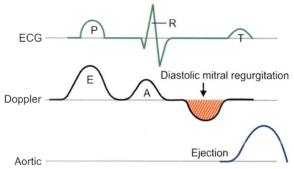

Fig. 6.5 The figure shows the effects of a too long PR interval. Diastolic mechanical flow from atrium to ventricle (the A wave) as a result of atrial contraction occurs slightly later. Similarly, following the QRS complex aortic ejection occurs after a definite and significant electromechanical delay interval. Because atrial filling has been completed and the ventricle has not yet started contracting, blood flows back into the atrium during diastole (diastolic mitral regurgitation). This results in increase left atrial pressure which gets reflected to the pulmonary veins leading to increased propensity of development of atrial fibrillation

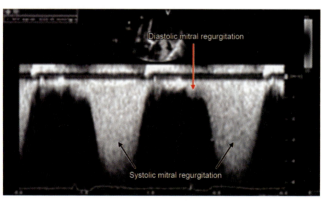

Fig. 6.6 The figure shows mitral regurgitation due to atrioventricular dyssynchrony

prolonged interatrial conduction time is often associated with PR interval prolongation depending on the condition of the AV nodal conduction. These AV conduction disorders probably originate from a discrete injury of atrial tissue, similar to sinus dysfunction also frequent in this population. A long PR will abolish the effect of delayed left atrial activation by delaying left ventricular activation. Conversely, if the AV conduction time remains in the normal range, a high grade interatrial conduction block may cause significant left heart AV asynchrony.

The interatrial conduction block is a direct marker for left atrial contractile dysfunction, with a linear relationship between the degree of electrical delay and the extent of left atrial dysfunction.[7] Besides the reduction or loss of atrial contribution and the proportional reduction of overall cardiac performance, delayed left atrial contraction may also induce major neurohumoral changes that contribute to lowering blood pressure through atrial reflexes activated by increased atrial stretch and pressure causing elevation of atrial natriuretic peptides.[10] These hemodynamic disorders are particularly important when interatrial conduction delay is long, shifting atrial systole after the beginning of ventricular contraction and against a closed mitral valve, resulting in a derangement similar to 1:1 ventriculoatrial conduction during ventricular pacing. In such a situation, atrial contraction provokes sudden and major atrial distension and induces AV regurgitation that may be felt by the patient as painful neck vein pulsations and pulsatile headache. Right atrial pacing may reveal or enhance atrial conduction disorders depending on the site and rate of atrial pacing. Ishikawa et al. determined a critical PR interval of 0.23 ± 0.01 s, above which most patients will show some degree of diastolic mitral regurgitation, which can easily be identified by continuous-wave Doppler echocardiography.[9]

The main benefits that the selective sites for right atrial pacing should provide are: **(1)** a very short interatrial conduction delay and a significant decrease in P-wave duration; **(2)** a reduction in dispersion of atrial refractoriness; **(3)** a more homogeneous recovery of excitability and atrial activation; and **(4)** electrical atrial remodeling, with a gradual reduction in left atrial diameters and volume.[11]

Interatrial septal pacing modifies the atrial activation pattern and abbreviates the total atrial activation time judged by a significant decrease in P wave duration and shortening of interatrial conduction between the high right atrium and distal coronary sinus.[12] Consequently, a reduced propensity to AF can be expected from reduced dispersion of atrial refractoriness and a more homogeneous recovery of excitability. Pacing at this site can prevent AF initiation by premature beats by prolongation of the premature intervals of ectopics in relation to the maximal preexcitation of that critical area. As discussed earlier, there are many septal interatrial connections, including those around the fossa ovalis, in the triangle of Koch area, and in the coronary sinus, in addition to the Bachmann's bundle in the anterosuperior part of the atria. Pacing at these sites, at the Bachmann's bundle level or near the coronary sinus ostium, therefore, provides simultaneous and more synchronized activation of both atria. However, this process depends on the integrity of interatrial septal connections and the absence of conduction blocks at their level.

Selective Site: Right Atrial Septal Pacing

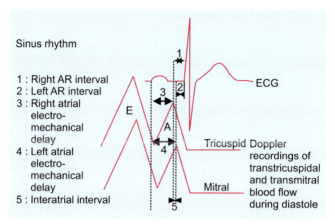

Fig. 6.7 Schematic representation of parameters based on synchronous electrocardiogram and pulse Doppler echocardiography recordings. (1 and 2) The right and left AR intervals correspond to the interval separating the atrial systoles and the ventricular depolarization. They were measured from the apex of the A wave to the onset of the QRS complex. (3 and 4) The right and left atrial electromechanical delays were measured from the onset of the P wave to the apex of the A wave. (5) The interatrial interval was defined as the difference between the right and left atrial electromechanical delays

In a study[13] atrial conduction was assessed with the following parameters in right atrial appendage pacing and atrial septal pacing (Fig. 6.7):
- P wave duration and PR interval.
- Right and left atrial electromechanical delays (RAEMD and LAEMD) measured from the onset of the P wave to the peak A wave on Doppler echocardiography, respectively, at the tricuspid and mitral annulus. The peak A wave is chosen because it is easier to locate than the onset of the wave.
- Interatrial interval, defined by the difference between the RAEMD and LAEMD.

They have found that during right atrial appendage pacing, P wave duration, PR interval, RAEMD and LAEMD are prolonged compared to sinus rhythm; conversely, the left AR interval is reduced. All these modifications may influence atrial vulnerability to arrhythmia (Fig. 6.8). Indeed, prolongation of the P wave duration increases the heterogeneity of the refractoriness, while a long PR interval may induce a reduction in the ventricular filling time and the possibility of diastolic mitral regurgitation. The prolongation of the RAEMD may be the result of a greater intra-atrial conduction delay in the Koch triangle; this phenomenon has been observed during the high atrium versus low atrial septal pacing and is associated with higher AF inducibility. As far as the reduction of the left AR is

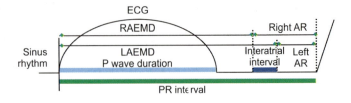
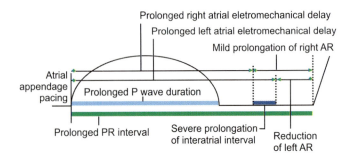
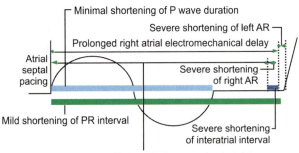

Fig. 6.8 Scaled schematic electrocardiogram representation of the relative modifications induced on P wave duration, PR interval, electromechanical delays, interatrial interval, and AR intervals. In sinus rhythm, the right atrial systole occurs before the left atrial systole and the right AR interval is longer than the left AR interval. The size of the bars represents the mean values of the two control groups. During atrial appendage pacing, P wave duration, PR interval, RAEMD and LAEMD are prolonged. The left AR interval is reduced. The prolongation of the P wave, PR interval and RAEMD and the shortening of the left AR interval could have harmful effects. During atrial septal pacing, the P wave is not prolonged, the PR interval is shortened and the prolongation of the RAEMD is attenuated. The undesirable effects of right atrial appendage pacing are avoided, except for the shortening of the left AR. A reduction of the right AR interval and a slight reversal of the two atrial systoles are also observed

concerned, it can lead to an aborted atrial emptying and can promote atrial arrhythmia.

The prevention of atrial arrhythmias by alternate site pacing or multisite atrial pacing is by several different mechanisms:

(1) Improvement of intra-atrial conduction: Patients with atrial arrhythmias exhibit prolonged intra-atrial conduction delays in response to an extrastimulus, compared with normal arrhythmia-free subjects which can be decreased or completely abolished by multi-site atrial pacing. In particular, right intra-atrial conduction delay observed after right atrial appendage stimulation can be abolished by septal, left atrial (coronary sinus), or biatrial pacing modes. This effect could be the result of early depolarization (preexcitation) of the low right atrium and/or of a **"collision effect"** in the case of multi-site pacing. Simultaneous right and left atrial pacing (biatrial pacing) increases atrial refractoriness and decreases the intra-atrial conduction delay after atrial ectopic beats originating away from a pacing site.[14] Furthermore, pacing from different atrial sites may at best compensate for the anatomic or functional block sites required to sustain a reentrant circuit.

(2) Coupling interval of atrial premature beats: Multisite pacing can increase the coupling interval of premature atrial depolarization in critical zones for initiation of sustained atrial arrhythmia, either because the atrial activation determined by the pacing site(s) is antidromic in relation to that of premature beats or pacing preexcites the reentry zone. The right atrial posteroseptal region, at Koch's triangle level, can be critical because of its properties of anisotropic conduction when AF is induced by a right atrial extrastimulus. Multisite pacing incorporating left atrial or coronary sinus stimulation, by preexciting this critical zone, reduces conduction delays in the right posterior interatrial septum, and abolishes AF induction by a high right atrial extrastimulus.[15]

Obviously, other critical zones can be involved in reentrant arrhythmia and multi-site pacing can prevent functional conduction blocks, by premature activation of the zone beyond the line(s) of block, thereby illustrating the difficulty of selecting the optimal pacing site in clinical practice.

(3) Homogeneous Atrial Depolarization: Multisite atrial pacing can make atrial repolarization more homogeneous and prevent functional conduction block(s) without changing the duration of action potentials or local refractory periods, even in regions where atrial activation is modified or in collision zones.[15] However, the reduction of local activation times and that of global atrial activation eventually reduces local and global repolarization times. In other words, homogeneity of activation is accompanied by a spatiotemporal homogeneity of repolarization. In this regard, the true biatrial pacing configuration (high right atrium-low left atrium) is more effective than the dual site right atrial configuration (high and low right atrium) in reducing global atrial repolarization time.

Left atrial pacing appears necessary as the duration of action potentials and left atrial refractory periods are usually longer than right atrial ones. Even pacing of the left atrium alone can reduce dispersion of atrial repolarization. Conversely, if the left atrium is activated late during right atrial pacing, dispersion of atrial repolarization is enhanced because longer left atrial activation times add up to the longest action potential durations and shorter right atrial activation times are combined with the shortest action potential durations. **(4) Timing of atrial systole:** In the presence of intra (inter-) atrial block, left atrial activation and systole may occur late, even during full ventricular systole.[16] Biatrial pacing preserves left atrioventricular (AV) synchrony by preempting left atrial contraction, and the improved hemodynamics reduce atrial stretch favoring AF.

When left atrial activation and contraction delay is associated with adverse symptoms various approaches may be considered to deal with left AV dyssynchrony. **In patients with long interatrial conduction time, adapted prolongation in PR interval and normal transmitral flow pattern:** In cardiac pacing, it is best to avoid needless ventricular capture because it tends to jeopardize the delicate balance between atrial conduction and AV conduction and induces the risk of left heart dyssynchrony with potential long-term consequences. In such situations septal atrial pacing contribute to a more homogeneous activation of both atria. Another alternative is to use special algorithms to prevent unnecessary ventricular capture in DDD pacing. **In patients with long interatrial conduction time requiring AV pacing:** For various reasons (excessive prolongation of PR interval or highest degree AV block, distal conduction disorders, need to capture the ventricle for hemodynamic reasons like pacing in hypertrophic obstructive cardiomyopathy or pacing in heart failure,

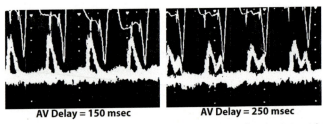

Fig. 6.9 Deleterious hemodynamic consequences of major intraatrial conduction delay in patients permanently paced in the DDD mode for conventional anti-bradycardia indication. Programming a standard AV delay value of 150 ms results in major AV dyssynchrony in the left heart (short filling time and single pulse mitral flow). Increasing the AV delay at 250 ms restores normal AV synchrony. AV = atrioventricular

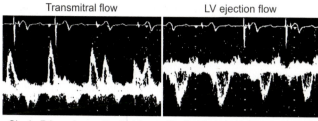

Fig. 6.10 Acute hemodynamic changes induced by biatrial synchronous DDD pacing as compared with standard DDD pacing standard DDD pacing in a patient with long interatrial conduction time. On the left panel switching from standard to biatrial pacing instantaneously corrects baseline atrioventricular dyssynchrony in the left heart. On the right panel switching from biatrial to standard DDD results in a dramatic impairment of the left ventricular systolic performance as indicated by a huge decrease in V max and velocity-time integral (VTI) of the aortic ejection flow

patients with a long interatrial conduction time may require AV pacing. The practical problem is to preserve effective left atrial contribution and prevent a dual chamber pacemaker syndrome. Septal atrial pacing may reduce AV asynchrony but may not suffice in the presence of high degree atrial conduction disorder. Consequently, the two possible solutions are available:

1. Traditional DDD pacing with a long paced AV delay up to 250–300 ms to restore the atrial contribution hidden by standard AV delays of 150–200 ms (Fig. 6.9). However, this maneuver lengthens the total atrial refractory period of the pacemaker and lowers the 2:1 point to the low level of 100–120 beats/min, thereby restricting exercise tolerance. This solution is acceptable only in elderly and inactive patients.
2. Biatrial synchronous DDD pacing: Aside from its probable antiarrhythmic effects, this pacing mode produces a significant hemodynamic benefit in difficult situations. By preempting the left atrial systole by 30–75 ms, it restores normal left AV synchrony and permits programming standard values for the AV delay (Fig. 6.10). Finally, the preferred hemodynamic indication for biatrial synchronous DDD pacing can involve patients with hypertrophic obstructive cardiomyopathy, long interatrial conduction delay, and normal-short PR interval.

In unpaced patients with long interatrial conduction time and normal or short PR interval: This rare situation is a problem mainly in patients with hypertrophic cardiomyopathy whose ventricular filling is highly dependent on left atrial contribution. The aim of treatment is to prolong the intrinsic AV conduction time just enough to restore normal timing of atrial and ventricular systole. Various pharmacologic agents can prolong the AV conduction time (atenolol plus verapamil at increasing doses). In refractory cases selective ablation of the AVN fast pathway lengthen the PR interval. This results in separation of the left atrial component of the P wave from the QRS.

Two different technical methods have been described for multisite atrial pacing: (1) biatrial synchronous pacing involves pacing both atria simultaneously with two leads, one in the right the atrium close to the sinus node, and the other one in the median or distal part of the coronary sinus, so as to selectively detect and pace the left atrium. Both atrial leads are to be connected to the atrial port of a DDD (R) pacemaker through a Y bifurcated adapter. A special "atrial resynchronization" algorithm is loaded into the memory of the device, which triggers instantaneous atrial synchronous pacing after every atrial event is sensed, either sinus beat or right or left atrial extrasystole. This AAT-like pacing mode results in permanent atrial resynchronization. (2) In the other technique, the alternative pacing site is the low posterior right atrium, close to the coronary sinus ostium, which is known to be a key area for arrhythmogenesis in patients with AF. The pacing technique proposed here consists of using a standard DDD (R) pacemaker with no specific algorithm. Both atrial leads (the high right atrium and coronary sinus ostium) are connected to the atrial port of the unit through a Y bifurcated adapter. In that technique, the two atrial pacing sites are simultaneously activated only during the paced atrial cycles. There is no pacing at any site on the sensed atrial cycles, either sinus beats or atrial extrasystoles. To compensate for this technical limitation, the investigators tried to permanently overdrive the intrinsic atrial rate by programming fast baseline pacing rates and sensor-driven pacing and by giving cardio-depressor drugs to reduce the intrinsic atrial rate. In fact, it appears that when both sites have been effectively captured, biatrial pacing and dual-site right atrial pacing have quasi-identical electrophysiologic effects,[17,18] with significantly reduced global activation time (P-wave duration) and homogenized local activation times at the crista terminalis, the His bundle area and the coronary sinus ostium region, as compared with spontaneous sinus rhythm and single site-atrial pacing at different pacing sites (high right atrium, coronary sinus ostium and distal coronary sinus). This indicates that the possible differences in the clinical effectiveness of the two methods of multisite atrial pacing are due to the specific characteristics of the pacing modes used (triggered mode with permanent atrial resynchronization in biatrial synchronous pacing and overdrive inhibited mode in dual-site right atrial pacing).

The synchronous biatrial pacing (**SYNBIAPACE**) study consisted of an intra-patient comparison of three different pacing modes according to a dual crossover design over periods of three months: 1) "inhibited" or no atrial pacing; 2) standard DDD pacing (70 beats/min) at a single high right atrial site; and 3) biatrial synchronous pacing (DDTA, 70 beats/min). Preliminary results[17] did not reveal any statistically significant difference between the three pacing modes in both the time to first recurrence and the total time spent in arrhythmia. Despite a trend in favor of biatrial synchronous pacing, these results did not warrant validation of atrial resynchronization as a sole means to prevent drug-refractory arrhythmia in patients with intra-atrial conduction delay.

Dual-site atrial pacing to prevent atrial fibrillation (**DAPPAF**) trial[18] showed the dual site right atrial pacing is safe and better tolerated than high right atrial and support pacing. In patients on antiarrhythmic dual site right atrial pacing and high right atrial pacing tend to prolong time to recurrent atrial fibrillation compared with support pacing.

IMPLANTATION

The two most investigated pacing sites within the interatrial septum are: (1) the anterosuperior part (the BB region) or high atrial septum and (2) the inferoposterior portion near the CS ostium (the Koch triangle region) or low atrial septum (Fig. 6.11). The area of the high RA septum involves the crista terminalis and Bachmann's bundle, is particularly difficult to pace with

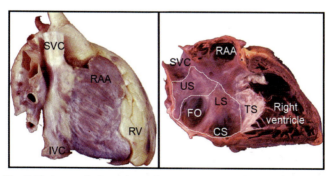

Fig. 6.11 Anatomical specimen showing an external view of the heart (A) and the anteroposterior view of the right atrial septum (B) The part of the atrial septum above the limbus fossa ovalis is known as upper (high) septum and the rest is lower septum. SVC = superior vena cava, IVC = inferior vena cava, TV = tricuspid valve, RAA = right atrial appendage, FO = fossa ovalis, CS = coronary sinus, US = upper septum, LS = lower septum

conventional tools. The conductive properties of the BB differ from those of the RAA, as it contains fibers with histologic characteristics of Purkinje tissue, conducting impulses slightly more rapidly than the surrounding myocardium. Pacing in the region of BB decreases P wave duration, increases symmetry of atrial activation, and decreases atrial activation and recovery time.

Bachmann's Bundle or High Atrial Septal Pacing

After having venous access to subclavian vein in Bachman's bundle pacing, the lead is first placed in the right atrial appendage (RAA). The position is observed in posteroanterior and left anterior oblique fluoroscopic view which serves as the reference position, before it is moved to the BB area. The target region for the implantation of the lead in Bachman's bundle pacing is a confluence of the right atrial roof and the interatrial septum. To locate the Bachman's bundle region, the atrial lead is gradually pulled from atrial appendage and positioned toward the superior septum until the lead deforms, defining the roof of the right atrium in a left anterior oblique (LAO) fluoroscopic view with the help of a hand-made stylet with a single right angle curve. The fluoroscope is then positioned in the right anterior oblique (RAO) view, and the screw is deployed. After 5 minutes the parameters are tested. Figure 6.12 illustrates the BB positioning in the posteroanterior (PA), left anterior oblique (LAO) and left lateral (LL) fluoroscopic views.

The implantation of the BB lead is based on the 2 criteria: (i) fluoroscopic position: in the posterior-anterior (PA) view, the tip of the lead lies slightly above the RAA location, and moves cranially in LAO view with minimal, only 'up-and-down' movements of the lead tip in PA view and in both left anterior oblique as well as left lateral view it faces posteriorly

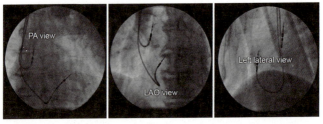

Fig. 6.12 Posteroanterior, left anterior oblique and left lateral fluoroscopic views of a patient with dual chamber pacemaker with ventricular lead placed in RV mid-septum and atrial lead placed near the Bachmann's Bundle. Note that atrial lead tip in left anterior oblique (LAO) as well as left lateral (LL) view faces posteriorly towards the spine

Selective Site: Right Atrial Septal Pacing

STEP 1 Position the atrial lead in the right atrial appendage with the help of conventional J-stylet. Now, work in left anterior oblique (LAO) view. Pull out the stylet.

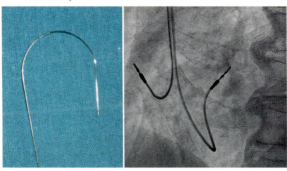

STEP 2 Change the shape of the same stylet to a 90 degree bend with the help of an artery forceps. Put the stylet into the lead. Slowly pull out the lead-stylet assembly keeping an anti-clockwise torque. Once the lead hinges to the target site with the lead tip facing posteriorly in LAO view deploy the screw and remove the stylet. Operator may has to reduce or increase the stylet tip length according to the heart size of the patient.

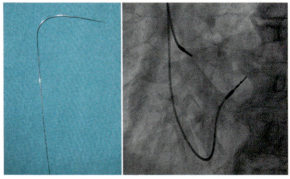

STEP 3 Give loop in the lead with the help of a straight stylet. Check the lead parameters after few minutes.

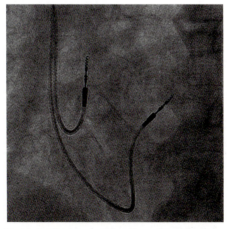

Fig. 6.13 Method of Bachmann's bundle pacing. Note the ventricular lead is positioned into the interventricular septum

towards spine; (ii) characteristic ECG findings (paced P-wave **positive** in leads I, II, and III, **starting immediately** with the pacing spike, and **shorter** than the sinus P-wave with paced P waves are expected to be 15–20 ms shorter than sinus P waves measured on the 12-lead electrocardiogram). The step-wise method of positioning of the atrial lead in the upper inter-atrial septum (Bachmann's bundle) is illustrated in the Figure 6.13.

Low atrial Septal Pacing

The selective site for low RA septum is the mouth or CS os. The usual target for lead attachment is just superior to the CS os. The right atrial appendage (RAA) position is associated with a typical windscreen-wiper movement of the lead in normal sinus rhythm, which is observed on fluoroscopy in the frontal view while an up and down movement of the tip of the lead is

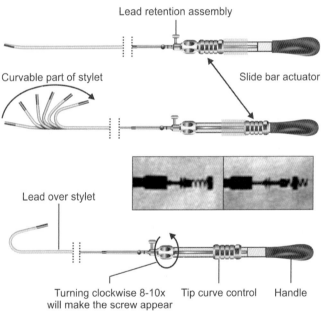

Fig. 6.14 (A) The stylet (Locator,, St. Jude Medical) can deflect the distal 40 mm of the bipolar active fixation lead (St. Jude) using a handle with a slide bar actuator at the distal end of the stylet. The bipolar lead passed over the stylet and attached to the handle with the lead retention assembly. Moving the slide bar over the handle causes a curve of the distal part of the lead. The amount of curvature depends on the distance the slide bar is withdrawn or advanced. (B) When the lead is fixed to the stylet with the retention screw, rotation of the lead retention assembly 8–10 times in a clockwise rotation advances the helix outside the lead tip. By rotating the handle of the stylet around its axis, the lead will also turn around its axes, maneuvering the curved stylet clockwise or counterclockwise in the atrium for active fixation in the atrial septum (From De Voogt WG, Van Mechelen R, Van Den Bos A, et al: A technique of lead insertion for low atrial septal pacing. PACE 28:639, 2005)

Selective Site: Right Atrial Septal Pacing

best appreciated for the low atrial septal (LAS) position in the LAO 45° view.

The leads in low atrial septal pacing are screwed in the atrial septum above the coronary ostium after having changed the original shape of the stylet to a 90° angle. At times, the selected site is almost inaccessible with conventional leads. Special J-shaped stylets are often required. Two types of delivery systems are now available for such difficult clinical situations. The first is a **steerable stylet** (Fig. 6.14). In its current design, the curves achieved by the stylet preclude access to some selective sites. A steerable stylet is connected to a handle with a slide bar. This activates and adjusts the curve. The stylet is actually inside a 0.0016-mm tube that is attached to the slide bar on the handle. The tube is passed down the pacing lead to be inserted. The lead is slipped over the tube and attached to the handle, and the desired curve is made with the lead in the

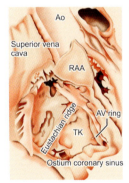
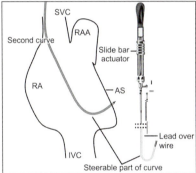

Fig. 6.15 (A) The triangle of Koch (TK) is situated in the lower part of the interatrial septum. The triangle is confined within the borders of the tricuspid valve annulus at the inferior and the eustachian ridge superiorly. The base of the triangle is formed by the coronary sinus ostium. The posterior part of the TK is a muscular part of the interatrial septum. In the superior part of the interatrial septum, there is separation of both atria by the interatrial grove. Pacing at that level does not pace both atria at the same time. In the middle of the IAS, the fossa ovalis is located. The fossa ovalis separates the interatrial septum in a superior part where Bachmann's bundle is located and an inferior region with the TK. (B) Before insertion of stylet and lead in the venous system, a second curve in the same plain as the extendable part should be made manually outside the patient to achieve more stability of the lead in the superior vena cava and/or high right atrial junction. The distance of the second curve to the lead tip is determined by estimation of the right atrial diameter on fluoroscopy. Ao= aorta; AS = atrial septum; AV = atrioventricular; IVC = inferior vena cava; RA = right atrium; RAA = right atrial appendage; SVC = superior vena cava .and TK = triangle of Koch. (From De Voogt WG, Van Mechelen R, Van Den Bos A, et al. A technique of lead insertion for low atrial septal pacing. PACE 28:639, 2005)

heart. The handle is also used to turn the lead around its axis, maneuvering the curve clockwise or counterclockwise (Fig. 6.15). The stylet can also be manually curved to achieve desired secondary curves, which can help achieve stability of the lead in the SVC. The stylet curves the distal to 4 cm of the pacing lead.

The second system is built on the concept of a **catheter delivery system**. A family of steerable catheters (**Selectsite**, Medtronic, Inc.) has been developed to guide pacing leads to selective sites as discussed in previous chapter. In these products, the 4F active-fixation lead is passed down the steerable catheter to the desired position for fixation. This lead is a simple cable and has no guiding stylet, being delivered by a guide catheter.

In our lab, none of the above mentioned delivery system is available. So, we have improvised an alternative technique (Figs 6.16 and 6.17). First, put an EP catheter (Decapolar/Quadripolar) into the coronary sinus. Using this catheter as a landmark take the atrial lead and pass it into the coronary sinus under fluoroscopy (LAO view) and the lead position is verified by sensed electrograms and paced electrocardiographic (ECG) configuration. The lead is then withdrawn to the coronary sinus ostium, and a secondary tip curvature of the stylet used to lodge it at the rim of the ostium, generally posteriorly. The up and down movement of the lead in LAO view in sinus rhythm and negative polarity of P wave in inferior leads with a shorter PR interval than sinus rhythm during pacing confirm the position in the lower atrial septum. The sensed voltage of the P-wave is usually larger in the LAS patients compared with the RAA patients.

However, we may experience pacemaker syndrome during coronary sinus pacing in some cases. Pacemaker

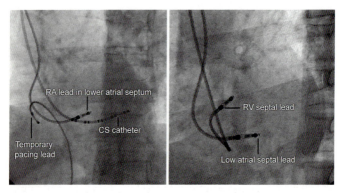

Fig. 6.16 (A) A decapolar catheter is positioned in coronary sinus to guide the atrial lead in lower atrial septum. (B) RV lead is positioned in interventricular septum and atrial lead in the lower atrial septum

Selective Site: Right Atrial Septal Pacing

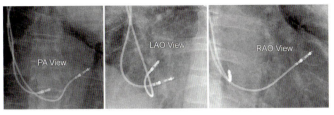

Fig. 6.17 Different fluoroscopic views of a patient with RV lead in the RVOT septum and RA lead in lower atrial septum

syndrome is a complex of adverse clinical, hemodynamic and electrophysiological signs resulting from disruption of appropriate atrioventricular (AV) synchrony. Typically pacemaker syndrome is described in patients with a single-chamber ventricular pacemaker and preserved ventriculo-atrial conduction, or a dual-chamber pacemaker with inappropriate AV delay timing; however, it has also been noted as a consequence of prolonged intra- or interatrial conduction times. Pacemaker syndrome during coronary sinus pacing can be related to a change in impulse propagation within the atria and earlier ventricular activation.

Single-site coronary sinus pacing results in several detrimental hemodynamic effects in the right heart because of significant prolongation of the electromechanical delay in the lateral RA wall, which results in retardation of RA contraction. It reverses the physiological right-to-left atrial contraction sequence, shortens the RA wave. RA contraction delay and earlier ventricular activation causes marked shortening of the right ventricular mechanical AV delay and a decrement in the right ventricular inflow.

The shorter the right ventricular mechanical AV delay, the greater is the RA wave diminution. Left heart mechanical AV delay is not shorter during coronary sinus pacing (because of appropriate timing of LA contraction), and left heart stroke volume is preserved. Bachmann's bundle pacing provided more physiological atrial contraction sequence and synchrony.

Local EGM and stimulation analysis, which is important for the recognition of far-field R-wave (FFRW) detection, can cause inappropriate mode switching. The height of any FFRW recorded on the atrial channel must be measured. During an implantation, FFRW analysis in sinus rhythm and normal atrioventricular (AV) conduction can be masked by the "current of injury" caused by the active fixation of the atrial septal lead. FFRW signals become superimposed on the current of injury (Fig. 6.18). To avoid this problem, FFRWs can be measured during VVI pacing, in which the wave can be seen to precede

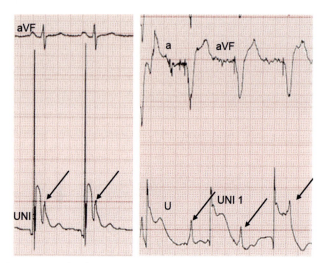

Fig. 6.18 Far field R-wave (FFRW) signals during implantation. The left panel shows at the top lead aVF and the bottom the unipolar acute atrial signal followed by the injury current. The FFRW (arrow) is superimposed on the injury current during sinus rhythm, ruling out correct measurement of its height. The right panel shows at the top lead aVF with ventricular pacing and atrioventricular dissociation in the same patient. The unipolar atrial channel at the bottom confirms the atrioventricular dissociation and displays FFRW (arrows) separated from the acute atrial signals. This condition allows better measurement of the FFRW voltages (Courtesy: De Voogt WG, Van Mechelen R, Van Den Bos A, et al. A technique of lead insertion for low atrial septal pacing. PACE 28:639, 2005)

the atrial complex, when ventriculoatrial (VA) conduction is present, or can be seen between beats during VA dissociation. FFRW voltages should be less than the P-wave voltage. If high FFRW voltages are found, lead repositioning should be considered. In addition, high FFRWs may also mean that the screw-in mechanism of the atrial lead is protruding into the ventricular myocardium.[19] This possibility can be evaluated with high-output pacing from the atrium, which produces simultaneous atrial and ventricular stimulation if the lead is in the ventricular myocardium. Malpositioning of an atrial septal lead can be deleterious, possibly causing pacemaker syndrome or, if high-rate atrial tachyarrhythmia therapy pacing is used, resulting in inappropriate, dangerously high ventricular rates.

Dual-site right atrial pacing may offer additional benefits and should be considered either as the primary mode or in patients unresponsive to single-site pacing. The first atrial pacing electrode is positioned using a curved stylet with primary and secondary curvatures in the lower atrial septum. The second atrial lead is passed and fixed in the high right

Selective Site: Right Atrial Septal Pacing

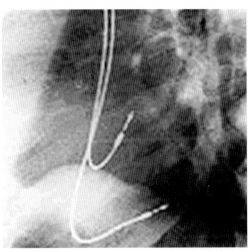

Fig. 6.19 Left lateral view demonstrating pacing lead positions at the Bachmann's bundle region and in the coronary sinus ostium area

atrium, usually in the right atrial appendage or Bachmann's bundle under fluoroscopic control (Fig. 6.19). Fluoroscopic appearances of high and low atrial septal pacing in comparison to right atrial appendage pacing are given in Figure 6.20.

Electrocardiographic Characteristics

During evaluation of a patient with atrial pacing, the 12-lead ECG yields important information about the site of pacing as well as the effect of pacing on atrial depolarization in term of duration and vectoral change. The atrial based pacing ECG should be evaluated on the following features:

- *Latency:* The latency is defined here as the interval from the pacemaker stimulus to the onset of the earliest paced P wave. The demonstration of latency requires a 12-lead ECG taken at fast speed (50 mm/sec) for diagnosis. Normally the spread of activation within each atrium and from right to left follow circumferential and longitudinal muscle bundles, but they are generally not considered to be part of the specialized conduction system. The sites of electrical connections between the right and the left atrium are the high septal right atrium or Bachmann's bundle, the region of Koch's triangle, with left posterior extension of the AV node, the fossa ovalis, and the coronary sinus level with connections between the coronary sinus muscle cover and the left atrium. In the right atrium, the crista terminalis and its medial extension favor the spread of activation in a longitudinal direction, whereas transverse conduction is limited. In the left atrium, circumferential muscle fibers along the mitral annulus as

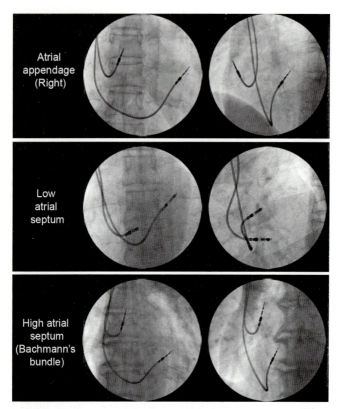

Fig. 6.20 Comparison of three atrial sites of pacing in fluoroscopic appearances in posteroanterior (PA) and Left anterior oblique (LAO). Note all 3 patients have right ventricular lead positioned in mid-septum or outflow tract septum. Also, note right atrial lead is looking posteriorly (towards the spine) in Bachmann's Bundle and low atrial septal pacing in comparison to right atrial appendage pacing where it faces anteriorly (towards the sternum)

well as longitudinal fibres propagate slowly the wave of depolarization. In **right atrial appendage** pacing, atrial muscle bundles take considerable time to propagate the stimulation from right atrial appendage to the right atrial free wall then to the crista terminalis and whole right atrium and subsequently to the left atrium across the atrial septum. So, there is a marked latency period and the paced P wave duration becomes prolonged specifically if there is inter and intra-atrial conduction delay. In **Bachmann's bundle pacing** (junction of the roof right atrium atrial septum), the wave of depolarization rapidly traverses to the left atrium via the bundle and excites the left atrium and in the right atrium via crista terminalis to the whole right atrium. So, there is no latency period and the P wave duration is short. In **low atrial septal pacing,** the latency period is also very short as the spread of activation from the pacing site rapidly traverses to the left atrium via coronary sinus musculature and simultaneously right atrium gets stimulated in a reverse direction by right atrial musculature.

- *P wave duration and vector:* The P wave normally appears entirely upright in leftward- and inferiorly oriented leads such as I, II, III, aVF, and V4 to V6. It is negative in aVR because of the rightward orientation of that lead and is variable in other standard leads. The part of the atrial septum on which the lead is screwed is determined according to the polarities of the paced P wave in aVF: total positivity, initial positivity, initial negativity, and total negativity corresponding to four distinct sites starting from the highest to the lowest part of the septum. When pacing from the **low atrial septum**, the P-wave vector is directed superiorly in the frontal plane (negative in lead II, III and aVF) as the spread of activation occurs in caudo-cranial direction while in the precordial leads the vector is directed anterior and to the right. The P wave duration is short as the left atrium starts depolarizing very early (simultaneously or may be earlier than the right atrium) thereby taking less time for total atrial depolarization. The typical P-wave morphology in **right atrial appendage** pacing shows an inferior vector in the frontal plane and the P-wave duration is prolonged (equal or more than the sinus P-wave duration). In **Bachmann's bundle pacing** the paced P-wave is positive in leads I, II, and III, starting immediately with the pacing spike (no latency), and shorter than the sinus P-wave (expected to be 15–20 ms shorter than sinus P waves). Both the atria get depolarized simultaneously as through the Bachmann's bundle the stimulus goes to the left atrium rapidly and the crista terminalis spread the activation longitudinally in the right atrium from the site of pacing resulting in shortest P wave.

- *P wave morphology in lead V1:* The P wave contour is normally smooth and is either entirely positive or entirely negative in all leads except V1 and possibly V2. In the short axis view provided by lead V1, which best distinguishes left- versus right-sided cardiac activity; the divergence of right- and left-atrial activation typically produces a biphasic P wave. The mechanisms of P wave morphological changes in pacing at different sites of right atrium are illustrated in Figures 6.21–6.24. The P wave in lead V1 in **low atrial septal pacing** is positive if monophasic this suggests that left atrium is unable to cancel the RA forces and terminally positive if biphasic suggesting that the left atrium negates the initial forces of the right atrium and the terminal forces are formed mainly by the right atrium. An alternative explanation is that

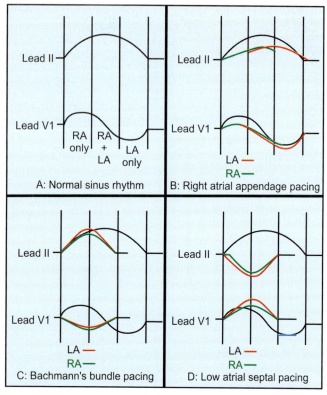

Fig. 6.21 Mechanism of changes in P wave morphology in different atrial sit pacing in comparison to normal sinus rhythm

the left atrium is depolarized prior to the right atrium when stimulated from the low atrial septum as suggested earlier. The typical morphology of the P-wave in lead V1 in **right atrial appendage** pacing is almost identical to sinus rhythm morphology with a terminal negative deflection, caused by the normal activation sequence of the atria, right before left.

In right atrial appendage pacing, the impulse traverses from the site of pacing to free wall and from there propagates through crista terminalis down to whole right atrium and simultaneously the wave of depolarization reach the interatrial septum from where it reaches left atrium by preferential conduction via Bachmann's bundle, along the limbus fossa ovalis, and proximal coronary sinus musculature. The whole process takes considerable amount of time leading to prolonged latency period and the P wave duration is also prolonged (equal or more than to sinus rhythm). The P wave voltage is slightly reduced.

In Bachmann's bundle pacing, the wave of depolarization rapidly crosses to the left atrium through the bundle itself, limbus fossa ovalis, along the proximal coronary sinus musculature,

Selective Site: Right Atrial Septal Pacing

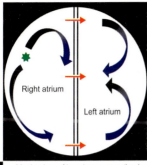

In right atrial appendage pacing, the impulse traverses from the site of pacing to free wall and from there propagates through crista terminalis down to whole right atrium and simultaneously the wave of depolarization reach the inter-atrial septum from where it reaches left atrium by preferential conduction via Bachmann's bundle, along the limbus fossa ovalis, and proximal coronary sinus musculature. The whole process takes considerable amount of time leading to prolonged latency period and the P wave duration is also prolonged (equal or more than to sinus rhythm). The P wave voltage is slightly reduced.

A Mechanism of impulse propagation in right atrial appendage pacing

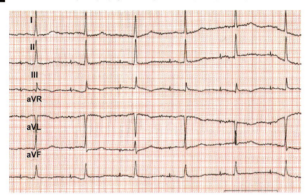

B 6 Lead surface ECG during right atrial appendage pacing. Note there is decreased amplitude of P waves. Also, note the long latency in lead II.

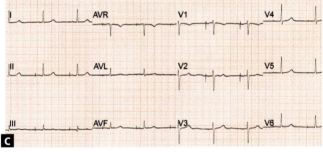

C

Fig. 6.22 Right atrial appendage pacing: (A) Spread of activation wavefront; (B) 6 lead surface ECG shows appearance of P wave during right atrial appendage pacing; (C) 12 lead surface ECG during right atrial appendage pacing

and extension from AV node. Along the crista terminalis the impulse gets propagated longitudinally in the right atrium. Thus, the left atrium gets stimulated simultaneously or may be little earlier with the right atrium and results in short and sharp P wave with minimal or no latency period.

In low atrial septal pacing, the depolarization wave front rapidly crosses to the left atrium along the musculature around the proximal coronary sinus. Both the atria get stimulated in a

Cardiac Pacing: A Physiological Approach

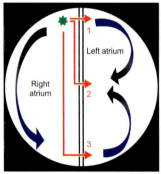

In Bachmann's bundle pacing, the wave of depolarization rapidly crosses to the left atrium through the bundle itself, limbus fossa ovalis, along the proximal coronary sinus musculature, and extension from AV node. Along the crista terminalis the impulse gets propagated longitudinally in the right atrium. Thus, the left atrium gets stimulated simultaneously or may be little earlier with the right atrium and results in short and sharp P wave with minimal or no latency period.

A Mechanism of impulse propagation in Bachmann's bundle pacing

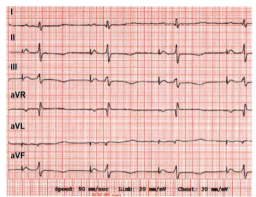

B 6 Lead surface ECG during Bachmann's bundle pacing. Note there is no latency period (P wave starts immediately after the pacing spike in lead II, III). Also, note the P waves are short and sharp.

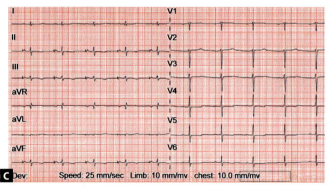

Fig. 6.23 Bachmann's bundle pacing: (A) Spread of activation wavefront; (B) 6 lead surface ECG shows appearance of P-wave during BB pacing; (C) Bachmann's bundle pacing; C: 12 lead surface ECG during Bachmann's bundle Pacing

caudo-cranial direction (reverse to normal sinus rhythm and just opposite of Bachmann's bundle pacing). So, it produces P-waves with superior axis (negative in inferior leads). As, the propagation time is short and both the atria get stimulated simultaneously, it produces narrow P-wave.

Selective Site: Right Atrial Septal Pacing

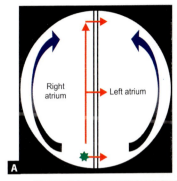

In low atrial septal pacing, the depolarization wave front rapidly crosses to the left atrium along the musculature around the proximal coronary sinus. Both the atria get stimulated in a caudo-cranial direction (reverse to normal sinus rhythm and just opposite of Bachmann's bundle pacing). So, it produces P waves with superior axis (negative in inferior leads). As, the propagation time is short and both the atria get stimulated simultaneously, it produces narrow P wave.

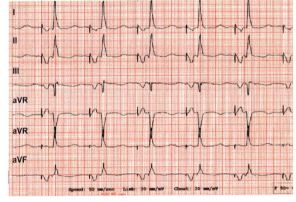

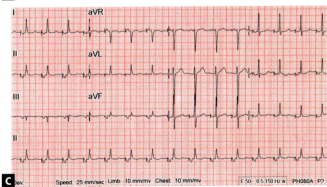

Fig. 6.24 Low atrial septal pacing: (A) Spread of activation wave-front; (B) 6 lead surface ECG shows appearance of P wave during LAS pacing; (C) 12 lead surface ECG during low atrial septal pacing

CONCLUSION

Low atrial septal pacing is a reliable technique and avoids the undesirable prolongation of atrial, interatrial, and AV conductions observed with conventional right atrial appendage pacing, particularly in patients with a long P wave before pacing or a previous history of AF. In patients with preserved but prolonged AV conduction, it may allow exclusive AAI pacing in more patients. However, it produces a slight reversal of atrial systoles and reduces AR and PR intervals. Thus for the moment, low atrial septal pacing can be proposed only to patients with prolongation of atrial, interatrial, and AV conductions. For patients with a history of previous AF but without long P wave duration or for patients with AV block and sinus bradycardia, it is preferable to wait for the results of the more randomized, controlled trials assessing the potential antiarrhythmic effect of septal pacing. Bachmann's bundle pacing is technically difficult but not impossible with conventional tools. It should be considered in all cases of inter- and intra-atrial conduction delay, especially with a history of atrial fibrillation. Single site Bachmann's bundle pacing provides the best atrial contraction synchrony in patients with atrial conduction abnormality. Dual-site right atrial pacing may offer additional benefits and should be considered in patients unresponsive to single-site pacing.

REFERENCES

1. Rosenqvist M, Isaaz K, Botvinick EH, et al. Relative importance of activation sequence compared to atrial ventricular synchrony in left ventricular function. Am J Cardiol. 1991;67:148.
2. Leclercq JF, DeSisti A, Fiorello P, et al. Is dual site better than single site atrial pacing in the prevention of atrial fibrillation? PACE. 2000;23:2101.
3. Bachmann G. The inter-auricular time interval. Am J Physiol. 1907; 1:1.
4. Roithinger FX, Cheng J, Sippen Groenewegen A, et al. Use of electroanatomic mapping to delineate transseptal atrial conduction in humans. Circulation. 1999;100:1791-97.
5. Skanes A, Krahn A, Yee R, et al. Progression to chronic atrial fibrillation after pacing: The Canadian trial of physiologic pacing. J Am Coll Cardiol. 2001;38:167-72.
6. Kindermann M, Schwaab B, Berg M, Frohlig G. The influence of right atrial septal pacing on the interatrial contraction sequence. Pacing Clin Electrophysiol. 2000;23:1752-7.
7. Goyal SB, Spodick DH. Electromechanical dysfunction of the left atrium associated with interatrial block. Am Heart J. 2001;142: 823-7.
8. Stefanadis C, Dernellis J, Toutouzas P. A clinical appraisal of left atrial function. Eur Heart J. 2001;22:22-36.
9. Ishikawa T, Kimura K, Miyazaki N et al. Diastolic mitral regurgitation in patients with first-degree atrioventricular block. PACE. 1992;15:1927-31.
10. Strangl K, Weil J, Seitz K, et al. Influence of AV synchrony on the plasma levels of atrial natriuretic peptide (ANP) in patients with total AV block. PACE. 1988;11:1176-81.
11. Ogawa M, Kumagai K, Gondo N, et al. Novel electrophysiologic parameter of dispersion of atrial repolarization: Comparison of

different atrial pacing methods. J Cardiovasc Electrophysiol. 2002; 13:110-7.
12. A. G. Manolis, A. G. Katsivas, C. Vassilopoulos, et al. Prevention of atrial fibrillation by inter-atrial septum pacing guided by electrophysiological testing, in patients with delayed interatrial conduction. Europace. 2002;4:165-74.
13. Jean Sylvain Hermida, Christophe Carpentier, Maciej Kubala, et al. Atrial septal versus atrial appendage pacing: feasibility and effects on atrial conduction, interatrial synchronization, and atrioventricular sequence. PACE. 2003;26:26-35.
14. Padeletti L, Porciani MC, Michelucci A, et al. Interatrial septum pacing: a new approach to prevent recurrent atrial fibrillation. J Interv Card Electrophysiol. 1999;3:3543.
15. Padeletti L, Porciani MC, Michelucci A, et al. Interatrial septum pacing: a new site to pace simultaneously both atria on patients with paroxysmal atrial fibrillation. In: Antonioli GE (ed). Pacemaker Leads 1997. Bologna, Italy, Monduzzi Editore, 1997; pp. 229-32.
16. Yu WC, Chen SA, Tai CT, Feng AN, Chang MS. Effects of different atrial pacing modes on atrial electrophysiology: implicating the mechanism of biatrial pacing in prevention of atrial fibrillation. Circulation. 1997;96:2992-6.
17. Mabo P, Paul V, Jung W, Clementy J, Bouhour A, Daubert C. Biatrial synchronous pacing for atrial arrhythmia prevention: the SYNBIAPACE study (abstr). Eur Heart J. 1999;20:4.
18. Fitts SM, Hill MRS, Mehra R, et al. Design and implementation of the dual site Atrial Pacing to Prevent Atrial Fibrillation (DAPPAF) clinical trial. J Intervent Clin Electrophysiol. 1998;2:139-44.
19. De Voogt WG, Van Mechelen R, Van Den Bos A, et al. A technique of lead insertion for low atrial septal pacing. PACE. 2005;28:639.

CHAPTER 7

Case Discussion

CASE 1

A 72-year-old hypertensive, smoker, non-diabetic gentleman presented with history of recurrent syncope. He was diagnosed to have sick sinus syndrome and he was advised permanent pacemaker implantation (Fig. 7.1).

A dual chamber pacemaker implantation was done with a passive fixation RV apical ventricular lead and an active fixation atrial lead in right atrial appendage (Fig. 7.2).

Let us observe the electrocardiographic changes in this patient during DDD pacing (Fig. 7.3).

With RV apical pacing QRS duration increased to 135 msec (vs 74 msec in sinus rhythm). The morphology of QRS complex shows left bundle branch block (LBBB) pattern and left-axis deviation. This electrical dyssynchrony (QRS duration of more than 120 msec) eventually leads to mechanical dyssynchrony and reduced left ventricular systolic function. Wider the baseline QRS more is the electrical dyssynchrony. Moreover, we know left bundle branch block is an independent predictor of cardiac morbidity and mortality, particularly in patients with systolic heart failure (HF).[1,2] Not all patients with RV apical pacing develop the adverse hemodynamic consequences. In the Most study, only about 10% of patients had HF during follow-up and were more likely to have a lower ejection fraction (EF), myocardial infarction, and a worse New York Heart Association functional class compared with patients who did not experience HF.[3] The pattern of mechanical dyssynchrony of RV apical pacing induced LBBB differs significantly from intrinsic LBBB.[4] The mechanical activation pattern of the left ventricle (LV) depends in intrinsic LBBB on the level of block in the conduction system and in induced LBBB on the position of RV lead within the right ventricle. This mechanical activation pattern also affects the pattern of LV dyssynchrony. In pacing-induced LBBB, the mid- and apico-septal regions of LV are in the majority of patients the earliest activated regions, whereas

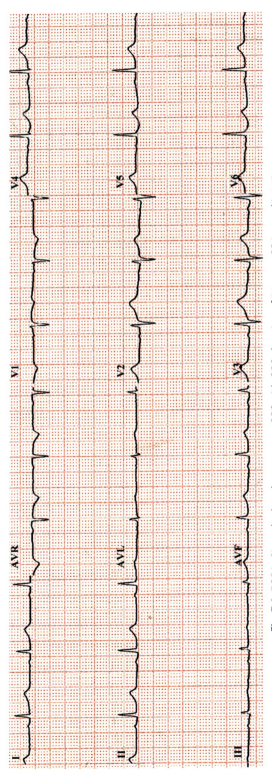

Fig. 7.1 ECG in Sinus rhythm shows narrow QRS with QRS duration of 74 msec. PR interval is 148 msec

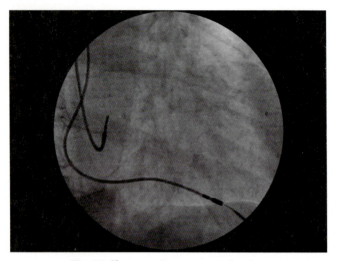

Fig. 7.2 Fluoroscopic anteroposterior view

in intrinsic LBBB the basal-septal segment is most frequently the earliest activated region. Furthermore, there are differences in latest activation sites between these two groups: in pacing-induced LBBB one of the lateral segments (apico-lateral, mid-lateral, and basal-lateral) is in 75% the latest activated segments, and in contrast in intrinsic LBBB the lateral wall is only in 35% of patients the latest activated segment. In pacing-induced LBBB, activation vector is directed from apical to basal and from right to left. In contrast, in patients with intrinsic LBBB, activation vector is usually directed from basal to apical and from septal to lateral. Also, note the P-wave morphology during right atrial appendage pacing. The amplitude of P-wave during pacing is reduced to half of its sinus rhythm amplitude. This probably indicates weaker wave of depolarization which leads to weaker force of atrial contraction during ventricular filling. So, the ventricular filling is hampered partially. This also leads to heterogeneous electrical activation pattern in both the atria which increases the propensity for development of atrial fibrillation, especially in the patients with preexisting atrial (intra and inter-) conduction disorder. So, this is **clearly not physiological.**

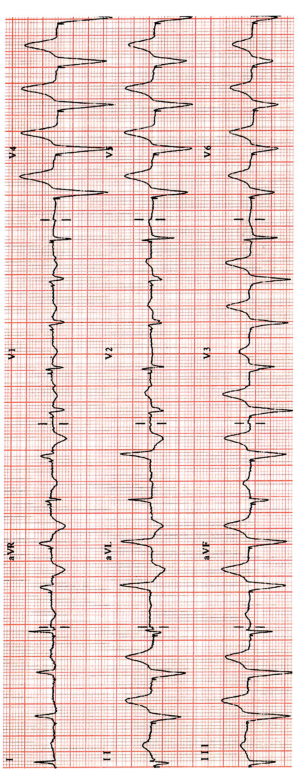

Fig. 7.3 ECG during DDD pacing. QRS duration is 135 msec with intermittent fusion beats

REFERENCES

1. Baldasseroni S, Opasich C, Gorini M, et al., and the Italian Network on Congestive Heart Failure Investigators. Left bundle branch block is associated with increased 1-year sudden and total mortality rate in 5,517 outpatients with congestive heart failure: a report from the Italian network on congestive heart failure. Am Heart J. 2002;143:398-405.
2. Schneider JF, Thomas HE Jr., Kreger BE, et al. Newly acquired left bundle branch block: the Framingham study. Ann Intern Med. 1979;90:303-10.
3. Sweeney MO, Hellkamp AS. Baseline and post-implant risk scores for predicting heart failure hospitalization during pacemaker therapy for sinus node dysfunction. Heart Rhythm. 2005;2 Suppl 2:S75-6.
4. Abdul Ghani, Peter Paul H.M. Delnoy, et al. Assessment of left ventricular dyssynchrony in pacing-induced left bundle branch block compared with intrinsic left bundle branch block. Europace. 2011;13:1504-9.

CASE 2

A 65-year-old gentleman non-diabetic, normotensive presented with symptomatic 2:1 AV block. A dual chamber pacemaker (Medtronic, Model - Adapta) implantation was done. Right ventricular lead was placed in the RVOT septum. Right atrial lead was placed in the right atrial appendage.

Note in both the view right ventricular lead tip points posteriorly towards the spine and the right atrial lead points anteriorly towards the sternum (Figs 7.4 and 7.5). Now, let us look at the Paced ECG in DDD mode at pacing rate of 100 beats per minute (Fig. 7.6).

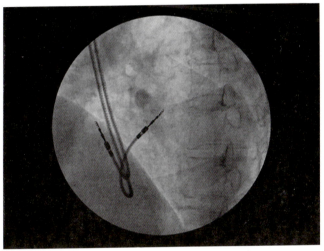

Fig. 7.4 Fluoroscopic left anterior oblique (LAO) view 30 degree

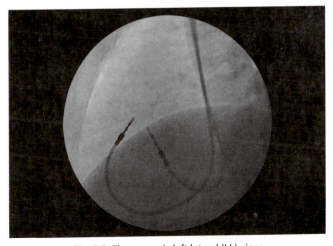

Fig. 7.5 Fluoroscopic left lateral (LL) view

144 Cardiac Pacing: A Physiological Approach

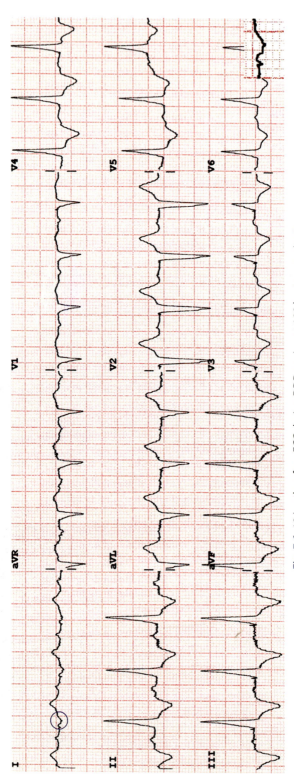

Fig. 7.6 12 Lead surface ECG during DDD pacing at 100 beats per minute

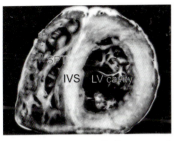 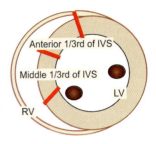

Fig. 7.7 Anterior 2/3rd of interventricular septum in parasternal short axis view at papillary muscle level (mid-ventricular level) is the ideal site for RV lead attachment in RV septal pacing

Dominant R wave in inferior leads indicate RVOT position of the lead. Early precordial transition and lack of notching on R wave in the inferior leads confirm septal location of the lead. Morphology in lead I suggest location of the RV lead in the anterior part of the interventricular septum (site 3) (see Fig. 11, chapter 4).[1] Note the QRS duration is 115 msec.

If we look at the interventricular septum in a cross sectional view, the attachment of the septo-parietal trabeculation is anteriorly. So, Leung and colleagues[2] have proposed that the attachment of a true right ventricular septal lead should be on the anterior and middle third of the interventricular septum on echocardiographic parasternal short axis view at mid-ventricular level (at the level of papillary muscles).

REFERENCES

1. Dixit S, Gerstenfeld EP, Callans DJ, Marchlinski FE. Electrocardiographic patterns of superior right ventricular outflow tract tachycardias: distinguishing septal and free-wall sites of origin. J Cardiovasc Electrophysiol. 2003;14:1-7.
2. Arnold CT Ng, Christine Allman, Jane Vidaic, Grad D Health, Hui Tie, Andrew P Hopkins, Dominic Y Leung. Long-term impact of right ventricular septal versus apical pacing on left ventricular synchrony and function in patients with second- or third-degree heart block. Am J Cardiol. 2009; 103:1096-101.

CASE 3

A 65-year-old gentleman has undergone dual chamber pacemaker implantation for symptomatic sinus node disease. An attempt was made to position the ventricular lead in the interventricular septum (Fig. 7.8).

Let us look at the 12 lead surface ECG during VVI pacing. His ECG during VVI pacing shows (Fig. 7.9):
- Dominant R wave in inferior leads indicate RVOT position.
- Absence of notching in R wave in inferior leads excludes free wall location.
- Late precordial transition does not favor septal position.

The above features suggest the probable location of the lead is not truly septal but may be little towards the anterior wall. Now, let us look at the RV lead position in the fluoroscopic left lateral view.

The RV lead in left lateral fluoroscopic view points upward confirming the anterior wall location of the RV lead (Fig. 7.10). Here lies the importance of the left lateral view. Mond and his colleagues suggested left lateral view as the specific view (100% specific) for confirmation of the septal location of the RV lead.[1] However, achieving routine left lateral view during pacemaker implantation is not possible because of sterility reason. But, 40 degree left anterior oblique view can easily be performed during lead implantation. Forty degree has been chosen as it is near maximum orientation in the oblique position that can be

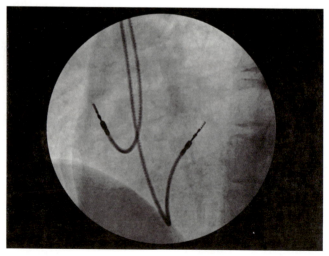

Fig. 7.8 Fluoroscopic left anterior oblique view shows posteriorly facing RV lead tip suggesting septal location of the lead

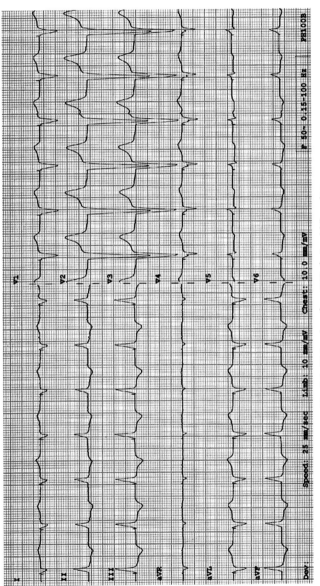

Fig. 7.9 12 Lead surface ECG during VVI pacing

achieved without compromising the sterile field. In an another study, Prof. Mond indicated that lead tip angulation between 0 to 60 degree in 40 degree LAO view is highly suggestive of septal attachment of the lead.[2] Angulation of 80 to 100 degree suggests anterior wall location and 120 to 140 degree indicates free wall location of the RV lead. Sixty to eighty degree suggests transition zone between septal and anterior wall location. Hundred to hundred and twenty degree is the transition between anterior and free wall location of the RV lead (Fig. 7.11).

Now, let us reanalyze the RV lead tip angulation of this patient in LAO 40 degree fluoroscopic projection.

So, RV lead tip angulation in this patient in 40 degree LAO projection is 80 degree (Fig. 7.12). It means the transition zone between septal and anterior location of the lead (**Template zone 1**).

Let us look at the previous patient (Case 2).

Here, RV lead tip angulation is 45 degree, highly suggestive of true septal location of the RV lead attachment (Fig. 7.13). In my opinion, we have to try to position the RV lead with a tip angulation of less than 40 degree (**template zone 3:** 0 to 40 degree) to be absolutely confident about the septal location of the lead tip.

However, factors such as pulmonary and vertebral column disease can distort the positioning and orientation of the heart in the mediastinum, thus potentially altering the lead position in the LAO view. But, it should be obvious with the PA or RAO

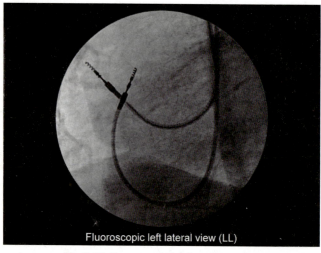

Fig. 7.10 Fluoroscopic left lateral view (LL)

Case Discussion 149

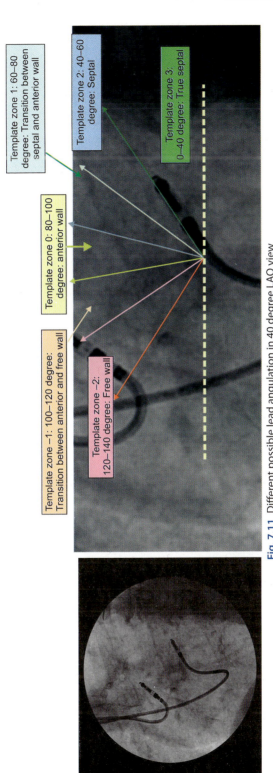

Fig. 7.11 Different possible lead angulation in 40 degree LAO view

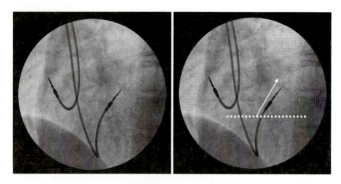

Fig. 7.12 RV lead tip angulation in 40 degree LOA view is 80 degree

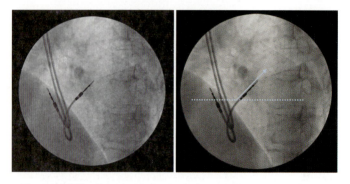

Fig. 7.13 RV lead tip angulation in 40 degree LOA view is 45 degree

views and, thus, taken into account when observing the LAO fluoroscopic view.

REFERENCES

1. Mc Gavigan AD, Roberts-Thomson FC, Hillock RJ, Stevenson IH, Mond HG. Right ventricular outflow tract pacing: radiographic and electrocardiographic correlates of lead position. PACE. 2006:29:1063-8.
2. Harry G Mond, Alexander Feldman, Saurabh Kumar, et al. Alternate site right ventricular pacing: defining template scoring. PACE. 2011;34:1080-6.

CASE 4

A 72-year-old hypertensive gentleman presented with history of recurrent syncope. His sinus rhythm ECG shows bifascicular block (right bundle branch block with left anterior hemi block) with prolonged PR interval (Fig. 7.15). A dual chamber pacemaker implantation was done. Right ventricular lead was placed in the RVOT septum and the position was confirmed by fluoroscopic left lateral view (Fig. 7.14). Right atrial lead was placed in the Bachman's bundle area (upper inter-atrial septum).

Although fluoroscopic left lateral view confirms septal position of the leads, pacing at the interventricular septum fails to significantly narrow the QRS duration (130 msec vs 144 msec) (Fig. 7.16). Paced rhythm shows late precordial transition with some degree of fusion. Late precordial transition probably indicates severe infra-Hisian disease. Failure of QRS narrowing indicates probable disease of Purkinje-myocardial junction.

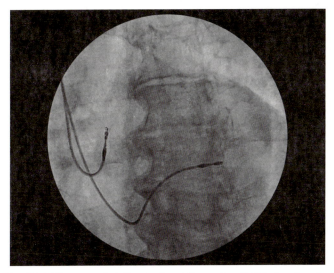

Fig. 7.14 Fluoroscopic left anterior oblique view (LAO) showing the position of the leads. Note both the lead tip is facing posteriorly towards the spine. Also, note the RV lead tip angulation is about 10 degree which confirms the septal location of the lead tip

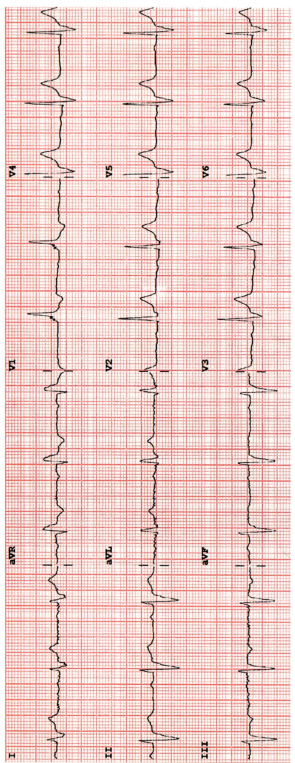

Fig. 7.15 Sinus ECG shows RBBB with LAHB with prolonged PR. QRS duration is 144 msec

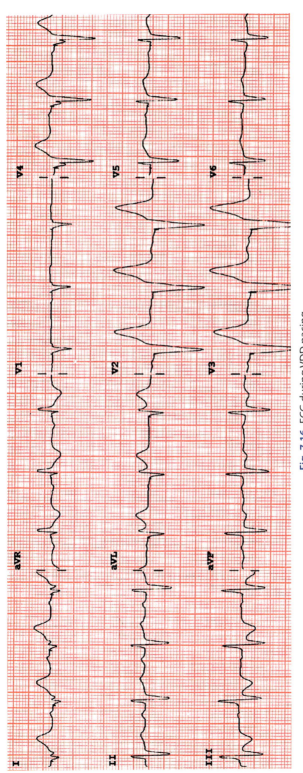

Fig. 7.16 ECG during VDD pacing

CASE 5

A 80-year-old hypertensive, post-CABG patient presented with history of recurrent syncope. His sinus rhythm ECG shows left bundle branch block in limb leads and with right bundle branch block in precordial leads (also known as **Masquerading bundle branch block**) (Fig. 7.18). A dual chamber pacemaker implantation was done. Right ventricular lead was placed in the RVOT septum and the position was confirmed by fluoroscopic left lateral view. Right atrial lead was placed in the right atrial appendage (Fig. 7.17).

His paced ECG shows significant QRS narrowing (111 msec vs 140 msec). But precordial leads do not show early transition. Rather it shows negative concordance (Fig. 7.19). So, in sinus rhythm ECG shows RBBB and paced rhythm shows LBBB. However, the clinical consequence of this change in ventricular electrical activation sequence is not completely known.

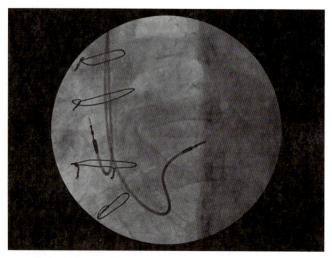

Fig. 7.17 Fluoroscopic left anterior oblique view (LAO) 40 degree showing the position of the leads

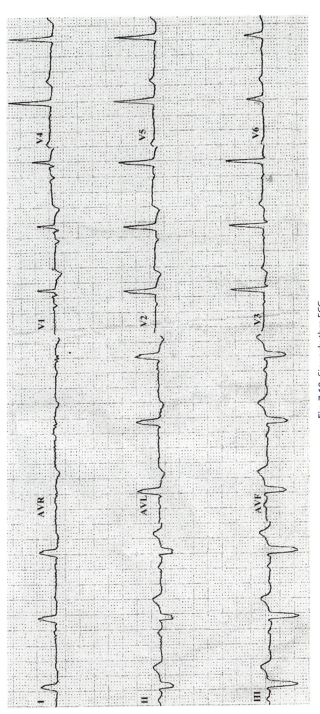

Fig. 7.18 Sinus rhythm ECG

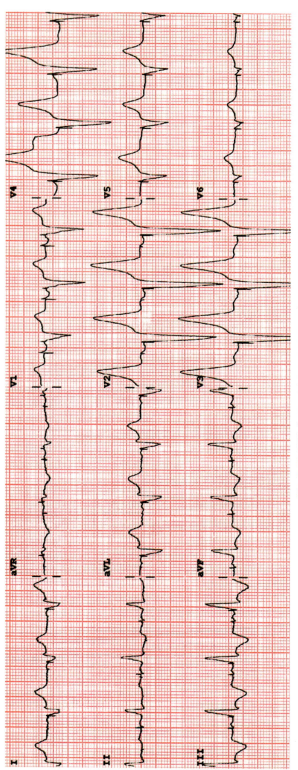

Fig. 7.19 ECG during DDD pacing at 80 bpm

CASE 6

A 70-year-old gentleman presented with severe sinus node disease (Fig. 7.21). A dual chamber pacemaker (Boston Scientific, Model – Ingenio DR) was implanted. Right ventricular lead was placed in the Para-Hisian area and the right atrial lead was placed in the Bachman's bundle area (upper inter-atrial septum) (Fig. 7.20). Both the leads (Fineline II Sterox EZ) have a body diameter of 5.1 F (1.7 mm) with a helix length of 1.6 mm.

In Para-Hisian pacing,, the helix of the lead probably reaches the His bundle at the crest of the muscular ventricular septum, where the bundle emerges from the central fibrous body. This captures simultaneously the His bundle and the surrounding myocardium showing a "preexcitation-like" pattern in the ECG. The feasibility of capturing adjacent myocardium permits a bifocal RV pacing. This has two beneficial effects over Direct His bundle pacing while maintaining the physiological ventricular activation; (1) avoid risk of His bundle block induced by the trauma and injury caused by the screw-in lead, (2) in case of progression of conduction system disease avoids future problems related to a high pacing threshold and/or a conduction block below the Hisian pacing site.[1] In this event, the threshold of RV capture may be equal, higher or lower to the threshold of His bundle capture.

The septal atrial lead permits (1) a very short interatrial conduction delay and a significant decrease in P-wave duration; (2) a reduction in dispersion of atrial refractoriness; (3) a more homogeneous recovery of excitability and atrial activation; and (4) electrical atrial remodeling, with a gradual reduction in left atrial diameters and volume.[2]

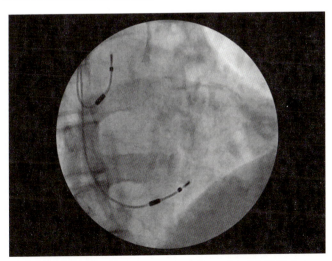

Fig. 7.20 Fluoroscopic rightt anterior oblique view (RAO) 30 degree showing the position of the leads

158 Cardiac Pacing: A Physiological Approach

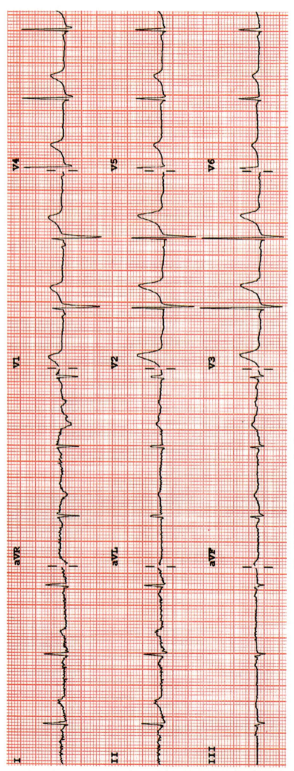

Fig. 7.21 ECG in sinus rhythm with rate of 72 bpm. QRS duration is 81 msec

With the Para-Hisian pacing, as the Hisian conduction axis is penetrated, it results in a narrow QRS (< 120–130 msec) with the **electric axis concordant** with the non-paced sinus QRS and as the high muscular septum around the His bundle is stimulated it results in a preexcitation-like pattern (Figs 7.22 and 7.23). The notches in the QRS complex in some precordial leads probably reflect the bifocal nature of RV stimulation.

The main purpose of permanent cardiac pacing is to maintain an adequate cardiac rhythm, and restore the physiology of the normal excitatory-conductive physiology of the heart as much as possible. In true sense physiological pacing, must: (1) maintain the correct stimulation-contraction sequence in the right and left atria; (2) maintain the synchrony between right and left ventricles; (3) maintain the sequence between the atria and ventricles; and (4) help increase the cardiac rate according to metabolic need.

In my understanding, there are two categories of patients who require permanent pacemaker implantation. Followings are the two categories:

- *Patients with low presumed pacing burden:* patients with paroxysmal excitation and/or conduction diseases who need very low rate of pacing: in this kind of patients, atrial and ventricular leads can be placed at any site including conventional sites (RAA and RVA). In addition different algorithms that decrease the frequency of ventricular pacing (e.g. SafeR, MVP, AV search hysteresis) can be employed.
- *Patients with high presumed pacing burden:*
  - *Baseline narrow QRS (QRS duration ≤ 120 msec):* These patients need **optimal physiological pacing** and this should be performed with: (1) an atrial lead actively fixed on the inter-atrial septum; and (2) a ventricular lead actively fixed at the para-Hisian region.
  - *Baseline wide QRS (QRS duration > 120 msec):*
    - *Patients with preserved left ventricular systolic function:* In these patients we should initially perform His-bundle pacing by a mapping EP catheter and watch for the electrical resynchronization (QRS duration ≤ 120 msec). If QRS significantly narrows down, we should perform **optimal physiological pacing** (para-Hisian area for right ventricular lead and interatrial septum for right atrial lead). If QRS duration do not narrows down, we should perform **septal pacing** for the ventricular stimulation to minimize fluoroscopic time.
    - *Patients with left ventricular systolic dysfunction:* Patients with electro-mechanical desynchronization in addition to left ventricular systolic dysfunction

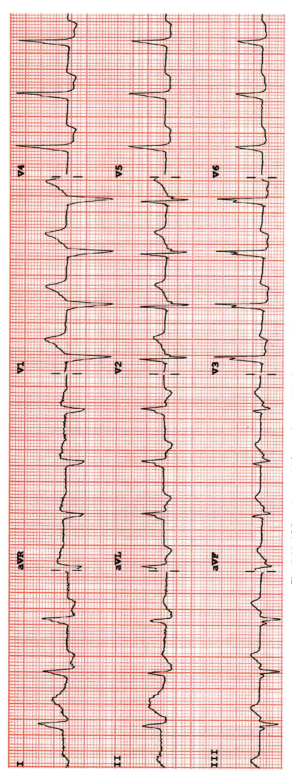

Fig. 7.22 VVI pacing at 90 bpm shows QRS duration of paced rhythm is 111 msec

Case Discussion

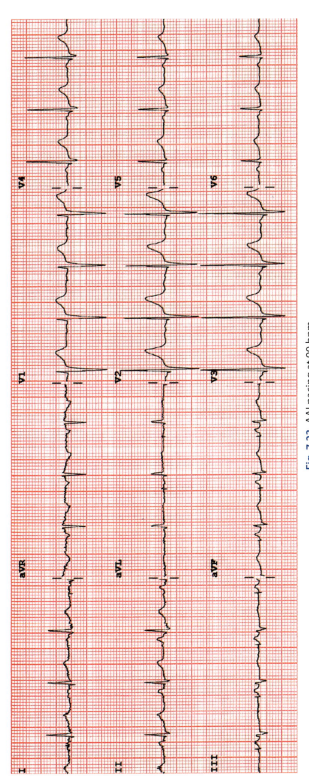

Fig. 7.23 AAI pacing at 90 bpm

should receive **resynchronization therapy (CRT)** with biventricular pacing (atrial, right and left ventricular leads). In absence of dyssynchrony patient should receive **optimal physiological pacing.**

REFERENCES

1. Eraldo Occhetta, Mirian Bortnik, Paolo Marino. Future easy and physiological cardiac pacing. World J Cardiol. 2011;3(1): 32-9.
2. Padeletti L, Porciani MC, Michelucci A, et al. Interatrial septum pacing: a new approach to prevent recurrent atrial fibrillation. J Interv Card Electrophysiol. 1999;3:3543.

CHAPTER 8

Introduction to Cardiac Resynchronization Therapy

INTRODUCTION

Heart failure (HF) is a clinical syndrome that results from any functional or structural cardiac disorder that impairs the ability of the ventricles to fill with or eject blood. Symptoms include fatigue, poor exercise tolerance, dyspnea (exertional or resting), and signs and radiographic evidence of pulmonary and systemic congestion.[1] Standardized clinical criteria for the diagnosis of HF have been described, such as Framingham criteria, the Boston, and National Health and Nutrition Examination Survey Criteria.[2-4] Other tools, such as echocardiography and measurement of B-natriuretic peptide (BNP), also are used for diagnosis. Effective use of diuretics, vasodilators, and inotropes to stabilize acute heart failure relies on matching the most appropriately tailored therapy to specific clinical profiles. Diuretics seems to be most beneficial in patients who have substantial volume overload, often seen in patients who have normal systolic blood pressure. Vasodilator therapy seems to have its greatest usefulness in patients who have acute pulmonary edema associated with an elevated systolic blood pressure and is recommended as first-line therapy in this group. Inotropes are effective in restoring hemodynamic stability in patients who have cardiogenic shock and need emergent enhancement of cardiac contractility to achieve clinical stabilization. But, this may lead to increased short- and long-term mortality.[5]

Neurohormonal activation plays a key role in the initiation and progression of chronic heart failure by influencing cardiac remodeling process. Increased tissue and plasma levels of neurohormones occur in patients with left ventricular dysfunction even when they are at an asymptomatic stage without overt heart failure. The renin-angiotensin-aldosterone system, sympathetic nervous system, endothelin system, arginine-vasopressin system, and natriuretic peptide contribute significantly to the pathogenesis of heart failure. The most important therapeutic advance during the past decade is the development of agents that inhibit neurohormonal activation system. By altering the natural biologic responses that are involved in the pathophysiology of heart failure, neurohormonal blockade has been an important foundation of several drugs in treating heart failure. They relieve symptoms of heart failure, reduce hospitalization, and prolong survival in patients with heart failure from left ventricular systolic dysfunction. The compendium of evidence suggests that angiotensin-converting-enzyme (ACE) inhibitors should remain drug of first choice for treating patients who have congestive heart failure but that angiotensin receptor blockers (ARBs) are suitable and equally effective alternatives.[6-8] In symptomatic congestive heart failure (CHF) patients, the addition of ARB to ACE inhibitors likely diminishes morbidity further, particularly the morbidity of multiple heart failure hospitalizations.[9] Aldosterone blockade with either spironolactone or eplerenone is effective in reducing total mortality in patients who have systolic left ventricular dysfunction and signs of heart failure. The combination of ACE inhibitor or ARB and aldosterone blocker is more effective in correcting the pathophysiology of heart failure than either alone. Four beta-blockers (bisoprolol, carvedilol, metoprolol, and nebivolol) are known to reduce the mortality of patients with heart failure due to left ventricular systolic dysfunction. COMET trial clearly shows that carvedilol is superior to metoprolol.[14] The lessons from CARMEN are clear in that the combined treatment of beta-blockade with carvedilol and ACE inhibition should be considered when heart failure is detected in a patient.[10] The order of administration is at the discretion of the clinician, and may relate to baseline characteristics such as heart rate and blood pressure. The agents that inhibit other neurohormonal system are also available with their beneficial effects as add on therapy. Recently published PARADIGM-HF trial showed the superior efficacy of combination of valsartan and neprilysin inhibitor in comparison to enalapril in term of cardiovascular mortality.[11]

Diabetes is associated with a twofold to fivefold increase in the risk of heart failure, independent of hypertension, body mass index, or coronary artery disease, and the risk is greater in women than men. Chronic hyperglycemia leads to glycosylation and cross linking of proteins, premature aging of collagen, and premature stiffening of major arteries lead to systolic hypertension. The "cardiotoxic triad" of diabetic cardiomyopathy, hypertension with left ventricular hypertrophy, and coronary artery disease leads to ventricular dysfunction, which in turn stimulates the renin-angiotensin and sympathetic nervous system, leading to further injury to the myocardium, more ventricular hypertrophy, loss of cardiomyocytes to apoptosis, further increases in ventricular fibrosis, and worsening of left ventricular dysfunction. Diastolic dysfunction in diabetics is predicted by only two risk factors, elevated HbA1c levels and microalbuminuria. Therefore, treatment of diabetes and hypertension prevents initiation and worsening of heart failure in this population.

Subsets of patients with systolic left ventricular dysfunction who have associated ventricular conduction delay are at highest risk for HF progression and poor overall outcome. The mechanism for this phenomenon is thought to be due to asynchronous and inefficient contraction of opposing areas of the ventricular myocardium. More importantly, restoring synchronization, either via simultaneous pacing of the RV apex and the left ventricular free wall or with timed LV free wall activation, can lead to a significant hemodynamic improvement.

The normal pattern of electrical activation of the ventricular myocardium, once the impulse passes through the atrioventricular (AV) node, starts in the His bundle, followed by simultaneous activation of the right and left bundles of the Purkinje system, and it finally proceeds into the myocardium. The Purkinje system is electrically isolated from the rest of the myocardium until it reaches its exit points at the Purkinje-myocardial junctions. As a result, typical left ventricular myocardial activation occurs from apex to base, simultaneously in the septum and in the left ventricular free wall, and is described as synchronous. Due to tight electromechanical coupling of the myocardium, synchronous ventricular activation is followed by synchronous ventricular contraction. In the setting of left bundle branch block (LBBB), interventricular conduction delay (IVCD), or right ventricular pacing, the activation of the LV is not synchronous. This results from slower conduction of the electrical impulse through the myocardium as compared to the Purkinje system. As a consequence, the activation of the entire left ventricular myocardium takes almost twice as long, with the posterolateral segments being activated latest. This dyssynchronous activation pattern leads to increased arrhythmia susceptibility. Left ventricular chamber hypertrophy, dilation, and reduced efficiency in the face of reduced coronary reserve lead to increased ischemia susceptibility, creating a vicious cycle that perpetuates this process into more advanced heart failure. Cardiac resynchronization therapy (CRT) has been shown to reverse this deleterious process. Synchronized pacing has been shown to improve left ventricular function without increasing oxygen demand, suggesting that the improvement is related to better efficiency of the left ventricular chamber.

INDICATION

Conventionally, cardiac resynchronization therapy is indicated in patients with heart failure with *symptoms despite optimum medical treatment with New York Heart Association (NYHA) functional class III or IV, left ventricular ejection fraction of less than 35%, and prolonged QRS duration* (≥120 msec). Multisite Stimulation in Cardiomyopathy–Sinus Rhythm (MUSTIC-SR) enrolled patients with QRS duration of **150 msec** or more while Pacing Therapies in Congestive Heart Failure (PATH-CHF) I and II used QRS duration of **120 msec** or more for inclusion in the trial. MIRACLE (Multicenter InSync Randomized Clinical Evaluation) and MIRACLE-ICD trials included patients of heart failure with QRS duration of **130 msec** or more. Both Cardiac Resynchronization in Heart Failure (CARE-HF) and Comparison of Medical Therapy Pacing and Defibrillation in Heart Failure (COMPANION) trials used patients of QRS duration of 120 msec or more.

All these studies demonstrate that CRT alone reduced all-cause mortality in patients with advanced symptoms of heart failure that was refractory to conventional medical therapy. The reduction in mortality is primarily due to a decrease in the progression of heart failure.

These CRT trials also give the following informations:
- Survival benefits seem to be largely a result of a decrease in progressive heart failure. CARE-HF, designed to assess mortality benefit in patients with CRT-P only, did demonstrate a mortality reduction even without defibrillation capability.
- Most patients improve NYHA functional class by at least one grade, which is very appealing to most patients with refractory heart failure symptoms.
- The mortality benefit of CRT is significant when compared to other mortalities, i.e. one death prevented for every five patients receiving CRT.

In an effort to expand the scope of cardiac resynchronization therapy for the patients of heart failure different trials have been conducted targeting the three basic variables.[12-23]
1. QRS duration.
2. NYHA class.
3. Left ventricular ejection fraction.

New York Heart Association Class

Resynchronization Reverses Remodeling in Systolic Left Ventricular Dysfunction (REVERSE) is a prospective, multicenter, randomized, double blind, parallel controlled clinical trial followed 610 patients with NYHA class I or II heart failure, left ventricular ejection fraction ≤40%, and a QRS duration ≥120 ms for a maximum of 2 years.[12] All patients were implanted with a CRT device with or without ICD and were then randomized to CRT-ON or CRT-OFF. The primary end point was the percentage of patients with worsened clinical composite response. Patients were considered worsened if they died, had a HF hospitalization, crossed over to the other study arm because of HF, or moved to a more severe NYHA class. The primary clinical end point (the percentage of patients with worsened clinical composite score) did not meet statistical significance at 12 months. However, at 24 months, the proportion of patients with worsened clinical response was statistically different.

Multicenter Automatic Defibrillator Implantation Trial-Cardiac Resynchronization Therapy (MADIT-CRT), on the other hand, enrolled 1820 patients with an EF of ≤30%, QRS duration of ≥130 ms, and NYHA class I or II heart failure for an average duration of 2.4 years.[13] Patients were randomized to be implanted with either a CRT device with ICD (CRT-D) or an ICD only so that there was no blinding of randomized treatment arm. The primary end point was all-cause mortality or occurrence of first HF event, defined as either a hospital admission for HF or outpatient treatment of HF requiring intravenous therapy. The primary end point reached statistical significance, as did the secondary end point of LV reverse remodeling. In the CRT-D group, 17.2% of subjects experienced death or a HF event, whereas 25.3% reached the primary end point in the ICD-only group.

The major statistically significant findings from these studies are a 41% reduction in risk of first HF event in MADIT-CRT and a 53% risk reduction in time to first HF hospitalization in REVERSE. Moreover, both trials show significant LV reverse remodeling with CRT. Although an independent mortality benefit was not observed in either trial, the investigators set an ambitious goal for such a short follow-up period. The totality of evidence provides reason to view the results with optimism rather than dismissal. Subgroup analysis showed that the patients with wider QRS (>150 ms) showed a statistically significant benefit compared with the subjects with shorter QRS in either trials. In REVERSE, the clinical benefit was also significantly greater among nonischemic cardiomyopathy patients and the group with EF <27%. The MADIT-CRT investigators observed a greater response to CRT among women, but similar results were found among ischemic and nonischemic patients.

Biventricular versus Right Ventricular Pacing in Heart Failure Patients with Atrioventricular Block (BLOCK-HF) is a treatment, randomized, double-blind, active control, parallel assignment, safety/efficacy study to determine if CRT applied at earlier stages of functional limitation, NYHA I and II in addition to class III patients, with lesser degrees of left ventricular (LV) systolic dysfunction, ejection fraction ≤50%, in patients requiring pacing for AV block, will delay progression of heart failure.[14] The results show superiority of biventricular pacing over conventional right ventricular pacing in patients with atrioventricular block and left ventricular systolic dysfunction with NYHA class I, II, or III heart failure.

The Resynchronization/Defibrillation for Ambulatory Heart Failure Trial (RAFT) assessed 1798 patients receiving a CRT-D device to determine total mortality and hospitalization for CHF over a mean period of 40 months period. This large trial has enrolled patients with NYHA class II failure, LVEF ≤30% by multiple gated acquisition or LVEF ≤30% and LVEDD > 60 mm by echocardiogram, QRS duration ≥120 ms; optimal heart failure pharmacological therapy; and ICD indication for primary or secondary prevention.[15] Result shows that among patients with NYHA class II or III heart failure, a wide QRS complex, and left ventricular systolic dysfunction, the addition of CRT to an ICD reduced rates of death and hospitalization for heart failure. But, this improvement was accompanied by more adverse events (device or implant related complication).

QRS Duration

Resynchronization Therapy in Normal QRS (RethinQ) Trial is a prospective, multicenter, randomized (1:1), double-blind, controlled clinical investigation, designed to assess the safety and efficacy of CRT-D in patients who are indicated for ICD therapy with NYHA III, narrow QRS duration (<130 ms), and evidence of mechanical dyssynchrony as measured by echocardiography/TDI.[17] CRT did not improve peak oxygen consumption in patients with moderate heart failure, a QRS interval of less than 130 msec, and mechanical dyssynchrony. However, a subgroup of patients with a QRS interval of 120 msec to 130 msec did benefit from CRT.

The objective of the DESIRE study was to determine CRT benefit in patients with a narrow QRS < 120 ms, and to evaluate the value of dyssynchrony assessment to identify potential responders to CRT.[18] Baseline QRS duration did not predict response to CRT. The investigators concluded that in the patients presenting with chronic HF and a QRS width of less than 150 ms, the presence of one or more simple indices of mechanical dyssynchrony at baseline 2D-echo examination, but not QRS duration, predicted the response to CRT at 6 months of follow-up.

Evaluation of Screening Techniques in Electrically Normal, Mechanically Dyssynchronous Heart Failure Patient Receiving CRT (ESTEEM-CRT) is a single-arm feasibility study that includes NYHA class III patients with QRS duration <120 ms, evidence of ventricular mechanical dyssynchrony as measured by TDI echocardiographic techniques, and an ICD indication.[19] Sixty-eight patients received a CRT defibrillator, exercise testing, and echo exams, and 47 of these patients underwent invasive hemodynamic testing at implant. Follow-up was at 6 and 12 months. The patients with a narrow QRS and mechanical dyssynchrony as defined in this study did not improve as measured by acute hemodynamics, chronic exercise performance, or reverse remodeling.

Echocardiography Guided Cardiac Resynchronization Therapy (EchoCRT) is a prospective randomized controlled clinical trial to assess the clinical impact of CRT in patients with advanced heart failure (NYHA class III) and a narrow QRS complex who show mechanical dyssynchrony as assessed by echocardiography and enrolled 809 patients.[20] The result shows that compared to optimal pharmacological therapy and an ICD, the addition of CRT does not improve clinical outcomes assessed by the combined endpoint of all-cause mortality and heart failure hospitalization and it may increase mortality in patients with systolic heart failure patients with a QRS duration <130 msec.

Left Ventricular Ejection Fraction

The PACE trial, a prospective double-blind, multicenter study, compared apical RV pacing with CRT in patients with bradycardia and a preserved LV ejection fraction (EF >45%) in 177 patients.[21] The trial evaluated LV function and measurements of remodeling over 12 months. The results of the study demonstrated significant and substantial reductions in LVEF and increases in end-systolic LV volumes in the RV pacing group during the 1-year follow-up and the evidence of deterioration in LV function was not observed in the group with CRT pacing. But, what amount of benefit would justify the modest increased risk at implantation as well as the increase cost of a device with shorter longevity. Patients with infrequent episodes of bradycardia requiring a back up pacemaker would not be candidates for CRT. However, if there is AV block and expectation of pacemaker dependency, a device that results in chronic RV pacing will be likely to put the patient at risk for adverse remodeling and it may begin soon after the implantation and progress. However, isolated sinus node dysfunction without AV block may not required an RV lead, and the PACE trial results do not support implantation of a CRT in this population.

Biventricular pacing for atri**o**ventricular bl**o**ck to **p**revent **c**ardia**c** **d**esynchronization (BIOPACE) trial randomized 1810 patients with AV block to either RV pacing or BiV pacing to determine if the latter approach could prevent some of these deleterious effects irrespective of LV systolic functional status. After a mean follow-up of 5.6 years, the groups had a similar rate of the composite endpoint that included time-to-death or first hospitalization due to heart failure, with a nonsignificant trend in favor of BiV pacing.[22]

As a result of these trials, the original 2005 guideline recommendations for cardiac resynchronization therapy have been expanded to less symptomatic patients but also limited to some extent on the basis of QRS morphology and/or QRS duration. Based on these observations, recommendations for the use of cardiac resynchronization therapy are substantially revised in 2012.[23] According to these new cardiac resynchronization therapy guidelines, indications for cardiac resynchronization therapy include patients who have an LVEF of 35% or less, sinus rhythm, LBBB with a QRS duration of 120 milliseconds or longer, and NYHA class II, III, or ambulatory IV symptoms while receiving optimal medical treatment (Table 8.1).

However, the Heart Failure Society of America, the Heart Rhythm Society and the European Society of Cardiology have published their guidelines recently. Although there are a few distinctions among the guidelines, a vast majority of recommendations put forth are concordant. The initial indications for CRT have evolved to incorporate the degree of QRS prolongation, QRS morphology, presence of atrial fibrillation, and lower NYHA class to provide a more nuanced

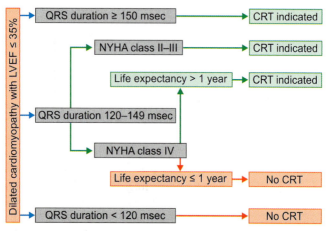

Fig. 8.1 Practical algorithm for CRT indication

Introduction to Cardiac Resynchronization Therapy

Table 8.1 ACC/AHA guidelines for cardiac resynchronization

Class	Indication	Level of evidence
I	CRT is indicated for patients who have an LVEF of ≤35%, sinus rhythm, LBBB with QRS duration of ≥ 150 msec, and NYHA class II, III, or ambulatory IV symptoms while receiving guideline-directed medical therapy.	Level of evidence A for NYHA class III/IV, level of evidence B for NYHA class II.
IIa	• CRT can be useful for patients who have an LVEF of ≤35%, sinus rhythm, a non-LBBB pattern with QRS duration of ≥ 150 msec, and NYHA class III, or ambulatory IV symptoms while receiving guideline-directed medical therapy.	Level of evidence A.
	• CRT can be useful for patients who have an LVEF of ≤35%, sinus rhythm, LBBB with QRS duration of 120 to 149 msec, and NYHA class II, III, or ambulatory IV symptoms while receiving guideline-directed medical therapy.	Level of evidence B.
	• CRT can be useful for patients with atrial fibrillation and an LVEF of ≤35% while receiving guideline-directed medical therapy if (1) patient requires ventricular pacing or otherwise meets the criteria for CRT and (2) atrioventricular nodal ablation or pharmacological rate control will allow almost 100% ventricular pacing with CRT.	Level of evidence B.
	• CRT can be useful for patients receiving guideline-directed medical therapy who have an LVEF of ≤35% and are undergoing placement of a new or replacement device with an anticipated requirement for significant (>40%) ventricular pacing.	Level of evidence C.
Class IIb	• CRT may be considered useful for patients who have an LVEF of ≤35%, sinus rhythm, a non-LBBB pattern with QRS duration of 120-149 msec, and NYHA class III, or ambulatory IV symptoms while receiving guideline-directed medical therapy.	Level of evidence B.
	• CRT may be considered useful for patients who have an LVEF of ≤35%, sinus rhythm, a non-LBBB pattern with QRS duration of ≥150 msec, and NYHA class II symptoms while receiving guideline-directed medical therapy.	Level of evidence B.
Class III	• CRT is not recommended for patients with NYHA class I or II symptoms and a non-LBBB pattern with QRS duration <150 msec.	
	• CRT is not indicated for patients whose co-morbid conditions and/or frailty limit survival with good functional capacity to <1 year.	

Class I : Conditions for which there is evidence and/or general agreement that the test is useful or effective.
Class II : Conditions for which there is conflicting evidence and/or a divergence of opinion about the usefulness or efficacy of performing the test.
Class IIa : Weight of evidence or opinion is in favor of usefulness or efficacy.
Class IIb : Usefulness or efficacy is less well established by evidence or opinion.
Class III : Condition for which there is evidence and/or general agreement that the test is not useful or effective and in some cases may be harmful.
Level A : Recommendations are derived from data from multiple randomized clinical trials.
Level B : Recommendations are derived from a single randomized trial or non-randomized studies.
Level C : Recommendations are based on the consensus opinion of experts.

approach to patient selection. Figure 8.1 summarizes these adjustments.

To summarize these recommendations followings are the recommendations for CRT implantation at the present moment:

Class I

- LVEF ≤35%,
- LBBB with QRS duration ≥150 msec
- NYHA functional class II to IV ambulatory.

Class IIa

LVEF ≤35%, NYHA functional class II to IV ambulatory with 1 of the following:
- LBBB with QRS duration 120–149 msec
- Non-LBBB with QRS duration ≥ 150 msec, or
- Ventricular pacing expected > 40%.

Class IIb

- LVEF ≤ 35%, Non-LBBB, with 1 of the followings:
  - QRS duration 120–149 msec with NYHA functional class III–IV ambulatory.
  - QRS duration ≥ 150 msec with NYHA functional class II.
  - Atrial fibrillation, QRS duration ≥ 120 msec with NYHA functional class II–III.
- LVEF ≤ 35%, LBBB with QRS duration ≥ 150 msec, NYHA functional class I.

Atrial tachyarrhythmias play a major role in CRT patients. AV junctional ablation is most preferred choice for controlling ventricular rate in patients with atrial fibrillation. Implantation of CRT following AV node ablation gives similar benefit to the patients of congestive heart failure as in patients of CRT in sinus rhythm. Ventricular rate control can also be possible with pharmacological agents and aim of CRT is to achieve the highest possible percentage of biventricular pacing. In absence of AV nodal ablation, pharmacological ventricular rate control should achieve biventricular capture of more than 80% and with this response to CRT is comparable with CRT in sinus rhythm.

Electrical Activation Sequence

In patients with heart failure, due to functional and structural alterations (cardiac remodeling) abnormal impulse generation and propagation is observed frequently. Sinus node functional abnormality and pathologic AV conduction incompetence are frequently observed in patients with heart failure. More than approximately one-third of heart failure patients present with ventricular conduction disturbances, left bundle branch block being the most common.

Left bundle branch block is a complex electrical disease and can result from block or conduction delays (fixed or functional) in any of several sites of the left-sided intraventricular conduction system, including the main left bundle branch or its subdivisions or, less commonly, within the fibers of the distal His bundle. The electrical impulse is conducted essentially through the working myocardium with slow conduction properties, rather than through the rapid specialized conduction system. As a result, during abnormal electrical conduction the time required for complete activation of the atrial and ventricular muscle is much longer than during physiologic conduction and furthermore a pathologic and asynchronous activation pattern occurs.

Depending on the substrate (ischemic vs. nonischemic dilated cardiomyopathy) the left ventricular endocardial activation pattern may differ. In nonischemic dilated cardiomyopathy, conduction delay resides entirely within the ventricular septum, and LV endocardial activation is rapid after single-point breakthrough. But, in ischemic dilated cardiomyopathy activation is slowed across regions of scar throughout the left ventricle. In both situations the posterior or posterolateral basal left ventricle is the latest activated region.

Thus, two most important factors for left ventricular endocardial activation sequence are:
1. *Transseptal conduction*
2. *Left ventricular transmural conduction* which is the result of presence and location of functional or fixed block. At least three patterns of delayed LV activation have been characterized:
    - Transseptal delay with or without LV endocardial delay
    - Normal transseptal conduction with slow conduction velocities in periinfarct regions and globally slow in nonischemic dilated cardiomyopathy
    - Slowed U-shaped activation around a line of functional block on the anterior wall. Total LV endocardial activation time in patients with LBBB is much longer (80–150 ms) than in patients without conduction delays (50–80 ms).

Significantly prolonged trans-septal conduction times through a diseased left bundle branch result in midseptal LV or septoapical breakthroughs and unidirectional wavefront propagation throughout the left ventricle. Rapid trans-septal conduction times typify conduction through septal branches of the His-Purkinje system, with basal breakthroughs from the anterior or posterior fascicle and bidirectional wavefront propagation from base to apex and high septum. Breakthrough from both fascicles results in a double wavefront that fuses on the posterolateral wall. Single-site breakthrough from the high septum caused by right-to-left muscular conduction (no conduction system present) results in a single wavefront that propagates from base to apex.[24] The pattern of septal activation may affect ventricular mechanics differently. High septal activation may result in simultaneous RV and LV activation in opposite directions, and papillary muscle activation may be influenced by the earliest site of LV activation.[25] The pattern of LV endocardial and epicardial activation is also influenced by the location and size of lines of fixed or functional conduction block. Fixed conduction block is caused by replacement of normal myocardium by interstitial fibrosis. The physiologic basis for functional conduction blocks has not been elucidated but could relate to stretch, heart rate, and spontaneous diastolic depolarization.

Anterior locations of the line of functional block are characterized by a U-shaped LV activation pattern, more prolonged QRS duration, and longer time to LV breakthrough (Figs 8.2A and B).[26] Late activation of the posterior or posterolateral basal left ventricle occurred by wave front propagation around the line of block using the apical or inferior LV walls. The activation front in these cases cannot cross directly from the anterior and superior region to the lateral wall due to a block to the conduction; this wave front reaches the lateral or posterolateral regions of the LV by propagating inferiorly around the apex, giving rise to a very characteristic and unique "U-shaped" discontinuous activation pattern. LV activation ultimately ends at the basal region of the lateral or posterolateral wall, near the mitral valve annulus. Local unipolar electrograms confirm the presence of fragmented, double, or multiphasic components in the anterior region where the wave front is not able to cross.

The conduction block is best represented by a line (line of block) that generally parallels the septum, directed from the base toward the apex, in the anterior or anterolateral region of the LV. Functional behavior of this line of block is demonstrated by a change in its location during ventricular pacing at different sites, with different cycle lengths and AV delays. Interestingly, this functional conduction block can be easily recognized by unipolar signals used by noncontact mapping and is not identified by bipolar electrograms used by contact mapping. This may suggest that the largest conduction delay is located

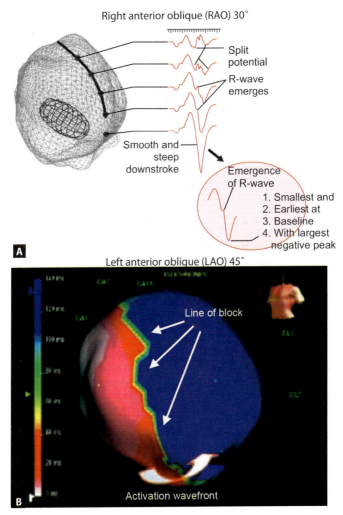

Figs 8.2A and B Intracardiac noncontact electrograms showing fragmented, multiphasic signals possibly indicating a reduction of conduction velocity and inability to propagate throughout anterior region with four criteria for identifying location and length of line of block. (A) Unipolar isochronal map, acquired with noncontact mapping system, of the LV showing the anterior location of functional line of block; (B) (Modified from Auricchio A, Fantoni C, Regoli F, et al. Characterization of left ventricular activation in patients with heart failure and left bundle branch block. Circulation: 2004;109:1133-39 with permission)

more intramurally than subendocardially; therefore it is conceivable that a functional block to the conduction emerges from anisotropic conduction due to disarray of intramyocardial layers of tissue, each with potentially different characteristics of conduction.

Lateral locations of the line of block are characterized by less prolonged QRS duration and shorter time to LV breakthrough

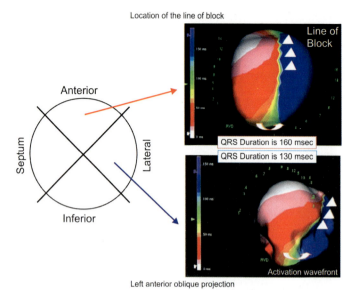

Fig. 8.3 Relation between QRS duration and LV activation sequence as assessed by unipolar isochronal maps. In patients with LBBB, a functional conduction block determines a discontinuous, U-shaped LV activation pattern. In patients with LBBB and QRS duration below 150 ms the conduction block is usually located in a more lateral position (upper right panel). In contrast, patients with LBBB and QRS longer than 150 ms consistently display an anterior location of the line of block (lower right panel) (Modified from Auricchio A, Fantoni C, Regoli F, et al. Characterization of left ventricular activation in patients with heart failure and left bundle branch block. Circulation: 2004;109:1133-39 with permission)

(Fig. 8.3).[26] Lines of conduction block do not correlate with regions of wall motion abnormality or scarring. Some lines of block arose only during pacing and were site dependent (functional), whereas other lines of block could not be manipulated with pacing maneuvers, indicating these were caused by slow or absent conduction (fixed). Latest activation most often occurred in the posterior or posterolateral basal wall, but was also observed in the anterior and inferior walls in some patients.

The transmural electrical activation processes in heart failure patients with LBBB have been further characterized recently. By combining conventional catheter mapping technique and three-dimensional noncontact mapping system, the epiendocardial ventricular activation sequence (i.e. the transmural activation sequence limited to the regions adjacent to the epicardial anterior and lateral coronary veins) has been evaluated[27] (Figs 8.4A and B). By comparing the timing of the earliest detectable ventricular epicardial activation, recorded at the anterior vein, with the time of the earliest LV

Introduction to Cardiac Resynchronization Therapy

endocardial activation by noncontact mapping, it has been shown that in patients with a short endocardial breakthrough time or trans-septal time, the transmural activation sequence at the anteroseptal region showed an endo- to epicardium sequential activation timing. In contrast, in patients with a prolonged trans-septal time, the transmural activation timing was reverted, as the epicardium was activated earlier than the endocardium. Notably, total LV endocardial activation time was significantly longer in patients with a short trans-septal time and an endo- to epicardium sequential activation timing than in those with a prolonged trans-septal time and a reversed epi- to endocardium timing. This can probably be explained by the fact that patients with a short transseptal time present with more pronounced disease of the working myocardial tissue and better preserved conduction capacities through the proximal specialized conduction system. Indeed, many patients with an ischemic cardiomyopathy demonstrate this type of conduction abnormality. However, the outcome and response to both

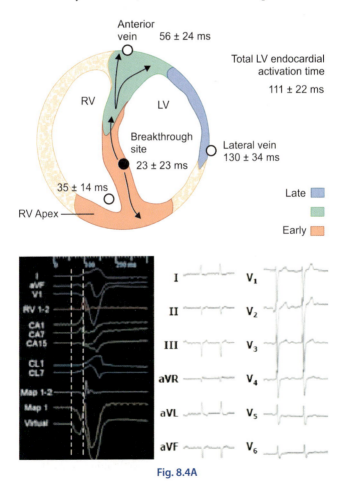

Fig. 8.4A

Cardiac Pacing: A Physiological Approach

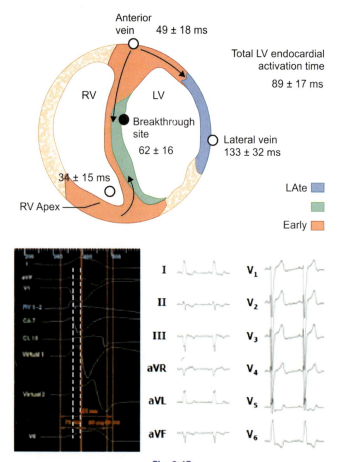

Fig. 8.4B

Figs 8.4A and B Transmural electrical activation sequence as assessed by combining conventional catheter mapping and noncontact mapping techniques. In the lower panel, along with surface ECG, intracardiac bipolar recordings of RV (RV_{1-2}), unipolar LV noncontact (virtual) electrograms, as well as epicardial unipolar recordings acquired through microcatheters inserted into the anterior (CA) and lateral (CL) epicardial veins are shown. In patients with a relatively short time to LV endocardial breakthrough (A), an endo- to epicardium activation timing in the anteroseptal region of the LV occurs. In contrast, in patients with prolonged time to LV endocardial breakthrough, an epi- to endocardium activation timing is recorded (B) (Modified from Fantoni C, Regoli F, Kawabata M, Klein HU, Auricchio A. Reversed transmural activation timing in patients with heart failure and left bundle branch block. Eur Heart J 2004 (suppl): 2320 with permission)

pharmacological and nonpharmacological therapies of these two groups are not characterized differently.

Despite similar surface electrocardiographic appearances, left ventricular electrical activation patterns during LBBB are highly heterogeneous and unpredictable (Table 8.2).

Table 8.2 Patterns of left bundle branch block (LBBB)

Characters	QRS duration is 120 – 150 msec	QRS duration of more than 150 msec
Location of Delay	Confined specifically to specialized conduction system.	Additional conduction delay in diseased myocardium.
Trans-septal conduction and line of block	Short trans-septal time and lateral location of line of block	Prolonged trans-septal conduction and anterior line of block
Total LV endocardial activation time	Significantly longer	Shorter
Transmural activation	Endo-to-epicardial activation sequence at the anteroseptal region.	Reversed, epi-to-endocardial activation sequence (Epicardial activation sequence).

Mechanoenergetics

The subset of patients with dilated cardiomyopathy with wide QRS complex in sinus rhythm (namely LBBB) shows dyssynchrony at multiple levels and can be (i) interatrial, (ii) atrioventricular, (iii) interventricular, (iv) intraventricular, and (v) intramural (Fig. 8.5). Such electromechanical decoupling results in disordered mechanical events, occur in isolation or in various combinations at any level, and degrade cardiac pump function. Most studies have emphasized that the importance of intraventricular dyssynchrony as the major contributing factor to progressive HF and a predictor of response to CRT.

Significant interatrial conduction delays may occur in myopathic atria. When interatrial conduction delay is too long, the atrial systole occurs after the beginning of ventricular contraction and against a closed mitral valve. In such a situation, atrial contraction provokes sudden and major atrial distension and induces AV regurgitation. This causes increased LA pressures, retrograde flow in the pulmonary veins, and counter-physiologic neurohormonal responses termed pseudopacemaker syndrome.[28]

Normally intrinsic atrioventricular interval results in atrial contraction just before the pre-ejection (isovolumetric) period of ventricular contraction. Properly timed atrial contraction maximizes LV filling and thereby its output. Too early atrial contraction causes a loss of the booster pump function of the atrium. Moreover, early atrial contraction may initiate early mitral valve closure, which limits ventricular diastolic filling

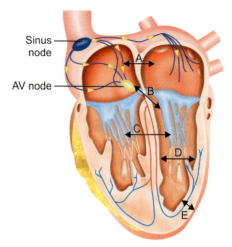

Fig. 8.5 Levels of mechanical dyssynchrony. The figure shows the levels of dyssynchrony within the heart: (A) interatrial, (B) atrioventricular, (C) interventricular, (D) intraventricular, and (E) intramural mechanical dyssynchrony

time. Three factors collaborate to achieve optimal closure of the AV valves. *First*, the ending of transvalvular flow at the end of the atrial contraction makes the valvular leaflets approach one another. *Second*, at the beginning of ventricular contraction, the annulus of the AV valves contracts, as do the papillary muscles that hold the leaflets. *Finally*, simultaneously, at the start of ventricular contraction, ventricular pressure rises above atrial pressure, and the valves close. When these factors are malaligned, an opportunity for diastolic and systolic mitral regurgitation is created. Appropriately timed AV coupling maintains a low mean atrial pressure, increases LV filling time, maximizes preload and pump function, and positions the mitral valve for closure during the isovolumetric phase of ventricular systole. Delayed coupling displaces atrial contraction earlier in diastole. Atrial contraction occurs during ventricular filling, which shortens diastolic filling time, and in extreme situations, occurs immediately after or coincident with the preceding ventricular contraction. This situation is aggravated by ventricular conduction delay (as occurs in LBBB), which increases ventricular ejection time and delays diastolic filling, increasing the probability of collision with atrial contraction. Atrial contraction before completion of venous return reduces preload stretching of the left ventricle, which reduces ventricular volume and contractile force. Delayed AV coupling reduces diastolic filling time and may result in diastolic mitral regurgitation when elevated LV end-diastolic pressure exceeds LA pressure. Partial closure of the mitral valve may also occur, further shortening diastolic filling time. Severe

AV decoupling coexists with ventriculoatrial (VA) coupling. In extreme conditions LA contraction occurs immediately after, within, or preceding the LV contraction, causing reversal of the left-sided AV contraction sequence, which initiates counterphysiologic circulatory and neurohumoral reflexes. Atrial fibrillation disrupts atrial coupling (atrial desynchronization) and eliminates AV coupling (AV uncoupling).

Normally, the synchronous mechanical activation and ventricular contraction is the result of rapid and homogeneous LV electrical activation with minimal temporal dispersion throughout the wall. This result in coordinated myocardial segment activation maximizes ventricular pump function. The various regions differ in the time of onset of contraction and in the pattern of contraction. In LBBB the earliest ventricular depolarization is recorded over the anterior RV surface and generally latest at the posterior or posterolateral basal LV surface. Regions that are activated early also start contracting early. Because of the vigorous contraction, the late-activated regions impose loading on the earlier activated territories, which now undergo systolic paradoxical stretch.[29] This reciprocated stretching of regions within the LV wall causes a less effective and energetically less efficient contraction. The poorer contractility is reflected by decreases in stroke work and rate of increase of LV pressure, and a rightward shift of the LV end-systolic pressure-volume relationship which results in left ventricular dilatation. So, the left ventricle operates at a consistently larger volume. The combination of these effects leads to a lower LV ejection time and EF (Fig. 8.6). The local differences in contraction pattern in the patients with LBBB imply a redistribution of mechanical work, perfusion, and oxygen demand within the LV wall. Asymmetrical hypertrophy

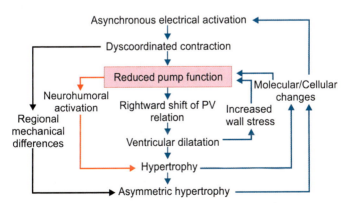

Fig. 8.6 Mechanisms of ventricular remodeling and progressive reduction in pump function during right ventricular apex pacing. PV = pressure-volume

in patients with LBBB is most likely due to the redistribution of workload, as evidenced by the regional differences in circumferential shortening in systole and external work. Regional differences in macroscopic hypertrophy are related to regional differences in myocyte diameter without differences in regional collagen content, indicating that the hypertrophy is due to a proportional increase of myocyte and collagen volume. The late-activated, most-hypertrophied regions show the most pronounced cellular derangements, such as down-regulation of proteins involved in calcium homeostasis and impulse conduction leading to dystrophic calcifications and disorganized mitochondria and myofibrillar cellular disarray. The reduced septal perfusion during LBBB appears to be the result of autoregulation following a reduction in local oxygen demand in early activated myocardium (so, can be considered as "functional").

Mitral regurgitation complicates and affects the prognosis of patients with dilated cardiomyopathy, and is usually associated with incomplete mitral leaflet closure (apically displaced coaptation with failure of the mitral leaflets to reach the level of the mitral annulus and without apparent intrinsic cusp abnormalities). Left ventricular (LV) dilation can potentially causes geometric changes in the mitral leaflet attachments. During systole, mitral regurgitation is due to combined effect of reduced force to close the leaflets and geometric changes in the mitral leaflet attachments, causing augmented chordal tension and leaflet tethering. But, tethering is a potential mechanism of mitral regurgitation in terms of restricted leaflet opening during diastole as well, when the question of systolic dysfunction is no longer present. **Severe functional mitral regurgitation**, defined as regurgitant volume (RV) of more than 30 mL or effective regurgitant orifice of more than 0.2 cm^2 or vena contracta (VC) of more than 0.4, is associated with two fold increase in the risk of adverse events after adjustment for LVEF and restricted mitral filling pattern in patients with heart failure due to dilated cardiomyopathy. A recent study suggested that severity of FMR is an independent predictor of adverse events in patients with heart failure due to dilated cardiomyopathy.[30]

In patients with heart failure, both atria are usually enlarged with widespread substitution of functioning myocardial cells by regions of fibrosis and scars as a result of apoptotic processes, repeated ischemic events and chronic inflammation, induced by increased mechanical stress and consequent metabolic changes. Atrial stretch leads to alteration in gene expression which may result in pathologic ion channel function. This leads to abnormal transmembrane currents and action potentials that constitute the pathophysiological base for so-called "electrical atrial remodeling", and is responsible for abnormal and slow conduction. As the sinus node extends over a variably large area of the right atrium, it is often involved by these pathologic alterations.[31] Patients with heart failure usually present with an abnormally caudal localization of the sinus node complex, due to loss of functioning myocardial cells in the upper regions of the right atrium. Structural alterations, abnormal loading conditions, and imbalanced neurohumoral influences account for the sinus node function impairment which results in increased intrinsic sinus cycle length, prolonged sinus node recovery time and slowed sinoatrial conduction velocity.[32] All together these phenomena lead to important derangement of sinus node function with consequent bradycardia and chronotropic incompetence, which may favor the onset and persistence of focal or reentrant atrial arrhythmias including atrial fibrillation and atrial flutter.

Assessment of Dyssynchrony

Ventricular dyssynchrony is a state of uncoordinated electrical activation of the heart resulting in different portions of the ventricle contracting at different times which results in a highly inefficient contractile state as opposed to the normal heart (in which all segments contract nearly simultaneously). Cardiac resynchronization therapy uses in addition to a right ventricular and a right atrial lead, a left ventricular lead positioned on the lateral wall (most commonly) of the left ventricle either endovascularly via the coronary sinus or epicardially via direct surgical placement. This leads to near simultaneous stimulation of both the ventricle. The measurement of QRS duration by the surface ECG (an electrical event which provides only a crude estimation of myocardial activation) can be used as an indirect evidence of ventricular dyssynchrony.[33] Echocardiography seems to be more reliable tool in assessing the severity of mechanical dyssynchrony and its impact on cardiac hemodynamics in a quantitative manner. The advent of newer echocardiographic technologies including spectral tissue Doppler imaging (TDI), color TDI, and post-processing of color-TDI such as strain, strain rate, tissue tracking etc. enabled us to have a more comprehensive, precise and quantitative assessment of global and regional cardiac function, in particular systolic dyssynchrony. Various nonechocardiographic techniques including magnetic resonance imaging (MRI) and nuclear imaging technique allow assessment of dyssynchrony and also provide information about the location and extent of scar tissue, especially in the region of presumed LV pacing site. Despite the obvious advantages of this imaging technique, at present the QRS duration still remains the main selection criterion for CRT implantation in currently available guidelines.[34,35] However, proper assessment of the patients undergoing CRT implantation using these techniques is essential to decrease the number of nonresponders.

Echocardiographic Assessment

The subset of patients with dilated cardiomyopathy with wide QRS complex in sinus rhythm (namely LBBB) shows two components: an electrical conduction disturbance and subsequent mechanical dyssynchrony. The impairment of left ventricular (LV) performance and energy consumption is seen with the development of an electrical conduction delay. The left ventricle is activated slowly through the septum from the right side and the LV endocardial activation time may exceed 100 ms.[36] LV pre-ejection pressure is lower than the right ventricular. The septal motion is abnormal. This results in an uncoordinated contraction sequence and delays LV ejection at the expense of diastolic filling.[37] As the electrical conduction disturbance in patients with advanced heart failure may involve the complete conduction system from the sinus node to the Purkinje fibers, the atrioventricular and ventricular conduction can be similarly affected and three different levels of dyssynchrony can be observed.

Atrioventricular Dyssynchrony (A Delay Between Atrial and Ventricular Contraction)

Atrioventricular dyssynchrony in a case of dilated cardiomyopathy occurs due to delayed ventricular activation in relation to the atria as a result of prolongation of the PR interval in sinus rhythm. It results in mitral valve incompetence with the occurrence of late diastolic regurgitation and a reduced ventricular filling time (limiting diastolic stroke volume). Moreover, atrial systole can occur simultaneously with early passive filling, with a further reduction of ventricular filling. The total diastolic filling interval (dFT = E wave duration + A wave duration) is shortened, mainly owing to a reduction in E wave duration. In the presence of severe AV dyssynchrony, the dFT typically measures < 40–45% of the corresponding cycle length and the E wave and A wave are fused (Fig. 8.7).

The aim is to increase the diastolic filling time to a maximum (above 50–60% of the corresponding cycle length) without early termination of atrial filling by premature mitral valve closure and to eliminate diastolic mitral regurgitation.[38] The delay between atrial filling and the onset of the LV pressure rise

Introduction to Cardiac Resynchronization Therapy

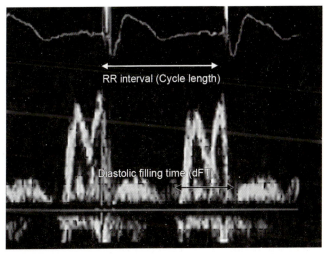

Fig. 8.7 Measurement of atrioventricular dyssynchrony: Cycle length is the measurement of RR interval and the diastolic filling time (dFT) is the sum of E and A wave depolarization. In this patient of dilated cardiomyopathy with LBBB is 30% (dFT/RR interval × 100) which indicates AV dyssynchrony

may also cause inversed AV flow during this period, with the occurrence of diastolic mitral regurgitation.

Interventricular Dyssynchrony

The delayed LV contraction and relaxation induces interventricular dyssynchrony and affects mainly the interventricular septal motion, which reduces LV ejection. Conversely, the earlier onset of RV contraction results in RV ejection occurring during the LV end-diastolic phase. Moreover, the higher RV pressure reverses the trans-septal pressure gradient and displaces the septum into the LV. Total ventricular activation time in the healthy human lasts about 60–80 msec, corresponding with QRS duration of 70–80 msec. The interventricular septum is activated from left to right and LV pressure rises slightly before right ventricular (RV) pressure. Under these normal conditions, RV and LV outflow occur almost simultaneously and the interventricular mechanical delay (IVMD) between the ventricles is close to zero (<25 msec). This parameter is defined as the difference between the LV and RV pre-ejection intervals (LV-PEI, RV-PEI), measured by standard pulsed-wave Doppler echocardiography as the interval between the onset of the QRS and the onset of aortic or pulmonary outflow ejection (Fig. 8.8). An IVMD above 40–50 msec in a patient with a dilated ventricle, low ejection fraction, and a broad QRS supports the indication for CRT, but

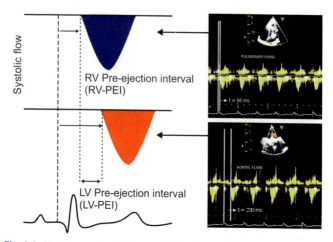

Fig. 8.8 Measurement of Interventricular dyssynchrony: interventricular mechanical delay (IVMD) is defined as the difference between the LV and RV pre-ejection intervals. LV pre-ejection interval is measured as the interval between the onset of the QRS and the onset of aortic outflow ejection and RV pre-ejection interval is measured as the interval between the onset of the QRS and the onset of pulmonary outflow ejection by standard pulsed-wave Doppler echocardiography. An IVMD above 40 msec is considered to be significant. In this index case it is 164 msec. LV-PEI of more than 140 msec indicates significant delay as an isolated parameter. In this patient it is 230 msec

a lower IVMD in this population does not necessarily imply that this potentially lifesaving therapy is not indicated. The IVMD correlates to QRS duration and is typically increased to >40 msec in patients with a QRS width of >150 msec. Some investigators advocate the use of the LV-PEI as an isolated parameter to identify possible CRT candidates and for post-implant optimization and suggest a cut-off value of >140 msec.[39]

Intraventricular (or LV) Dyssynchrony

Probably most important level of dyssynchrony to be evaluated in the context of CRT is within the left ventricle. It induces regions with early and delayed contraction which contribute to a reduction of systolic performance, an increase in end-systolic volume and wall stress, a delayed relaxation, and a reduction in LV efficiency. The most precise methodology for identification and quantitative assessment of this intraventricular level of dyssynchrony is probably TDI. However, intraventricular dyssynchrony may also be assessed by standard echocardiographic techniques, such as M-mode echocardiography by measuring septal-to-posterior wall motion delay. The septal-posterior wall motion delay (SPWMD) is measured between the first maximum systolic

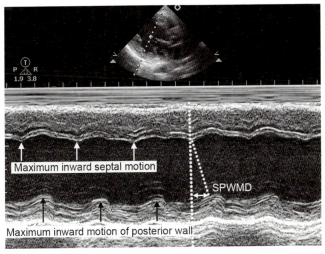

Fig. 8.9 Measurement of interventricular dyssynchrony: Septal-posterior wall motion delay (SPWMD) is measured from M-mode picture from parasternal long axis view as the distance between the first maximum systolic inward motion of the septum and the maximum inward motion of the posterior wall. A value of more than 130 msec indicates significant intraventricular delay

inward motion of the septum and the maximum inward motion of the posterior wall (Fig. 8.9). Baseline SPWMD > 130 msec predicted the CRT related LV reverse remodeling effect and long-term clinical improvement.[40] Effective CRT should reduce the SPWMD below the cut-off value of 130 msec and frequently the SPWMD will be close to zero.

Others

In LBBB, the interventricular septum typically shows a characteristic abnormal relaxation pattern with a multiphasic motion pattern. Another typical feature of dyssynchrony is the late-systolic counterclockwise rocking motion of the LV in the apical four-chamber view (apical shuffle).

The myocardial performance index (MPI, also referred to as "Tei-Index") is a combined systolic and diastolic Doppler derived index for the assessment of global LV performance which correlates well with invasive measurements of LV systolic and diastolic function. It is calculated as the sum of the isovolumic contraction time (IVCT) and the isovolumic relaxation time (IVRT) divided by LV ejection time. The sum of IVCT and IVRT is obtained by subtracting LV ejection time from the interval between cessation and onset of the mitral inflow velocity (Fig. 8.10).

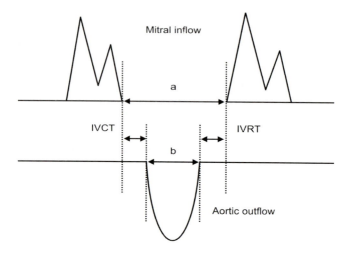

Fig. 8.10 Evaluation of the myocardial performance index by Doppler echocardiography of mitral inflow and aortic outflow. The interval between cessation and onset of mitral inflow (a) minus the LV ejection time (b) represents the sum of the isovolumic time intervals (IVCT + IVRT). MPI = (a − b)/b

In patients with normal LV function, the MPI measures < 0.5, values > 0.8 indicate significantly depressed LV performance. In a series of 32 heart failure patients recruited from the PATH-CHF I trial, the average MPI during intrinsic conduction (mostly LBBB) was 1.21 ± 0.5 and correlated to reduction of baseline LV peak +dP/dt in a nonsimultaneous measurement.[41] CRT resulted in an immediate reduction of the MPI to 0.85 ± 0.3. Hemodynamic responders showed a significantly higher improvement in MPI than hemodynamic nonresponders.

Poor RV function, either owing to very advanced biventricular heart failure or to concomitant pulmonary disease, is regarded as a poor prognostic marker for CRT. Prospective data on CRT patients with evidence of concomitant RV failure are scarce, but many single-center observations suggest that patients with a significantly dilated right ventricle with poor systolic function and elevated RV pressures do benefit less from CRT than patients with normal RV function. If the RV is severely dilated and if there is evidence of severe pulmonary hypertension (RV systolic pressure > 45–55 mm Hg), however, then it is less likely that such a patient will benefit significantly from CRT and therapeutic alternatives such as heart transplantation should be considered.

Advanced Echocardiographic Assessment

Newer echocardiographic technologies have permitted a more comprehensive and quantitative assessment of global and regional cardiac function, in particular systolic dyssynchrony. Tissue Doppler imaging (TDI) is a special form of Doppler echocardiography used to detect the direction and velocity of the contracting or relaxing myocardium. This is achieved by suppressing the high-pass filter but setting the threshold filter so that the low frequency, high amplitude myocardial signals will be detected. The application of TDI generates 2D TDI images from which "myocardial velocity curves" are constructed by placing the sampling window into the region of interest, typically the myocardium within a particular segment of the ventricle. The myocardial velocity curve can either be constructed online by spectral pulse TDI, or reconstituted offline from the 2D color-TDI image. To assess cardiac function and dyssynchrony, TDI can be performed at apical four-chamber, two-chamber and three chamber (or apical long-axis) views to examine the long-axis motion of the heart; or alternatively the parasternal short-axis views for circumferential fiber function. It is well known that most myocardial fibers, particularly those in the endocardial and epicardial layers, are aligned longitudinally and only a small proportion of middle layer fibers are aligned circumferentially and a helical structure of alignment has been suggested for left ventricular (LV) myocardial fibers in humans. In the event of heart failure with LV dilatation, however, the helical structure will criss-cross in a more horizontal manner. This implies the potential importance of examining circumferential motion. In apical views, the myocardial velocity curve consists of systolic myocardial velocities indicative of an isovolumic contraction phase and an ejection phase, both of which are positively or apically directed. During diastole, it consists of an isovolumic relaxation phase (negative or biphasic profiles), and early diastolic and late diastolic relaxation, which are negatively directed (Fig. 8.11).

Spectral pulse TDI has an excellent temporal resolution with highly robust signals. TDI signals are generated online from 2D color-TDI images when the Doppler sampling window is placed on the region of interest. The 2D color-TDI cine loops of multiple beats can be stored digitally for offline analysis. This allows the comparison of multiple segments from each view simultaneously, and is a much quicker way of assessing myocardial function and synchronicity. However, adequate technical attention is mandatory, however, to obtain optimal image quality that supports offline analysis. From the 2D color images, interrogation of regional motion can be performed by creating the M-mode image through the line of interest, the so-called color M-mode TDI image. Although this method has been used to identify regional dyssynchrony, it is largely a qualitative technique and has been superseded by quantitative

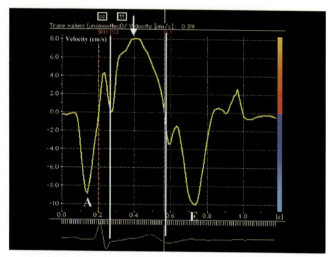

Fig. 8.11 Tissue Doppler image in the apical four-chamber view of a normal subject. The velocity profile during one cardiac cycle obtained at the base of the interventricular septum. The solid lines mark the duration of systole (310 ms), and the arrow indicates the peak systolic velocity (8 cm/s). The diastolic filling of the LV is reflected in the E-wave (E) and A-wave (A)

TDI methods based on spectral pulse Doppler and offline 2D color-TDI technologies. Color M-mode TDI might be helpful, however, for identifying the point of change in motion direction when assessing septal-to-posterior wall motion delay.

Assessment of mechanical dyssynchrony by TDI has many limitations, mainly because of its 2-dimensional nature, the angle dependency of the ultrasound signal, and the resulting signal noise. Consequently, apical segments cannot be analyzed, and TDI can only provide information on the systolic myocardial contraction of the basal and midsegments in the longitudinal direction. More important, because the magnitude and direction of the velocity vector change simultaneously, it is conceivable that the velocity component measured by TDI would reach its maximum value because of changes in direction alone without any changes in magnitude, which would considerably affect its ability to identify the time to peak velocity accurately.

The principles of indices of mechanical dyssynchrony are, however, to examine for variation of timing of contraction in different regions of the LV (intraventricular dyssynchrony) or between the left and right ventricle (interventricular dyssynchrony). Technically the following principles of quantitative assessment of dyssynchrony can be considered:
- The time from the beginning of the QRS complex to onset of systolic velocity.

- The time from the beginning of the QRS complex to peak systolic velocity in ejection phase (Ts).
- The time from the beginning of the QRS complex to peak post-systolic shortening velocity.

Displacement imaging is derived from the temporal integration of the myocardial velocity curve (i.e. velocity–time integral) from TDI data. It illustrates the cumulated amount of myocardial excursion during different periods of the cardiac cycle and presents it on a "curve" format throughout a cardiac cycle. When the amount of myocardial displacement is presented semiquantitatively by trans- can serve as a surrogate marker of reduced systolic dyssynchrony. The superiority of displacement mapping to tissue Doppler velocity in CRT assessment has, however, not been confirmed. Strain mapping is another postprocessing mapping of TDI data that calculates the amount (expressed as a percentage) of myocardial deformation in a cumulated manner throughout the cardiac cycle. To assess systolic dyssynchrony, the time to minimal (or maximal depending on direction) strain at different regions can be measured. Strain rate imaging reflects the rate of change of strain in the cardiac cycle (i.e. the slope of the strain curve). Therefore, it measures the rate of deformation of the myocardium. Theoretically, both strain and strain rate imaging are superior to tissue Doppler velocity and displacement mapping as translational motion from passive motions can be eliminated, such as respiration and tethering of adjacent segments. Current technical limitations, including artifacts and random noise, outweigh the theoretical advantages of strain rate imaging. The use of time to peak negative strain rate has not been found to be useful for predicting CRT response.

Tissue synchronization imaging portrays regional dyssynchrony on 2D images by transforming the Ts of tissue Doppler velocity data into color codes, which allows immediate visual identification of regional delay in systole at orthogonal walls. In addition, the quantitative measurement of regional delay is possible. At present, it is recommended that quantitative analysis be performed by measurement from the myocardial velocity curve (which is same as those from TDI) rather than directly from the color-coded TSI images to avoid technical errors during sampling. Note that the principle of dyssynchrony assessment is identical between TDI velocity and TSI.

Non-Doppler 2D-strain imaging derived from speckle tracking is a newer echocardiographic technique for obtaining strain and strain rate measurements. It analyzes motion by tracking speckles (natural acoustic markers) in the 2D ultrasound image. These acoustic markers are equally distributed throughout the myocardium and their size is about 20 to 40 pixels. These markers ("stable" speckles) within the ultrasonic image are tracked from frame to frame by special software. The integration and calculation of such data allows the measurement of regional cumulative deformation (i.e. strain). This tool has the advantage of being independent of angle, and allows the measurement of longitudinal and transverse strain in apical views as well as circumferential and radial strain in short-axis views.[42]

Real-time 3D-echocardiography is another technology that provides a comprehensive model of assessing systolic dyssynchrony in multiple regions of the LV in a "wide-angle" volume-rendered cine loop that is captured from only four to seven continuous beats. Assessment of systolic dyssynchrony is based on offline reconstruction of regional volumetric curves in a segmental model as defined by the American Society of Echocardiography. With TDI, the time to peak systolic velocity is measured, whereas with real-time three-dimensional echocardiography (RT3DE) the time to minimal regional volume is assessed. RT3DE acquisition of the LV is fast and accurate with high spatial resolution. Contrary to TDI, RT3DE provides simultaneous evaluation of intraventricular mechanical dyssynchrony of all LV segments. Furthermore, RT3DE allows identification of mechanical dyssynchrony of LV segments that may not be adequately imaged by TDI. Finally, RT3DE provides information of systolic contraction based on 3D endocardial motion, which is a result of radial thickening and longitudinal and circumferential shortening. In theory, this should be more in agreement with the anatomic patterns of myocardial fibers and therefore will likely give a more complete and accurate assessment of intraventricular mechanical dyssynchrony.[43] Current limitations of RT3DE are its low temporal resolution (15-35 volumes per second) and high dependence on image quality.

Most of the studies that applied advanced echocardiographic technologies to patients receiving CRT focused on the assessment of systolic dyssynchrony, because electromechanical delay resulting in regional dyssynchrony is believed to be the primary abnormality in heart failure with prolongation of QRS duration. Quantitative dyssynchrony assessment is a new horizon of echocardiography with continuous and rapid evolution. Assessment of systolic dyssynchrony in heart failure is more difficult than in any other cardiac disease or in normal patients. So, there is a long learning curve for the physicians before they can acquire all the essential skills and then apply them to clinical practice. The Predictors of Response to CRT (PROSPECT) study, a prospective multicenter trial tested 498 patients with standard CRT indications in 53 centers in Europe, the United States and Hong Kong. Twelve echocardiographic parameters of dyssynchrony, based on both conventional and tissue-Doppler based method, were evaluated after site training in acquisition methods and blinded core laboratory analysis.[44] The investigators concluded that despite promising preliminary data from prior single-center studies, echocardiographic measures of dyssynchrony aimed at improving patient selection criteria for CRT do not appear to have a clinically relevant impact on improving response rates when studied in a multicenter setting. Thus, at present, the echocardiographic parameters assessing dyssynchrony do not have enough predictive value to be recommended as selection criteria for CRT beyond current indications. However, these advanced echocardiographic modalities can be used for identifying latest activated region of left ventricular wall and target the area for LV lead placement.

Nonechocardiographic Assessment

Various nonechocardiographic, noninvasive imaging techniques may play a role in the selection of patients for CRT. Positron emission tomography (PET) is the only imaging technique that allows quantitative assessment of myocardial blood flow and metabolism. It also gives us the idea of presence, extent and location of scar and viable myocardium. However, it cannot assess the left ventricular dyssynchrony. Single photon emission computed tomography (SPECT) assesses left ventricular dyssynchrony and detect the extent and location of viability and scar tissue. It also gives information relating to myocardial blood flow, metabolism and innervation. Tagged magnetic resonance imaging is a three-dimensional imaging technique that permits characterization of LV mechanical activation sequence and detection of the latest activated segments. It evaluates the left ventricular shortening in the circumferential and longitudinal directions or the thickening in the radial direction. Particularly, the assessment of LV circumferential shortening provides superior accuracy than longitudinal shortening to predict favorable response to CRT. Despite recent technical advances, this imaging technique is not widely available. Contrast-enhanced MRI allows the precise delineation of scar tissue. The mechanism underlying the hyperenhancement seems to be related to the interstitial space between collagen fibers, which is larger in scar tissue than in the densely packed myocytes in normal myocardium, and the contrast agent will be trapped in these areas in infarcted tissue. The main limitations of MRI techniques are that data acquisition and analysis are time-consuming and that repeat analysis after CRT implantation is not possible in patients with pacemakers.

Computed tomography (CT) techniques permit noninvasive imaging of the venous anatomy, which may be useful in the decision of whether LV lead implantation can be performed transvenously or whether a surgical approach is needed. However, it does not allow assessment of cardiac dyssynchrony, or assessment of perfusion, metabolism, innervation, viability, or scar tissue. Therefore, nonechocardiographic techniques may have additional value in the selection and evaluation of patients undergoing CRT, but further studies are needed.

Effects of Cardiac Resynchronization Therapy

Cardiac

Cardiac resynchronization therapy has two immediate effects, electromechanical reconstitution (ventricular activation sequence) and chamber timing. CRT restores coordinated contraction by minimizing the conduction delay (restores interventricular and intraventricular coupling). The mechanisms of beneficial effects of CRT are summarized in Figure 8.12. It reduces left-sided AV decoupling and improves diastolic performance and ultimately improves LV pumping function. These acute beneficial hemodynamic effects may lead to even more beneficial long-term effects, because many adverse molecular and cellular derangements elicited by chronic RV apical pacing or LBBB appear to be reversible. The beneficial effects of CRT are maintained for many years, whereas many pharmacologic therapies tend to lose effectiveness over time. The best explanation of this lasting benefit is that it largely restores the normal electromechanical coupling of the heart with LBBB.

Atrioventricular resynchronization in CRT improves LV pump function by the following mechanisms:
- Lengthened diastolic filling time.
- Optimized filling pattern.
- Diminished mitral regurgitation.

The dominant therapeutic effect of CRT during atrial-synchronous LV or biventricular pacing is the immediate positive effect on ventricular mechanics and is due to reduction of intraventricular delay. The acute improvement in pump function is indicated by the followings:
- Increase in left ventricular pumping efficiency (Myocardial performance index).
- Increase in systolic blood pressure.
- Increase in pulse pressure, stroke volume, and stroke work.
- Increases in LV +dP/dt max
- Decrease in left ventricular end systolic volume.
- Synchronization of displacement of tissue metabolism.

Introduction to Cardiac Resynchronization Therapy

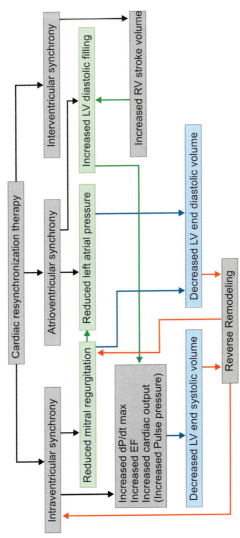

Fig. 8.12 Mechanisms of action of cardiac resynchronization therapy

Moreover, unlike the inotropic effects of dobutamine, systolic augmentation with ventricular resynchronization increases efficiency of conversion of myocardial oxygen consumption to mechanical work. This positive contractile response demonstrates a modestly positive correlation with increasing baseline QRS duration and is strongly correlated with baseline mechanical dyssynchrony. Conversely, neither improved contractility nor reverse volumetric remodeling requires QRS narrowing during LV or biventricular pacing. These acute improvements in ventricular mechanics are maintained chronically and are accompanied by reverse volumetric remodeling of the LV. Abrupt discontinuation of LV pacing results in immediate reduction in indices of improved contractility and regression of reverse remodeling over several weeks, as well as recurrence of mitral regurgitation. The indices of chronic improvement in cardiac function by CRT are follows:

- Increase in left ventricular ejection fraction (LVEF) by 5–15%.
- Decrease in left ventricular volume and mass (Systolic/Diastolic) >15% (10–30%).
- Decrease in sizes of left atrium, right atrium and right ventricle.
- Decrease in tricuspid regurgitation and pulmonary arterial pressure.
- Reduced mitral orifice size.
- Regression of asymmetric hypertrophy.

Maximally effective ventricular resynchronization occurs at the midpoint of the interventricular (V-V) interval, which is the conduction time from RV to LV pacing site during native activation. A single optimum AV delay will achieve maximally effective ventricular resynchronization by advancing LV activation sufficiently to minimize the V-V interval. The AV delay and the V-V interval have an interactive relationship. During LBBB, the right ventricle is activated by right bundle branch conduction before the left ventricle, and the time difference between RV and LV activation is the interventricular conduction delay. Biventricular pacing at short atrioventricular delay results in complete replacement of intrinsic activation, allowing complete control of chamber timing with sequential ventricular stimulation. Intermediate atrioventricular delay results in fusion among right bundle branch conduction, RV paced activation, and LV paced activation. Long atrioventricular delay results in "pure" fusion between right bundle branch conduction and LV paced activation since LV pre-excitation is still possible because of interventricular conduction delay.

Mechanical resynchronization reduces mechanical load heterogeneity throughout the left ventricle. Sustained improvement in ventricular mechanics results in regression of adverse LV remodeling, termed *reverse remodeling*. Evidence of greater baseline electromechanical asynchrony and acute mechanical resynchronization appears to be necessary for reverse remodeling to occur, and the greater the reduction in asynchrony, the higher the probability of remodeling.

In many patients, CRT reduces functional mitral regurgitation, which likely accounts for immediate reduction in symptoms in advance of possible reverse volumetric remodeling. This can be due to the following factors:

- Correction of left-sided atrioventricular (AV) timing, which helps position the mitral leaflets in the coaptation plane before isovolumetric systole. If the AV time is too long, the leaflets begin to drift back toward the atrium and out of the coaptation plane.
- Improved contractility reduces functional mitral regurgitation instantaneously and is quantitatively related to an increase in LV dP/dt max and transmitral pressure.
- Earlier delivery of the posterior apparatus in isovolumetric systole.
- Reverse volumetric LV remodeling reduces functional mitral regurgitation chronically by reducing LV volumes and sphericity, which reduces tethering forces on the mitral valve.

Extracardiac

Cognitive impairment and related negative consequences (self-care, quality of life, morbidity, and prognosis) have been largely documented in patients with heart failure. Low cardiac output and autonomic deregulation are the primary pathogenic mechanism. The preservation or improvement in cognitive performance is a significant outcome of CRT in patients with congestive heart failure.[45] Notably, the cognitive reserve theory, which outlines a discrepancy between cerebral pathology and cognitive impairment in heart failure patients, has led to hypothesize that the impact of CRT is not strictly connected to an improvement of ejection fraction. The response is highly varied and unpredictable, based not only on cardiovascular physiology but also on neural physiology.

During recent years, it has been recognized that endothelial dysfunction has a crucial role in the development of symptoms in congestive heart failure. One of the most important contributing factors is the reduction in the availability of nitric oxide (NO). Possible mechanisms are the reduction in flow, which leads to less shear stress in conductance and resistance arteries, and release of increased amount of reactive oxygen species (ROS), which rapidly inactivate NO. Endothelium-dependent vasodilatation is increased within 2 months of cardiac resynchronization therapy.[46]

Heart failure is associated with increased plasma level of neurohormones. Cardiac resynchronization therapy effectively reduces the circulating neurohormones in CHF patients which is associated with better long-term outcome in this patients population of patients. Reduction of NT-Pro BNP level along with left ventricular reverse remodeling better predicts the effect of CRT.[47]

The incidence of different arrhythmias is also reduced following CRT implantation, probably because of improvement of the heterogeneous electrical activation of left ventricle which is seen in patients of dilated cardiomyopathy.

REFERENCES

1. Hunt SA, Baker DW, Chin MH, et al. ACC/AHA guideline for the evaluation and management of chronic heart failure in the adult: executive summary. A report of the American College of Cardiology/American Heart Association Task force on practice guidelines (Committee to revise the 1995 Guideline s for the Evaluation and Management of Heart Failure). J Am Coll Cardiol. 2001;38:2101-13.
2. McKee PA, Castelli WP, McNamara PM, et al. The natural history of congestive heart failure: the Framingham study. N Engl J Med. 1971;285:1441-6.
3. Collins S, Storrow AB, Kirk JD, et al. Beyond pulmonary edema: diagnostic, risk stratification, and treatment challenges of acute heart failure management in the emergency department. Ann Emerg Med. 2008;51:45-7.
4. Wang CS, Fitzerald JM, Schulzer M, et al. Does this dyspneic patient in the emergency department have congestive heart failure? JAMA. 2005;294:1944-56.
5. Munger MA. Management of acute decompensated heart failure: treatment, controversy, and future directions. Pharmacotherapy 2006;26:131S-8S.
6. Flather MD, Yusuf S, Kober L, et al. Long-term ACE-inhibitor therapy in patients with heart failure or left ventricular dysfunction: a systematic overview of data from individual patients. ACE-Inhibitor-Myocardial Infarction Collaborative Group. Lancet. 2000;355:1575-81.
7. Heart Failure Society of America (HFSA) practice guidelines. HFSA guidelines for management of patients with heart failure caused by left ventricular systolic dysfunction—pharmacological approaches. J Card Fail. 1999;5:357-82.
8. Hamroff G, Katz SD, Mancini D, et al. Addition of angiotensin II receptor blockade to maximal angiotensin-converting enzyme inhibition improves exercise capacity in patients with severe congestive heart failure. Circulation. 1999;99:990-2.

Introduction to Cardiac Resynchronization Therapy

9. Jong P, Demer C, McKlevie RS, et al. Angiotensin receptor blockers in heart failure: meta-analysis of randomized controlled trials. J Am Col Cardiol. 2002;39:463-70.
10. Poole-Wilson PA, Swedberg K, Cleland JGF, et al for the COMET Investigators. Comparison of Carvedilol and Metoprolol on clinical outcomes in patients with chronic heart failure in the Carvedilol Or Metoprolol European Trial (COMET): randomized controlled trial. Lancet. 2003;362:7-13.
11. John JV McMurray, Milton Packer, Akshay S. Desai, et al. Angiotensin–Neprilysin Inhibition versus Enalapril in Heart Failure. NEJM. 2014:371(11):993-1004.
12. Linde C, Gold M, Abraham WT, Daubert JC. Rationale and design of a randomized controlled trial to assess the safety and efficacy of cardiac resynchronization therapy in patients with asymptomatic left ventricular dysfunction with previous symptoms or mild heart failure–the REsynchronization reVErses Remodeling in Systolic left vEntricular dysfunction (REVERSE) study. Am Heart J. 2006;151:288-94.
13. Moss AJ, Brown MW, Cannom DS, et al. Multicenter Automatic Defibrillator Implantation Trial-Cardiac Resynchronization Therapy (MADIT-CRT): design and clinical protocol. Ann Noninvasive Electrocardiol. 2005;10(Suppl 4):34-43.
14. Curtis AB, Adamson PB, Chung E, et al: Biventricular versus right ventricular pacing in patients with AV block (BLOCK HF): clinical study design and rationale. J Cardiovasc Electrophysiol. 2007:18:965-71.
15. Tang AS, Wells GA, Talajic M, et al. Resynchronization-Defibrillation for Ambulatory Heart Failure Trial Investigators; Cardiac resynchronization therapy for mild-to-moderate heart failure. N Engl J Med. 2010:363:2385-95.
16. Yu CM, Abraham WT, Bax J, et al., PROSPECT Investigators. Predictors of response to cardiac resynchronization therapy (PROSPECT) – study design. Am Heart J. 2005;149:600-5.
17. John F Beshai, Richard A Grimm, Sherif F Nagueh, et al for the RethinQ Study Investigators. Cardiac-Resynchronization Therapy in Heart Failure with Narrow QRS Complexes. N Engl J Med. 2007;357:2461-71.
18. Serge J Cazeau, J-Claude Daubert, et al. Responders to cardiac resynchronization therapy with narrow or intermediate QRS complexes identified by simple echocardiographic indices of dyssynchrony: The DESIRE study. European Journal of Heart Failure10. 2008;273-80.
19. Leon AR NI, Herrman K, Stucky M, Galle E, Donahue T Chronic evaluation of CRT in narrow QRS patients with mechanical dyssynchrony from a multi-center study: ESTEEM-CRT. Heart Rhythm: 2008; 5:S23-S24.
20. Funck RC, Blanc J-J, Mueller H-H, et al. for the BioPace Study Group. Biventricular stimulation to prevent cardiac desynchronization: rationale, design, and endpoints of the 'Biventricular Pacing for Atrioventricular Block to Prevent Cardiac Desynchronization (BioPace)' study. Europace. 2006; 8: 629-35.
21. Ruschitzka F, Abraham WT, Singh JP, et al. Cardiac-resynchronization therapy in heart failure with a narrow QRS complex. N Engl J Med. 2013:369:1395.

22. Fung JW-H, Chan JY-S, Omar R, et al. The Pacing to Avoid Cardiac Enlargement (PACE) trial: clinical background, rationale, design, and implementation. J Cardiovasc Electrophysiol. 2007;18:735-9.
23. Tracy CM, Epstein AE, Darbar D, et al. ACCF/AHA/HRS focused update of the 2008 guidelines for device-based therapy of cardiac rhythm abnormalities: A report of the American College of Cardiology Foundation/American Heart Association Task Force on Practice Guidelines and the Heart Rhythm Society [corrected]. Circulation. 2012 ;26:1784.
24. Rodriguez LM, Timmermans C, Nabar A, et al. Variable patterns of septal activation in patients with left bundle branch block. J Cardiovasc Electrophysiol: 2003:14:135-41.
25. Jia P, Ramanathan C, Ghanem RN, et al. Electrocardiographic imaging of cardiac resynchronization therapy in heart failure: observation of variable electrophysiologic responses. Heart Rhythm: 2006:3:296-310.
26. Auricchio A, Fantoni C, Regoli F, et al. Characterization of left ventricular activation in patients with heart failure and left bundle branch block. Circulation: 2004:109:1133-9.
27. Fantoni C, Regoli F, Kawabata M, Klein HU, Auricchio A. Reversed transmural activation timing in patients with heart failure and left bundle branch block. Eur Heart J. 2004 (suppl): 2320.
28. Mabo P, Pouillot C, Kermarrec A, et al. Lack of physiological adaptation of the atrioventricular interval to heart rate in patients chronically paced in the AAIR mode. Pacing Clin Electrophysiol.1991;14:2133-42.
29. Prinzen FW, Augustijn CH, Arts T, Allessi MA, Reneman RS. Redistribution of myocardial fiber strain and blood flow by asynchronous activation. Am J Physiol. 1990; 259:H300-8.
30. Rossi A, Dini FL, Faggiano P, et al. Independent prognostic value of functional mitral regurgitation in patients with heart failure. A quantitative analysis of 1256 patients with ischemic and non-ischemic dilated cardiomyopathy. Heart. 2011; 97(20):1675-80.
31. Sanders P, Kistler PM, Morton JB, et al. Remodeling of sinus node function in patients with congestive heart failure. Reduction of sinus node reserve. Circulation. 2004;110:897-903.
32. Olgin JE, Kalman JM, Fitzpatrick AP, et al. Role of right atrial endocardial structures as barriers to conduction during human type I atrial fl utter: activation and entrainment mapping guided by intracardiac echocardiography. Circulation. 1995; 92:1839-48.
33. Bleeker GB, Schalij MJ, Molhoek SG, et al. Relationship between QRS duration and left ventricular dyssynchrony in patients with end-stage heart failure. J Cardiovasc Electrophysiol. 2004; 15:544-9.
34. Gregoratos G, Abrams J, Epstein AE, et al. ACC/AHA/NASPE 2002 Guideline update for implantation of cardiac pacemakers and antiarrhythmia devices – summary article: a report of the American College of Cardiology/American Heart Association Task Force on Practice Guidelines (ACC/AHA/NASPE Committee to Update the 1998 Pacemaker Guidelines). J Am Coll Cardiol. 2002; 40:1703-19.
35. Hunt SA, Abraham WT, Chin MH, et al. ACC/AHA 2005 Guideline update for the diagnosis and management of chronic heart failure in the adult: summary article: a Report from the American College

of Cardiology/American Heart Association Task Force on Practice Guidelines (Writing Committee to Update the 2001 Guidelines for the Evolution and Management of Heart Failure). J Am Coll Cardiol 2005; 46: 1116-43.

36. Vassallo JA, Cassidy DM, Marchlinski FE, et al. Endocardial activation of left bundle branch block. Circulation.1984; 69: 914-23.
37. Grines CL, Bashore TM, Boudoulas H, et al. Functional abnormalities in isolated left bundle branch block. The effect of interventricular asynchrony. Circulation. 1989;79:845-53.
38. Cazeau S, Bordachar P, Jauvert G et al. Echocardiographic modeling of cardiac dyssynchrony before and during multisite stimulation: a prospective study. Pacing Clin Electrophysiol. 2003;26:137-43.
39. John Sutton MG, Plappert T, Abraham WT, et al. Effect of cardiac resynchronization therapy on left ventricular size and function in chronic heart failure. Circulation. 2003;107:1985-90.
40. Pitzalis MV, Iacoviello M, Romito R, et al. Ventricular asynchrony predicts a better outcome in patients with chronic heart failure receiving cardiac resynchronization therapy. J Am Coll Cardiol. 2005;45:65-9.
41. Auricchio A, Stellbrink C, Sack S, et al. The Pacing Therapies for Congestive Heart Failure (PATH-CHF) study: rationale, design, and endpoints of a prospective randomized multicenter study. Am J Cardiol. 1999; 83: 130D-135D.
42. Michael Dandel, Hans Lehmkuhl, Christopher Knosalla, et al. Strain and strain rate imaging by echocardiography – Basic concepts and clinical applicability. Current Cardiology Reviews. 2009;5:133-48.
43. Sebastiaan A. Kleijn, Jeroen van Dijk, Carel C. de Cock, et al. Assessment of Intraventricular Mechanical Dyssynchrony and Prediction of Response to Cardiac Resynchronization Therapy: Comparison between Tissue Doppler Imaging and Real-Time Three-Dimensional Echocardiography. J Am Soc Echocardiogr. 2009;22:1047-54.
44. Eugene S. Chung, Angel R Leon, Luigi Tavazzi, et al. Results of the predictors of Response to CRT (PROSPECT) Trial. Circulation. 2008;117: 2608-16.
45. Riccardo P, Gian M M, Luca C, et al. Can Cardiac Resynchronization Therapy Improve Cognitive Function? A Systematic Review. PACE 2014;37:520-30.
46. Erik T, Angelique S, et al. Effect of cardiac resynchronization therapy on endothelium-dependent vasodilatation in the cutaneous microvasculature. PACE. 2012;35:377-84.
47. Georgette E H, Ulas H, Joep T, et al. Clinical, Echocardiographic, and Neurohormonal Response to Cardiac Resynchronization Therapy: Are they interchangeable? PACE. 2013;36:1391-401.

CHAPTER 9

Role of Pre-procedure ECG Analysis

INTRODUCTION

In recent years, cardiac resynchronization by biventricular pacing has become an accepted approach towards the management of patients with dilated cardiomyopathy having wide QRS complex with severe left ventricular dysfunction. However, approximately 18–30% of patients fail to respond clinically to cardiac resynchronization therapy (CRT).[1] The 12 lead pre-procedure surface ECG is an indispensable tool to avoid emergence of non-responders. Analysis of ventricular activation using the standard 12-lead surface ECG accurately predicts the probability of LV reverse volumetric remodeling during CRT in patients with heart failure and LBBB with ventricular dyssynchrony. The left ventricular reverse remodeling depends on the interactions between substrate conditions and pacing-induced changes in ventricular activation before and after CRT. The main responsible factors are activation wave front fusion and LV conduction delay (maximum left ventricular activation time, LVATmax). It is negatively influenced by LV scar volume (QRS score) on the baseline ECG. Longer left ventricular activation time (LVAT) and smaller LV scar volume on the baseline ECG predict higher probability of reverse remodeling.

ROLE OF SURFACE ECG

Proper assessment of the 12-lead surface ECG is an essential part of planning for CRT implantation to avoid risk of failure to respond clinically. The assessment should include:
- *Type of conduction delay:* Majority of patients with heart failure with left ventricular systolic dysfunction who benefit from CRT have left bundle branch block (LBBB). In presence of LBBB, the right ventricle is activated first followed by right-to-left transseptal myocardial activation of the left ventricle. This results in late activation of the left ventricular free wall. However, in patients with right bundle branch block (RBBB) have late activation of the right ventricular free

wall and outflow tract with or without concomitant delay in the left ventricular lateral wall. Patients with intraventricular conduction delay (IVCD) have delayed activation of either some or all of the right, left, or both ventricles. CRT attempts to activate both the right and left ventricles simultaneously. So, the patients with heart failure and left-sided conduction delay are more likely to benefit. Patients with RBBB or IVCD therefore may not respond to CRT as good as LBBB. Studies have shown that patients with IVCD have an intermediate echocardiographic and symptomatic response compared with LBBB and RBBB.[2,3] So, patients of heart failure with non-LBBB morphology do not respond well to CRT and patients with RBBB show worst response.

- *QRS duration:* Numerous studies have reproducibly demonstrated that baseline QRS duration of more than 150 msec is predictive of acute hemodynamic improvement with CRT, whereas patients with QRS duration of less than 150 msec are less likely to respond (Fig. 9.1).[4] Endocardial catheter mapping studies in humans with left bundle branch block (LBBB) showed that the minimum amount of time for electrical activation to proceed through the interventricular septum is about 40 milliseconds. It takes an additional 50 milliseconds for reentry into the Purkinje

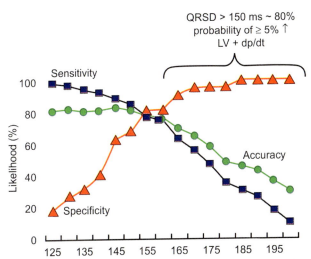

Fig. 9.1 Sensitivity, specificity and accuracy likelihoods are plotted for different QRS thresholds between 120 and 200 msec using acute hemodynamic data from PATH-CHF and PATH-CHF-II. Specificity curve indicates that 80% of non-responders have QRS duration less than 150 msec. Sensitivity curve indicates that 80% of responders have QRS duration more than 150 msec. Cardiac resynchronization therapy response is defined as more than 5% acute increase in LV + dP/dt

network and propagation through the anterosuperior and inferior walls. It takes another 50 milliseconds to activate the posterolateral wall. This produces a total QRS duration of 140 to 150 milliseconds. Any increase in anteroseptal or posterolateral wall thickness further increases QRS duration. Thus, most patients with a QRS duration of > 120 and <140 milliseconds do not have true LBBB.[5]

- *Myocardial scar burden:* Scar tissue is inexcitable. So, putting the left ventricular lead on a region of scar or near to the scar will not result in recruitment of adequate myocardial tissue during cardiac systole to give a satisfactory level of improvement. Chronic fibrosis (scar) from ischemic or nonischemic etiology creates regions of slowed conduction. Even in nonischemic cardiomyopathy the scar could be produced by the disruption of blood flow at a micro vascular level. In 1972, Selvester, et al. outlined detailed ECG and vectorcardiogram criteria developed from the computer simulations for localizing and quantifying MI size.[6] In 1977, Savage et al performed detailed postmortem histologic analyses of hearts with computer digitization of infarct location in patients with single well-circumscribed infarcts.[7] Despite the documented clinical utility, the QRS score did not develop widespread use likely because of the limitation of manual application of the 54 criteria. Thus, a series of studies investigated the use of a limited number of screening criteria and automation of the score. Anderson, et al. identified 3 criteria that achieved good sensitivities and specificity, among patients identified by coronary angiography and ventriculography:[8]
  - Q ≥30 milliseconds in aVF,
  - Any Q or R ≤10 milliseconds and ≤0.1 mV in V2,
  - R ≥40 milliseconds in V1.

A subsequent study showed that the screening criteria performed equally well in patients with anatomically documented single and multiple infarcts.[9] Similarly the criteria for scar estimation in patients with conduction disorder have been laid down.

The LBBB QRS score criteria are shown in Figure 9.2. The criteria for QRS scoring in the limb leads (I, II, aVL, and aVF) are similar to the criteria in other conduction types; however, the criteria are drastically different in the precordial leads. Selvester QRS score (LV scar volume) of more than 12% indicates poor outcome in term of LV reverse remodeling post-CRT.

Figure 9.3 shows a patient with nonischemic cardiomyopathy, LBBB, and anteroseptal scar. As opposed to normal conduction where anteroseptal scar would produce

Role of Pre-procedure ECG Analysis

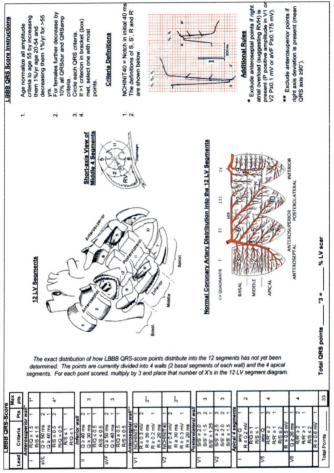

Fig. 9.2 Left bundle branch block QRS score criteria

a Q wave in V1 through V2, in LBBB, anteroseptal scar causes large R waves.

Recent MRI studies with late gadolinium enhancement have shown that many nonischemic cardiomyopathy patients have discrete scar. Cardiac MRI with late-gadolinium enhancement has been shown to accurately visualize and quantify MI and nonischemic fibrosis *in vivo*.[10] Two studies with small numbers of patients have compared the QRS score with MRI-estimated infarct and found a strong correlation.

- *Location of line of block:* Ventricular conduction blocks are the main barrier to achieve maximum ventricular activation fusion. Conduction blocks may be fixed or functional. Conduction blocks may exist at different levels within the ventricular myocardium (e.g., epicardium vs endocardium). Sequential ventricular activation is consistently observed

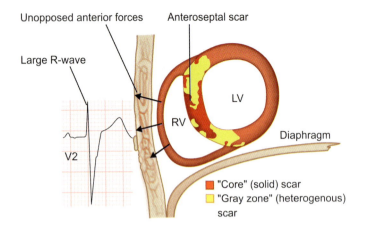

Fig. 9.3 Magnetic resonance imaging of nonischemic cardiomyopathy with LBBB and anteroseptal scar. In LBBB without any scar, electrical depolarization would begin in the endocardium of the RV on the free wall and on the septum. This results in electrical cancellation and either no deflection or a small R wave at the beginning of the QRS complex in leads V1 through V2. However, in the presence of anteroseptal scar, the electrical forces from the RV free wall are unopposed, leading to large R waves in the leads V1 through V2. The red shows the area of solid scar and yellow shows the "gray zone" that contains interspersed live and dead myocardium (*Courtesy*: Schmidt A, Azevedo CF, Cheng A, et al. Infarct tissue heterogeneity by magnetic resonance imaging identifies enhanced cardiac arrhythmia susceptibility in patients with left ventricular dysfunction. Circulation. 2007;115:2006).

during LBBB (RV → LV) and posterobasal left ventricle (near mitral valve annulus) is invariably the latest activated region. However, there is significant inter-patient variability in term of the location, orientation, and extent of conduction blocks, yielding distinct patterns of LV epicardial activation despite similar patterns on the surface ECG. Fixed conduction blocks are characterized by a boundary of activation delay that interrupts and redirects activation wave front propagation and are caused by ventricular scar. Functional conduction blocks during LBBB occur in absence of scar and the location of the line of block can be shifted with pacing maneuvers. These lines of functional block correlate with regional mechanical delay. To reduce LV conduction delay maximally, LV stimulation must occur distal to the line of conduction block; LV paced activation wave front must propagate out from the stimulation site; and R → L and L → R activation wave fronts must be properly timed to generate fusion. LV pacing from an early-activated site proximal to a line of block may worsen LBBB conduction delay. Fixed or functional lines of block may "jail" (electrically isolate) large regions of the left ventricle despite electrical resynchronization at the remote stimulation sites. Sequential BiV pacing (LV → RV) and increased LV voltage output (virtual electrode effect) are required to generate ventricular activation wave front fusion. The paced activation wave front from the left ventricle is broadly delayed because of conduction blocks, even though the conduction path between the two stimulus sites yields simultaneous conduction times.

Recently, 3 dimensional endo- and epicardial catheter mapping has revealed that the patients of left ventricular systolic dysfunction with LBBB with lesser QRS duration (≤ 150 msec) have conduction delay confined specifically to the specialized conduction tissue of the heart with a lateral location of the line of block and short trans- septal conduction time. Total left ventricular endocardial activation is significantly long in these patients with endo- to-epicardial activation sequence at the antero-septal region. On the contrary, patients with higher QRS duration (> 150 msec) exhibit prolonged transseptal conduction time and additional conduction delay in diseased myocardium with line of conduction block situated anteriorly. However, total left ventricular endocardial activation is shorter and there is reversed epi-to-endocardial activation sequence.[11,12]

- *Ventricular activation time:* Left ventricular (LV) conduction delay due to left bundle branch block (LBBB) causes regional heterogeneity in contraction and stretch (asynchrony), which reduces pump function and stimulates negative LV remodeling. Resynchronization of electromechanical activation induces "reverse" remodeling (LV volume reductions) and improved pump function (increased LV ejection fraction [LVEF]). At baseline, longer left ventricular activation time (LVATmax) has been seen to be significantly associated with left ventricular end systolic volume reduction, indicating that greater LV conduction delay is associated with higher probability of reverse remodeling, if it is assumed that delay is sufficiently corrected by CRT.[13]

RV activation time (RVAT) is measured as time (msec) between QRS onset and first notch in any of ≥ 2 adjacent leads. LV activation time (LVAT) is QRS duration minus RVAT (msec). For modeling purposes, the longest LVAT (LVATmax) recorded in any lead and region is used. Because multiple notches in the R and S wave during LBBB may occur because of myocardial scar, the first notch is assumed to indicate the transition between RV and LV depolarization. Notching in the first 40 msec of the S wave in V1 through V2 is excluded because this indicates scar in the QRS score (Fig. 9.4).

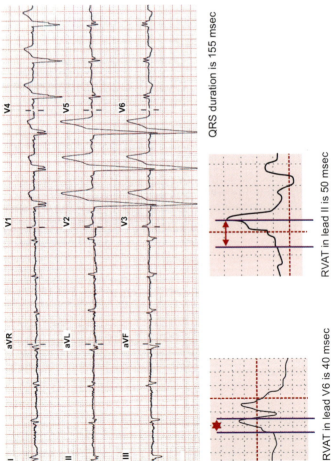

Fig. 9.4 Measurement of maximum left ventricular activation time (LVAT max): LVAT is calculated as QRS duration minus RVAT. In this patient LVAT max is 115 msec

A multivariable model identified 2 base-line and 2 post-CRT independent predictors of ≥ 10% reduction in end systolic left ventricular volume (ESV) at 6 months.[13] **Increasing LVATmax** was associated with a greater probability of ≥ 10% reduction in ESV up to 125 ms; for longer LVATmax, there was no further increase in probability of response. **Increasing QRS scores** were negatively associated with reverse remodeling for each 1-point increase from 0 to 4. After CRT, **increasing R amplitudes in V1 through V2,** indicating ventricular fusion, were associated with increased probability of reverse remodeling. This effect was not observed until the mean change in R amplitude was ≥ 4.5 times the baseline value. A second measure of ventricular fusion, **left axis deviation (LADEV) to right axis deviation (RADEV)**, was associated with increased probability of reverse remodeling.

CASE 1 (FIG. 9.5)

A 52-year-old lady of Dilated Cardiomyopathy with severe left ventricular systolic dysfunction (LVEF is 30%) presented to us with exertional dyspnea (NYHA class III) despite optimum medical therapy. Let us look at her ECG in sinus rhythm.

Her ECG showed:
- Complete **left bundle branch block** with QRS duration of **171 msec**.
- Sequential ventricular activation from right ventricle to left ventricle and registered as fragmented QRS complexes with RSR' configuration ("notch").
- LBBB **QRS score (myocardial scar burden) is 0**.
- Presumably, the conduction delay is due to delay in specialized conduction system as well as diseased myocardium. Transseptal conduction is prolonged with the **line of block situated anteriorly** and the conduction block is **functional.** Transmural activation of left ventricle occurs in reverse sequence (Epi-to-Endo).
- Right ventricular activation time in lead II is 45 msec and in lead V6 is 60 msec. Maximum left ventricular activation time **(LVAT max) is 126 msec.**

So, from the surface ECG, it is evident that this patient has all features favoring successful LV reverse remodeling. She received CRT with LV lead positioned in the lateral vein and RV lead in right ventricular apex. QRS duration during biventricular stimulation (simultaneous) was 128 msec. At 6 months post-CRT follow up, left ventricular ejection fraction improved from 30% to 40% and reduction in left ventricular end systolic volume was 28%.

Role of Pre-procedure ECG Analysis 211

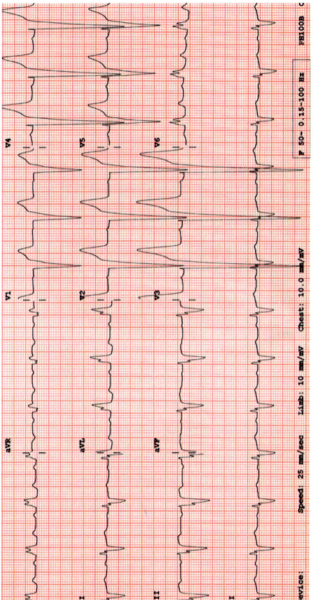

Fig. 9.5 Sinus rhythm ECG

CASE 2 (FIG. 9.6)

A 47-year-old gentleman presented with ischemic cardiomyopathy with severe left ventricular systolic dysfunction (LVEF is 32%) for CRT-D implantation.

His ECG revealed:
- **Left bundle branch block** with QRS duration of **160 msec**.
- Sequential ventricular activation from right ventricle to left ventricle and registered as fragmented QRS complexes with RSR' configuration ("notch").
- LBBB **QRS score is 4**. So, the myocardial scar burden is **12%**
- Presumably, the conduction delay is due to delay in specialized conduction system as well as diseased myocardium. Transseptal conduction is prolonged with the **line of block situated anteriorly** and the conduction block is **fixed** due to presence of scar. Transmural activation of left ventricle occurs in reverse sequence (Epi-to-Endo).
- Right ventricular activation time in lead II is 50 msec and in lead V6 is 45 msec. Maximum left ventricular activation time **(LVAT max) is 115 msec.**

Although the baseline ECG shows LBBB with wide (> 150 msec) QRS complex, the presence of significant scar burden (12%) can adversely influence probability of LV reverse remodeling. Presence of scar in the anterior wall (past history of anteroseptal wall myocardial infarction) and presumed anterior line of fixed conduction block mandate positioning of the LV lead in posterolateral vein of coronary sinus (away from the line of block). She received RV ICD lead in right ventricular apex. QRS duration during biventricular stimulation (LV first with VV delay of 40 msec) was 132 msec with tall R wave in lead V1 with right axis deviation from left axis deviation (pre-implant). So, in this case favorable factors for LV reverse remodeling are: 1) Increased LVAT max, 2) Increased R wave amplitude inV1 and V2 post-CRT, 3) Quadrant shift of QRS axis and the only adverse factor is high LBBB QRS score. Probability of LV reverse remodeling in his is intermediate (50 – 75%). Post-CRT 6 month follow up showed case marginal improvement in LVEF with dramatic symptomatic improvement.

Role of Pre-procedure ECG Analysis 213

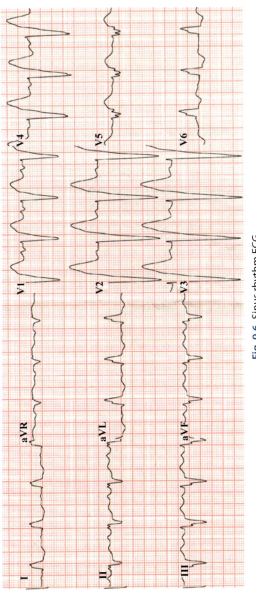

Fig. 9.6 Sinus rhythm ECG

REFERENCES

1. Ypenburg C, van Bommel RJ, Borleffs CJ, et al. Long-term prognosis after cardiac resynchronization therapy is related to the extent of left ventricular reverse remodeling at mid term follow-up. J Am Coll Cardiol. 2009;53(6):483-90.
2. Adelstein EC, Saba S. Usefulness of baseline electrocardiographic QRS complex pattern to predict response to cardiac resynchronization. Am J Cardiol. 2009;103:238-42.
3. Rickard J, Kumbhani DJ, Gorodeski EZ, et al. Cardiac resynchronization therapy in non-left bundle branch block morphologies. PACE. 2010;33:590-595.
4. Kadhiresan V, Vogt J, Auricchio A, et al. Sensitivity and specificity of QRS duration to predict acute benefit in heart failure patients with cardiac resynchronization. PACE. 2000; 23:555.
5. Vassallo JA, Cassidy DM, Marchlinski FE, et al. Endocardial activation of left bundle branch block. Circulation. 1984; 69:914.
6. Selvester RH, Wagner JO, Runin HB. Quantitation of myocardial infarct size and location by electrocardiogram and vectorcardiogram. In: Snellen HA, Hekmer HC, Hugenholtz PG, Van Bemmel JH, editors. Quantitation in cardiology. Baltimore: The Williams and Wilkins Company. 1972. p. 31.
7. Savage RM, Wagner GS, Ideker RE, Podolsky SA, Hackel DB. Correlation of postmortem anatomic findings with electrocardiographic changes in patients with myocardial infarction: retrospective study of patients with typical anterior and posterior infarcts. Circulation. 1977;55:279.
8. Anderson WD, Wagner NB, Lee KL, et al. Evaluation of a QRS scoring system for estimating myocardial infarct size. VI: Identification of screening criteria for non-acute myocardial infarcts. Am J Cardiol. 1988;61:729.
9. Sevilla DC, Wagner NB, Anderson WD, et al. Sensitivity of a set of myocardial infarction screening criteria in patients with anatomically documented single and multiple infarcts. Am J Cardiol. 1990;66:792.
10. Mahrholdt H, Wagner A, Holly TA, et al. Reproducibility of chronic infarct size measurement by contrast-enhanced magnetic resonance imaging. Circulation. 2002;106:2322.
11. Auricchio A, Fantoni C, Regoli F, et al. Characterization of left ventricular activation in patients with heart failure and left bundle branch block. Circulation. 2004:109:1133-9.
12. Fantoni C, Regoli F, Kawabata M, Klein HU, Auricchio A. Reversed transmural activation timing in patients with heart failure and left bundle branch block. Eur Heart J. 2004 (suppl): 2320.
13. Sweeney MO, van Bommel RJ, Schalij MJ, et al. Analysis of ventricular activation using surface electrocardiography to predict left ventricular reverse volumetric remodeling during cardiac resynchronization therapy. Circulation. 2010;121:626-34.

CHAPTER 10

Anatomy of Coronary Sinus

INTRODUCTION

The coronary venous system is used to access target areas and implant the LV pacing lead in cardiac resynchronization therapy (CRT). With experience and new implantation tools, physicians are increasingly inclined to place the lead in a specific location in contrast to earlier days when implanters used to select the available area. As a result, we need to study the patient's coronary venous circulation to determine the best way to direct the LV lead to the desired location. So, a set of good quality cine-angiogram (venogram) is important to know the detailed anatomy of coronary sinus.

ANATOMY

The heart is drained by the coronary sinus and its tributaries, the anterior cardiac veins, and the small cardiac veins. The coronary sinus and its tributaries return blood to the right atrium from the entire heart (including its septa) except for the anterior region of the right ventricle and small, variable parts of both atria and the left ventricle. The anterior cardiac veins drain an anterior region of the right ventricle and, when the right marginal vein joins this group, a region around the right cardiac border, and end principally in the right atrium. The small cardiac vein (Thebesian veins) open into the right atrium and ventricle and, to a lesser extent, the left atrium and sometimes the left ventricle. The larger veins accompany the major arteries, and drain into the coronary sinus (Fig. 10.1). The coronary sinus runs within the groove, lying between the left atrial wall and the ventricular myocardium, before draining into the right atrium between the sinus septum and the sub-eustachian sinus.

The anterior wall of the left ventricle and intraventricular septum is drained by branches of the anterior intraventricular vein (Fig. 10.2). These drain back to the mitral annulus and are joined by branches of the lateral venous system. Anterolateral, lateral, and posterolateral veins are frequently found. On the

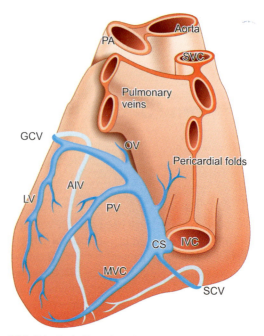

Fig. 10.1 Principal tributaries of coronary sinus viewed from back
Abbreviations: AIV, anterior interventricular vein; GCV, great cardiac vein; LV, lateral veins; PV, posterior vein of the left ventricle; MCV, middle cardiac vein; SCV, small cardiac vein; CS, coronary sinus; OV, oblique vein of the left atrium; SVC, superior vena cava; IVC, inferior vena cava; PA, pulmonary artery.

annulus, the vein is named the great cardiac vein. Where the great cardiac vein is joined by the main posterior lateral vein, the coronary sinus itself is formed. The coronary sinus in turn often receives a posterior venous supply in the form of a posterior vein and the middle cardiac vein. Throughout its course, the atrial musculature is drained into the venous system via various atrial veins. The most consistent atrial vein is one formed at the junction of the great cardiac vein and posterolateral vein and is called the vein of Marshall. This vein, also called the oblique vein, is a remnant of the left superior vena cava.

The **anterior interventricular vein** courses from the ventricular apex to the annulus just lateral to the anterior ventricular septum. Various tributaries drain the anterior wall of the left ventricle and parts of the anterior wall of the right ventricle. In the right anterior oblique projection, this vein is seen just behind the sternum and is the most anterior vein seen in this view. In about 30% of hearts, the proximal branch (apical) of the anterior intraventricular vein interdigitates and is continuous with similar branches of the posterior and middle

Anatomy of Coronary Sinus 217

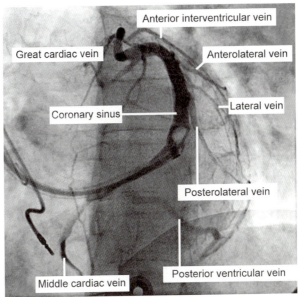

Left anterior oblique (LAO) view

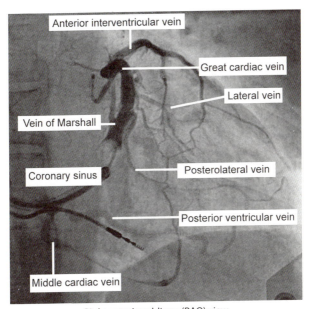

Right anterior oblique (RAO) view

Fig. 10.2 Various tributaries of coronary sinus

cardiac veins (Fig. 10.3).[1] Thus, a guide wire advanced apically into the anterior intraventricular vein in these patients will enter the middle cardiac venous system and through this vein reenter the coronary sinus and right atrium. The course of the anterior intraventricular vein is similar to the left anterior descending

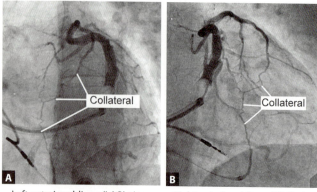
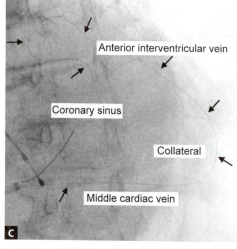

Figs 10.3A to C (A and B) LAO and RAO view of occlusive CS venogram showing collateral connection between anterior interventricular vein and middle cardiac vein. (C) A coronary wire has been passed from middle cardiac vein through the collateral to main CS body across the anterior interventricular vein in a different patient

coronary artery and the primary anterolateral tributary to the anterior ventricular vein is analogous to the first diagonal branch of the left anterior descending coronary artery.

Lateral cardiac veins are typically three distinct veins seen draining the lateral wall of the left ventricle.[1-3] The posterolateral vein is most consistent, often the largest, and occurs directly opposite the vein of Marshall. A smaller straight lateral vein and one or more anterior lateral veins can be seen. When the anterior lateral veins are large, draining into the great cardiac vein, the anterolateral tributary of the anterior interventricular vein is often small or absent. The great cardiac vein itself is the accompanying vein of the circumflex coronary artery and is usually superficial to the artery. Large multiple anastomoses between the various lateral veins, the posterior cardiac vein and the anterolateral tributary of the anterior intraventricular vein are frequently seen. The phrenic nerve typically courses lateral to the left atrial appendage, crossing superficial to the great cardiac vein forming variable relations with the lateral vein, posterior branches of the anterolateral vein and anterior branches of the posterolateral cardiac vein. Note that because of the thickness of the ventricular myocardium at this site, fairly large secondary tributaries of these lateral veins can be seen going intramyocardially. A pacing lead placed in one of the secondary tributaries will avoid stimulation of the phrenic nerve.

The **posterior ventricular vein** arises just distal to the middle cardiac vein and is often confused by implanters with the middle cardiac vein. In about one-quarter of patients, the middle cardiac vein and the posterior vein share a common cloacal ostium.[1-3] In even fewer patients, the posterior vein arises as a proximal tributary of the middle cardiac vein. The vein, regardless of the nature of its origin, courses directly to the lateral wall and accompanies the posterolateral branches of the right coronary artery. This is the only normally occurring tributary of the venous system whose main body runs parallel or nearly parallel to the annulus and its tributaries coursing from apex to base or vice versa.

Because of this course, it is frequently mistaken to be a branch of the middle cardiac vein. This vein, regardless of origin, can be consistently used to place a pacing lead to the lateral wall of the left ventricle, even when the posterolateral and lateral veins are absent, tortuous, or otherwise not amenable to implant. The distal branches of the posterior ventricular vein interdigitate with tributaries of the lateral venous system and are frequently related to the phrenic nerve at these sites. Because the ostium of this vein is very close to the ostium of the middle cardiac vein, selective cannulation of this vein can be difficult. Thus attempting to enter the vein from the right atrium directly will cause sub-selection of the middle cardiac vein and when sheaths are placed into the coronary sinus, the ostia of both the posterior vein and middle cardiac vein are covered, rendering these veins inaccessible. Understanding the anatomy of this vein allows its cannulation by placing the sub-selecting catheter or leads into the main body of the coronary sinus, withdrawing the sheath back to the right atrium and with clockwise torque engaging, upon withdrawal of the lead or catheter, the ostium of the posterior ventricular vein.[4]

The **middle cardiac vein** is nearly always present and is the largest proximal tributary to the coronary sinus. The ostium is located between the orifice of the small cardiac vein and the left posterior vein.[4] These two latter veins may arise as tributaries of the middle cardiac vein. The middle cardiac vein courses from apex to base on the posterior interventricular groove where it is accompanied by the posterior descending artery and covered by fat. Tributaries that drain the posterior and posterolateral left ventricle, as well as rightward tributaries that drain part of the posterior right ventricle, drain into the middle cardiac vein along its course in the posterior interventricular sulcus. Sometimes, the middle cardiac vein may arise as a separate ostium where its orifice can be found superior to the main orifice of the coronary sinus. Distal tributaries of the middle cardiac vein have numerous anastomoses near the apex with the apical tributaries of the anterior intraventricular vein and the lateral cardiac veins. The phrenic nerve does not have an anatomic relation (right or left phrenic nerves) with the middle cardiac vein. Pacing leads placed apically in the distal middle cardiac vein, however, may directly capture the left hemi-diaphragm.

Intraoperative hemodynamic studies suggest that left ventricular (LV) stimulation with a pacing electrode located in the mid portion of the LV free wall results in the greatest benefit. Fortunately, the venous drainage of the lateral wall tends to be extensive with interdigitating branches of all the main tributaries of the coronary sinus and great cardiac vein. The most direct anatomic drainage of this site is via the lateral, high posterolateral, or anterolateral veins. Sometimes cannulation of these veins can be difficult as typically the ostium and proximal tributary is nearly at right angles to the axis of the great cardiac vein.

The average length of the coronary sinus as defined above is 40–45 mm with an average diameter of 10 mm. The diameter of the coronary sinus is also highly variable and is dependent on the loading conditions on the heart, presence and extent of atrial myocardium within the coronary vein, and the presence of cardiac disease or previous cardiac surgery. It is at times slightly 'atrialized' coursing up to 10 mm atrial to the atrioventricular sulcus and thus not precisely on the annulus, along the left atrial myocardium. The coronary sinus lies in relation to the posterior mitral annulus and drains through the posteroseptal portion of the right atrium on the interatrial septum into the right atrium. Atrial myocardium forms the inner layers of the coronary sinus and extends into the coronary veins. This myocardial sleeve is always continuous in its entirety with the right atrial myocardium at the ostium and at variable portions and to a variable extent with the left atrial myocardium through interdigitations.[5]

Anatomy of Coronary Sinus

Several valves are present in the cardiac venous system. Consistently present is the Thebesian valve found at the ostium of the coronary sinus. Vieussens' valve is also frequently seen at the ostium of the primary posterolateral vein opposite to the opening of the vein of Marshall. Valves may be found in other ventricular and atrial veins. Rarely seen, but most common of the non-Vieussens' variety, is a valve at the ostium of the middle cardiac vein. The right ventricular venous drainage and portions of the interventricular septum are primarily through the Thebesian venous network directly into the right ventricle. The most proximal of the branches of the coronary venous system is the small cardiac vein which drains the posterior and posterolateral portions of the right ventricle and right atrium opening into the coronary sinus at its ostium in the right atrium.[6-8]

The **coronary sinus ostium** is almost always located on the posterior interatrial septum anterior to the eustachian ridge and valve and posterior to the tricuspid annulus. The valve usually extends to about one-third of the ostium but may sometimes nearly completely occlude the ostium. When nearly circumferential valves are found, multiple fenestrations are usually seen. When the circumference is only partially covered, it is usually the superior and posterior surfaces that are covered. Thus, entering the coronary sinus from an inferior and ventricular starting point avoids confronting the valve. Rarely the valve covers the inferior hemi-circumference, making it necessary to enter the coronary sinus from a superior route dragging the catheter sheath supero-inferiorly on the interatrial septum anterior to the eustachian ridge. Traversing the floor of the coronary sinus ostium in about one-third of normal hearts are extensions of the pectinate muscles that course from the lateral wall across the sub-eustachian isthmus and into the proximal coronary veins where they form part of the atrial myocardial sleeve.

Different anomalies of coronary sinus are absence of the coronary sinus, atresia of whole or part or a tributary of the coronary sinus, and hypoplasia of the coronary sinus. These anomalies are often associated with a persistent left superior vena cava. Coronary sinus diverticulae are malformations typically associated with the main tributaries of the coronary sinus and great cardiac vein and have been associated with epicardial accessory pathways.

VENOGRAPHY

Coronary angiogram should be done on a prior date to device implantation to ascertain the etiology of the dilated cardiomyopathy (idiopathic/ischemic) and with venous-phase images to have an initial idea about the coronary sinus anatomy. The occlusive CS venogram is the better way to understand the coronary venous anatomy for LV lead placement as it **1)** fully defines the coronary venous anatomy; **2)** collateral vessels are well visualized; **3)** retrograde filling of proximal veins is seen. Some implanting physicians prefer half-strength contrast to avoid contrast-induced nephropathy. However, limited visualization is obtained with occlusive CS venography using half-strength contrast agent. Full-strength contrast provides much better visualization of the venous system, both antegrade filling and retrograde filling. Full-strength contrast agent also visualizes venous collateral vessels that may be used for retrograde placement of the LV lead if the antegrade approach is problematic. Venous anomalies that may be important to lead placement also are better visualized. If the balloon does not occlude the mid-CS, it can be advanced further into a narrow portion of the CS and inflated. The vessels proximal to the occlusion can usually be seen as they fill retrograde. Alternatively, the balloon may be double-inflated. When imaging the coronary venous system, it is tempting to "jump ahead" after the first injection; for efficient, effective lead placement in every case, however, it is essential to obtain all three views (LAO, RAO and AP) to fully visualize the anatomy. In many cases, the critical anatomic information required is apparent in only one view. Without all views the implanter may work for hours on the basis of a false assumption about the venous anatomy. In some cases, despite adequate occlusive CS venograms, no lateral veins are identified but the anterior and middle cardiac vein are seen. Injection of the anterior or middle cardiac with the vein selector usually fills a lateral wall vein via collaterals vein. If more contrast is needed, the delivery guide is used. In some cases, contrast injection through a delivery guide into the body of the vein may not be helpful; in this case, the vein selector can be advanced into a small-branch vein. Contrast injection into the small branch will usually reveal a target vein to the lateral wall through collateral filling, with subsequent lead placement.

The variability of the venous anatomy may at first seem infinite, but there are basic patterns. Recognition of the venous pattern is important in selecting an approach to the target area and the type of lead. The venous anatomy can be classified according to the size of the vein that drains a particular area and characterized by the takeoff angle of the vein from the CS. The four patterns in the caliber of veins draining into the CS are as follows:

Anatomy of Coronary Sinus

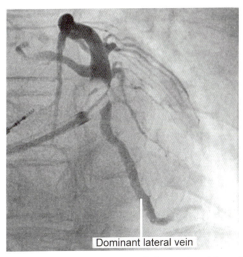

Fig. 10.4 Occlusive CS venogram in left anterior oblique (LAO) projection demonstrates mid-lateral dominance

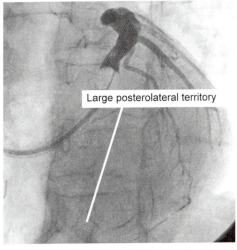

Fig. 10.5 Occlusive CS venogram in left anterior oblique (LAO) projection demonstrates posterior lateral dominance

1. *Mid-lateral dominant:* Largest coronary vein drains into the mid portion of the coronary sinus (Fig. 10.4).
2. *Posterior lateral dominant:* Largest coronary vein drains into the posterior part of the coronary sinus (Fig. 10.5).
3. *Balanced:* The lateral wall target veins are of approximately equal sizes (Fig. 10.6).
4. *Anterior lateral dominant:* The mid-lateral wall veins are small. The anterolateral vein is large and thus dominant (Fig. 10.7).

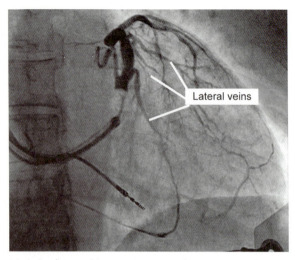

Fig. 10.6 Occlusive CS venogram in right anterior oblique (RAO) projection demonstrates almost equal sized lateral veins (balanced)

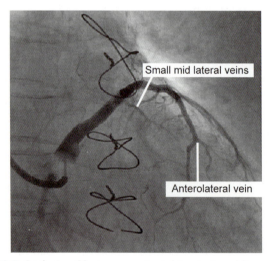

Fig. 10.7 Occlusive CS venogram in right anterior oblique (RAO) projection in a post-CABG patient demonstrates anterior lateral dominance

OTHER IMAGING MODALITIES

The preprocedural use of CT and MRI may facilitate patient selection as well as help plan and potentially select the tools for the implantation procedure. Multi-slice computed tomography (MSCT) at this stage is able to provide a fairly detailed perspective of the coronary venous anatomy. High-speed rotational coronary venous angiography (RCVA) is a novel imaging method that offers a multi-angle view of the coronary venous tree, using a rapid isocentric rotation over a wide arc. This technique acquires multiple images, thereby allowing an individualized LV lead implantation approach, using the views best suited for the anatomy. Intraprocedural echocardiography is evolving as a tool to aid in the process of localizing the coronary venous ostium to facilitate CS cannulation in difficult cases. The continued evolution of these imaging modalities will significantly increase the success of the implantation procedure, as well as aid in the development of superior technology and newer approaches for lead implantation.

TARGET VEIN AND TARGET SITE

The optimal placement of a left ventricular (LV) lead in a tributary of the coronary sinus is one of the most challenging technical aspects of cardiac resynchronization therapy (CRT) device implantation. Technically, the final position of the LV pacing lead depends on the anatomy of the cardiac venous system, the performance and stability of the pacing lead, and the absence of phrenic nerve stimulation. The primary therapeutic target of cardiac resynchronization therapy (CRT) is restoration of coordinated myocardial contraction and the current preferred method to achieve this is to position the LV lead at a lateral or posterolateral branch of the coronary sinus based on the results of early hemodynamic studies. Recent reports have challenged this view and suggest that there is great individual variation in the optimal LV pacing site. Singh, et al. have shown that the benefit from CRT is similar for LV leads positioned along the anterior, lateral, or posterior wall.[9] However, LV leads positioned in the apical region are associated with an unfavorable clinical outcome and favorable outcome in mid and basal region, suggesting that the apical lead location should be avoided in CRT (Fig. 10.8).

However, an integrated assessment of three factors is crucial to achieve a high favorable response rate and an improved clinical outcome:

- LV lead position should coincide with the **latest activated areas** of the left ventricle, since that location maximizes the hemodynamic benefits of CRT and provides superior long-term outcome.[10,11]
- The **presence of suitable tributaries** of the coronary sinus in the latest activated areas of the left ventricle is therefore mandatory.
- Evaluation of the **myocardial scar burden** is also an important consideration for achievement of an optimal result. The presence of transmural myocardial scar at the area

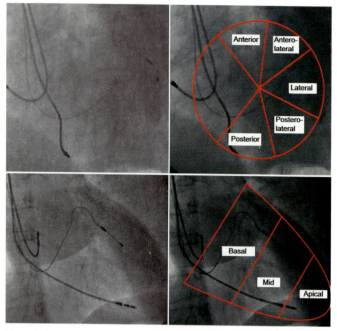

Fig. 10.8 Angiographic classification of left ventricular lead position. Top: Left anterior oblique (LAO) view used to divide the left ventricular wall along the short axis of the heart into different parts; anterior, anterolateral, lateral, posterolateral, and posterior. Bottom: Right anterior oblique (RAO) view representative of the long axis of the heart. This view enables segmentation of the heart into basal, mid-ventricular, and apical segments

targeted by the LV pacing lead reduces the beneficial effects of CRT on clinical outcome and cardiac performance.[12]

Several invasive and non-invasive imaging techniques have been proposed to identify the latest activated areas of the left ventricle. Three-dimensional non-contact LV endocardial mapping provides exact characterization of the LV activation sequence, indicating the latest activated LV regions where the LV pacing lead should preferably placed. The assessment of the latest activated LV areas can be also performed non-invasively by using echocardiographic techniques, such as tissue-Doppler imaging or two-dimensional speckle tracking imaging, and tagged magnetic resonance imaging. Ansalone et al demonstrated the role of echocardiographic tissue-Doppler imaging to identify the most delayed LV regions and to evaluate the effect of CRT on LV performance according to the LV lead position (at the latest activated areas or at remote areas).[10] Recently, two-dimensional speckle tracking echocardiography has been proposed as a valuable imaging tool to characterize the LV mechanical activation pattern and to identify the most delayed activated LV regions.[12] This echocardiographic imaging technique evaluates the active myocardial contraction in three orthogonal directions (radial, circumferential, and longitudinal). On the basis of radial strain–time curves obtained at the mid-ventricular short-axis images of the left ventricle, the most frequent latest activated areas were the posterior (36%) and the lateral (33%) regions. Finally, tagged magnetic resonance imaging is a three-dimensional imaging technique that permits characterization of LV mechanical activation sequence and detection of the latest activated segments.[13] Several methods and indices based on tagged magnetic resonance imaging have been proposed to quantify LV dyssynchrony. All of them evaluate the LV shortening in the circumferential and longitudinal directions or the thickening in the radial direction. Particularly, the assessment of LV circumferential shortening provides superior accuracy than longitudinal shortening to predict favorable response to CRT. Despite recent technical advances, this imaging technique is not widely available and incompatible with the CRT devices, limiting the evaluation of the effects of CRT on LV performance at follow-up.

The most common approach to evaluate the cardiac venous anatomy uses fluoroscopy just prior to implantation of the LV pacing lead. Particularly, to anticipate whether the LV pacing lead could be implanted in a lateral vein, the assessment of the cardiac venous anatomy with multi-detector row computed tomography or magnetic resonance may be of value. In patients without suitable lateral or posterolateral veins to host the LV pacing lead, a surgical implantation of the LV lead at the latest activated region may be preferred.

Finally, prior to implantation of the LV pacing lead, evaluation of location and extent of myocardial scar is crucial to achieve a high favorable response rate. Areas of fibrous myocardium are electrically and mechanically nonviable; therefore, pacing at those sites may be of little value. So, the implantation of an LV lead at an area with transmural myocardial scar may result in ineffective CRT. With the use of three-dimensional non-contact LV endocardial mapping systems, LV areas with extensive fibrosis or myocardial scar may be identified as areas of slow conduction. Lambiase, et al. demonstrated that positioning the LV pacing lead in areas of slow conduction resulted in prolonged LV activation time and dyssynchrony and, consequently, in less LV hemodynamic improvement.[11] Other non-invasive imaging techniques also provide information on myocardial scar burden (myocardial contrast echocardiography, single photon emission computed tomography, contrast-enhanced magnetic resonance).

Particularly, contrast-enhanced magnetic resonance provides accurate information on location and extent of myocardial scar.

The TARGET study (randomized, controlled) demonstrated the benefit of a targeted approach to LV lead placement in CRT, resulting in significant benefit defined by LV reverse remodeling, clinical status, and the long-term endpoint of combined death and heart failure-related hospitalization.[14] The study prospectively confirms the importance of the LV lead position in CRT outcomes and demonstrates the feasibility of LV lead targeting using speckle-tracking radial strain imaging as a modality to guide lead placement.

Therefore, the integration of information on the latest activated LV regions, venous anatomy, and myocardial scar may refine the patient selection for CRT and, consequently, may increase the favorable response rate. In addition, this information is of value to anticipate the strategy to implant the LV pacing lead (conventional transvenous approach or surgical approach). However, all these investigations put additional economic burden over the patients. So, in our practice we perform a conventional 2D echocardiography (though it has some limitations) and exclude or localize any visible myocardial scar tissue. Using tissue-Doppler imaging, we localize the most delayed activated myocardial segment. We get an initial idea about the coronary sinus anatomy from the venous-phase images of coronary angiogram done on a prior date to device implantation and finally select a suitable target vein integrating the information achieved from conventional and tissue-Doppler echocardiography.

REFERENCES

1. Ludinghausen M. Clinical anatomy of cardiac veins. Surg Radiol Anat. 1987;9:159-68.
2. Gensini GG, Digiorgi S, Coskun O, et al. Anatomy of the coronary circulation in living man; coronary venography. Circulation. 1965;31:778-84.
3. 29 Gilard M, Mansourati J, Etienne Y, et al. Angiographic anatomy of the coronary sinus and its tributaries. Pacing Clin Electrophysiol. 1998;21:2280-4.
4. Sethna DH, Moffitt EA. An appreciation of the coronary circulation. Anesth Analg. 1986;65:294-305.
5. Sun Y, Arruda M, Otomo K, et al. Coronary sinus-ventricular accessory connections producing posteroseptal and left posterior accessory pathways: incidence and electrophysiological identification. Circulation. 2002;106:1362-7.
6. Wit AL, Cranefield PF. Triggered and automatic activity in the canine coronary sinus. Circ Res. 1977;41:434-45.
7. Giudici M, Winston S, Kappler J, et al. Mapping the coronary sinus and great cardiac vein. Pacing Clin Electrophysiol. 2002;25:414-9.

8. Volkmer M, Antz M, Hebe J, et al. Focal atrial tachycardia originating from the musculature of the coronary sinus. J Cardiovasc Electrophysiol. 2002;13:68-71.
9. Jagmeet P Singh, Helmut U Klein, David T Huang, Sven Reek, Malte Kuniss, Quesada, et al. Left Ventricular Lead Position and Clinical Outcome in the Multicenter Automatic Defibrillator Implantation Trial-Cardiac Resynchronization Therapy (MADIT-CRT) Trial. Circulation. 2011;123:1159-66.
10. Ansalone G, Giannantoni P, Ricci R, Trambaiolo P, Fedele F, Santini M. Doppler myocardial imaging to evaluate the effectiveness of pacing sites in patients receiving biventricular pacing. J Am Coll Cardiol. 2002;39:489-99.
11. Lambiase PD, Rinaldi A, Hauck J, Mobb M, Elliott D, Mohammad S, et al. Noncontact left ventricular endocardial mapping in cardiac resynchronisation therapy. Heart. 2004;90:44-51.
12. Bleeker GB, Schalij MJ, van der Wall EE, et al. Posterolateral scar tissue resulting in non-response to cardiac resynchronization therapy. J Cardiovasc Electrophysiol. 2006;17:899-901.
13. Becker M, Franke A, Breithardt OA, Ocklenburg C, Kaminski T, Kramann R, et al. Impact of left ventricular lead position on the efficacy of cardiac resynchronisation therapy: a two-dimensional strain echocardiography study. Heart. 2007;93:1197-203.
14. Lardo AC, Abraham TP, Kass DA. Magnetic resonance imaging assessment of ventricular dyssynchrony: current and emerging concepts. J Am Coll Cardiol. 2005;46:2223-8.

CHAPTER 11

Implantation Technique

INTRODUCTION

Cardiac resynchronization therapy (CRT) is defined as the stimulation of the left ventricle or simultaneous stimulation of both the right and the left ventricle after atrial sensed or paced events. CRT requires permanent pacing of the LV wall and restores the synchronicity of the atrioventricular, interventricular, and intraventricular contractions, resulting in improved clinical outcomes and cardiac performance of advanced HF patients with wide QRS complex. Therefore, it involves positioning of a left ventricular lead (in addition to a right atrial and a right ventricular lead) on the lateral wall (preferably) of the left ventricle, epicardially either endovascularly via the coronary sinus or by direct surgical placement. This additional lead on the lateral wall of the left ventricle ensures nearly simultaneous stimulation of both the ventricle.

APPROACH

The preparation for a CRT implantation begins with insertion of a peripheral access line into a large or forearm vein on the side selected as the implantation site, prior to beginning the surgical preparation of the patient. This peripheral venous access is used for subclavian venography. Performing subclavian venography prior to a new implantation is a reasonable option; but is not a routine procedure. It should be strongly considered prior to an upgrading existing system to CRT by addition of only an LV lead. The venogram helps in localizing the cephalic and subclavian vein during a difficult puncture, demonstrating asymptomatic subclavian vein thrombosis (may be present in 10% to 15% of patients with multiple chronically implanted lead) or difficult and tortuous anatomy associated with scarring from previous insertion of pacing leads. The operator can opt to make three separate direct axillary or subclavian vein punctures or a cephalic cut down for one or both of the right heart leads, combined with a separate puncture for the

LV lead. Either right or left subclavian access can be chosen for implanting CRT system. Selecting right side has the advantage of ability to rotate imaging equipment to the left anterior oblique view without interfering with surgery and the ability to cannulate the CS ostium easily. However, right sided approach imposes a challenge to CS catheterization by requiring the guiding catheter to make two right-angle turns in opposite directions. We prefer left subclavian approach as it provides a more natural route for the curved guiding catheters to follow from the subclavian vein to the CS ostium. Furthermore, the ability to seat the guiding catheter deep in the CS to provide stability during venography and lead advancement appears greater from the left subclavian access site.

LEAD IMPLANTATION ORDER

Most of the patient assigned for CRT implantation have underlying intraventricular conduction system disease; mostly left bundle branch block (LBBB) pattern of activation. Trauma to the right bundle branch in these patients during rotation, advancement and manipulation of the guiding sheath in an attempt to enter the CS can produce high-degree atrioventricular (AV) block and asystole. So, most of the operators like to put the right ventricular (RV) lead before the left ventricular (LV) lead. However, we prefer to position the LV lead first as we believe in the concept of "Dialing-in" RV pacing lead after LV lead positioning coined by Heist and his colleagues (discussed later). So, we routinely prefer temporary pacing back up to avoid catastrophic event. The right atrial (RA) lead implantation can occur either before or after the LV lead implantation, at the discretion of the operator.

PLACEMENT OF LV LEAD

An effective technique for implantation of LV pacing lead requires an understanding of the anatomy of the failing heart and the coronary veins and the combination of standard pacing lead insertion skills with techniques common to interventional cardiology.
- Coronary sinus cannulation is the initial key step to successful CRT implantation. Manipulation of preformed guiding catheters with the tips curved to varying degrees may locate the CS ostium (Fig. 11.1). Counterclockwise rotation of the preshaped guide catheter directs the guide posterior in the atrium. When standard maneuvers with the preformed guiding catheter fails to find the CS ostium, using diagnostic catheter into the guiding catheter provides additional three-dimensional flexibility to locate the CS.

Inserting a multipurpose (MP), left internal mammary (LIMA), or Amplatz (AL) catheter in the available CS guiding catheter can help reach the CS in markedly abnormal right atrium (Fig. 11.2).

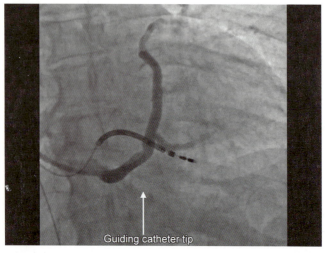

Fig. 11.1 Contrast injection through the guiding catheter cum long sheath. CS cannulation was done by rotating the sheath only

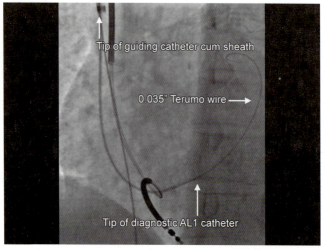

Fig. 11.2 Coronary sinus cannulation with the help of diagnostic coronary catheter

Implantation Technique

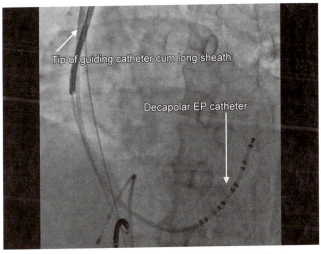

Fig. 11.3 EP approach of Coronary sinus cannulation

In EP approach, inserting a steerable mapping catheter (in our practice we use deflectable decapolar catheter) into a straight or preformed guide catheter allows the implanter to find the CS by changing the curve of the mapping catheter and gently advancing it until it follows the typical contour of the CS (Fig. 11.3). Fluoroscopic visualization, usually in the left anterior oblique view, confirms the position within the CS. Advancement of the guiding catheter over the mapping catheter places the guide in position for venography and lead advancement.

- Once the guide catheter sits at least 3–4 cm within the CS, one can insert the balloon-tip catheter (Swan-Ganz) into the position for contrast venography. Occlusive coronary sinus venography in at least 2 views (LAO and RAO) delineate all potential target veins, valves, strictures, collateral connections, and other specific anatomic details that permit optimal placement of LV pacing leads. The venogram should demonstrate all possible cardiac venous targets, the site at which each LV vein enters into the CS, and the course of each vein and its tributaries, from base to apex. The venogram in LAO view generates excellent views of the target vein as they enter the CS. It also removes the overlap between anterior/septal veins and antero-lateral veins. However, it usually foreshortens the view of the body of the tributary vein. Fluoroscopic RAO view best visualize the course of the target vein from the CS to the apex of the ventricle. Opacification of collaterals to posterior and posterolateral veins demonstrate potential target veins that would otherwise go unnoticed during injection of contrast beyond the point at which those veins enter the CS. Normal physiology dictates that all of the LV myocardium requires venous drainage. The inability to identify venous drainage from a large segment of the LV implies that venography failed to detect the tributary from that segment or collateral flow from one segment to a vein draining an adjacent segment or that failure to occlude the CS led to suboptimal contrast injection. Failure to utilize venography to guide LV lead implantation can diminish the chance of a successful implantation. One may fortuitously find LV veins without obtaining a venogram simply by probing for CS tributaries with a guide wire. However, the advantages of proper venography greatly outweigh its risk to the patient. Venography provides a roadmap to primary and secondary target veins. If the primary target fails because improper threshold of pacing or close proximity to the phrenic nerve, we can shift to secondary target vein.

- Once the target vein is selected, it is time to take a sub selective injection using either 5F JR or IMA catheter or various subselection catheters available from different companies. It gives detailed anatomy of the target vein, different collaterals from the target vein to other major tributaries of the coronary sinus and ideally it should be taken in RAO projection.
- The implanter should be prepared to select a LV lead that best fit with the available target vein. Several factors influence unpredictably in this choice, including coronary venous anatomy, phrenic nerve stimulation, and LV epicardial pacing thresholds. The initial choice of a LV lead focuses on the ostial take-off of the target vein, followed by an examination of the main body of the target vein. Often, these two considerations are in opposition, e.g. a tight ostial take-off accompanied by a large diameter vein. In this situation, a smaller diameter, flexible tip lead would be optimal for navigating the take-off, possibly assisted by a guide wire. An undesirable characteristic of smaller diameter leads, however, is that they tend to descend distally within larger target veins (apex seekers) until a matched cross-sectional diameter is encountered and fixation by wedging occurs. In contrast, a larger diameter, stiffer lead is more likely to achieve proximal fixation, which may reduce the chance of phrenic nerve stimulation, but may not be able to navigate the ostial take-off of the target vein. Currently available transvenous LV pacing leads may be either stylet driven or use over-the-wire (OTW) delivery similar to percutaneous coronary intervention (PCI). In general the smallest diameter leads are

unipolar and are delivered exclusively over a PCI guide wire. Larger diameter leads may accommodate a conventional stylet or a PCI guide wire (hybrids). In some cases, fixation relies primarily on "wedging" the lead tip into a distal site within the target vein such that the outer diameter of the lead closely approximates the inner luminal diameter of the vein. Some other current LV lead designs incorporate one or more tines, which may assist with fixation by catching on a valve or promoting thrombosis, but are probably otherwise irrelevant. Finally, some other LV leads have a self-retaining **cant** at the tip that has two intended purposes. The cant unfolds within the target vein simultaneously compressing the distal segment of the lead against the outer wall of the vein, improving fixation, and forcing the tip electrode against the epicardium, improving electrical contact for pacing. More recently, enhancements to lead design have been directed at combining the maneuverability of smaller diameter leads with the mechanical stability of large leads. This is achieved by incorporating reversible, **self-retaining S- or pigtail-shaped curves** at the lead tip, which increase the "effective" diameter of smaller leads for mechanical stability without degrading maneuverability. Another design incorporates deployable **"retention lobes"** which may provide superior mechanical stability, but may also be extremely difficult or impossible to extract. Figure 11.4 demonstrates some of these available LV lead from different companies.

Before attempting placement of an LV lead in the target vein, the ostium and proximal segment should be carefully examined in at least two fluoroscopic views (antero-posterior and left anterior oblique). The apparent origin of the target vein can be quite misleading particularly if it arises on the posterior wall of the CS, which is not easily visualized by any fluoroscopic view. The investment of additional contrast injections prior to attempted subselection of the target vein may avoid the selection of an inappropriate lead design for the anatomic situation and an excessively time consuming and futile effort. Some implanters recommend systemic anticoagulation with intravenous unfractionated heparin after CS cannulation but before attempted target vein subselection. The rationale for this recommendation is based on the common observation that extensive clots are often found on the tips and bodies of LV leads when they are removed and exchanged during attempted placement, raising the possibility that acute coronary vein thrombosis may prevent successful LV lead placement. Systemic anticoagulation is then reversed with intravenous protamine

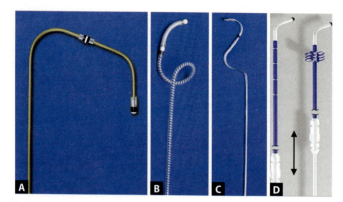

Figs 11.4A to D (A) Canted lead from medtronic (attain ability), (B) Pig-tail shaped lead from biotronik (Corox OTW BP), (C) S-shaped lead from St. Jude Medical (Quick Flex), (D) Lead with retention lobe from medtronic (Attain Starfix)

at the conclusion of the procedure, analogous to coronary arteriography or PCI. The approach with OTW leads involves placement of a PCI guide wire into the target vein over which the lead is tracked into the target vein. Occasionally the PCI guide wire can be manipulated into the target vein with minimal effort. When the unassisted PCI guide wire cannot be easily manipulated into the target vein, a guide catheter is employed. In general, the 4 French Judkins right coronary catheter (JR-3), an internal mammary artery (IMA) catheter, or Bern or Berenstein angiography catheters are effective for this purpose. Once the tip of the guide catheter has engaged the target vein ostium, the PCI guide wire is advanced as distally as possible into the vein and the guide catheter is withdrawn completely. This must be carried out under continuous fluoroscopic observation to be certain that the PCI guide wire is not inadvertently withdrawn from the target vein, or worse, the main body CS.

- In case of difficulties in delivering the LV lead into the target vein we have to adopt some of the following techniques of lead delivery.

BUDDY WIRE TECHNIQUE

This is used to advance a pacing lead beyond a tortuous area without the need for venoplasty. In this technique, a second extra-support angioplasty wire (the buddy wire) is used to straighten a tortuous or looped vascular segment, allowing the LV lead to pass more easily. Initially, a coronary sinus access catheter (same catheter used for selective angiography) is engaged into the mouth of the target vein. This provides a stable

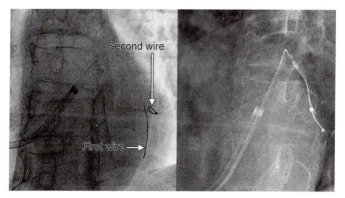

Fig. 11.5 Demonstration of buddy wire technique

platform to advance the stiff part of both the wires through the tortuous vein segment. The LV lead is delivered over floppier wire (tracking wire). With a stiff wire straightening the vein, the pacing lead encounters less resistance and can be advanced over the soft wire (Fig. 11.5).

RETROGRADE BUDDY WIRE TECHNIQUE

Severe tortuosity, in particular of the vein-sinus junction and angulation of the proximal vein, may prohibit successful delivery of the lead, despite the ability of a guide wire to successfully negotiate the course of the vessel. Although fluoroscopy shows the vessel to be straightened by the wire, it is unable to appreciate the changes in the vessel geometry induced by this distortion of the vessel. There may be bunching of endothelium in an accordion like fashion. Use of a second wire can facilitate lead delivery by a number of means. The wire can straighten out a highly tortuous vessel segment, lend additional support to the coronary sinus sheath, and act as a track to direct the lead away from the vessel wall. When difficulty is encountered at the vein/coronary sinus junction, this ability to serve as a track and deflect the advancing lead away from the wall, thereby avoiding bunched endothelium, could be of vital importance. However, the implanter may encounter friction due to the narrow internal diameter or binding due to development of thrombus within the sheath—both of which may potentially lead to loss of target vessel access or difficulty manipulating the pacing lead. Moreover, the tortuosity of the initial segment may prohibit successful delivery of even a single antegradely placed guide wire. In some instances, an implanter may not successfully advance a single wire beyond the junction of the vein and coronary sinus despite the use of a subselection sheath.

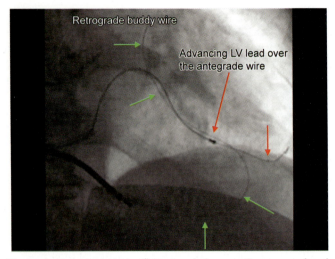

Fig. 11.6 Posterior anterior fluoroscopic images. Green arrowheads highlight the course of the guide wire that retrogradely enters the lateral vein and then into the CS body/ Red arrows indicate the course of the antegradely placed pacing lead and guide wire

Bridging collateral arising from the distal middle cardiac vein and extending to a lateral cardiac vein can frequently be identified during routine venography in the right anterior oblique view. The retrograde secondary wire can be advanced beyond the target vessel into the body of the coronary sinus and subsequently the right atrium. This distal positioning ensures that access within the vessel can be retained. A second coronary sinus sheath and anterograde guide wire can then be positioned. The retrograde wire serves not only as a fluoroscopic landmark for the junction of the lateral vein and the coronary sinus, but also serves to straighten vessel tortuosity (Fig. 11.6).

VENOPLASTY

If occlusive CS venography shows limited option for target veins we have to consider venoplasty of small or stenotic target veins. A delivery guide or angioplasty guide is placed at the os of the target vein. The lead would not follow despite the use of a buddy wire. A 2.5 or 3-mm balloon is advanced and inflated to 12 to 16 atm pressure. If contrast injection shows that the target vein is large enough to accept the lead, the lead is advanced. When phrenic pacing and high thresholds are encountered along the length of the target vein, placement of the LV lead in a branch vein can solve the problem. But, in many cases the branch veins are too small to accept the lead. Fortunately, the branch veins can be dilated to accommodate the LV lead. But, operator has to be extremely cautious of entering the pericardial space. When a vein cannot be entered antegrade, it can often be entered retrograde by dilating the collaterals between an adjacent vein and the target vein. Floppy angioplasty wire can be passed from one vein to another through a collateral vessel and reenter the CS through the second vein. When the collateral is too small or stenotic, the vein is first dilated with a smaller, 1.5 mm balloon, followed by a balloon that is large enough (2.5 or 3 mm) to allow the lead to advance. Subsequently the lead can be advanced. Inherent complication to this technique is dissection, perforation or rupture leading to loss of venous integrity. Clinical significance depends on the size and location (proximal or distal) of the disruption, as well as the pressure gradients. Unless there is a clinical event or contrast is injected, venous disruption will go undetected. Small peroration in patients with prior open heart surgery is less troublesome as the scar tissue that develops around the heart after cardiac surgery limits the bleeding from the low-pressure venous system. In patients without prior cardiac surgery, loss of venous integrity usually allows contrast to be extravasated into the pericardial space; however, development of tamponade is rare. In case of tamponade, successful drainage has no lasting adverse effects.

Let us look at the following occlusive CS venogram (Fig. 11.7).

In this case, the left ventricular lead could not be advanced into the target vein despite use of buddy wire technique because of its tortuosity. We could manage to advance the LV lead into the target vein using **balloon anchor technique.**

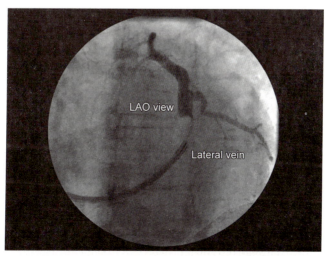

Fig. 11.7 Left anterior oblique view demonstrates severe tortuosity in the proximal part of the target vein

ANCHOR BALLOON TECHNIQUE

At first a coronary wire is placed in the target vein and advanced distally. Then, a coronary balloon (length should be ≥ 15 mm, diameter should be 3 to 4 mm and should be **compliant**). The diameter should be 3 to 4 mm, depending on how far distally the angioplasty wire and balloon are advanced into the CS. Coronary balloons have a hydrophilic coating, a low profile (small diameter), and a stiff proximal section. As a result, coronary balloons advance easily into the CS branch. Now, the balloon is inflated at 6 – 8 atm pressure as far distally in the CS branch vein as possible. With gentle traction on the balloon the sheath/guide is advanced over the balloon into the CS branch. If resistance is encountered, with maintained traction and gentle forward pressure is applied with careful clockwise and counterclockwise torque to more favorably align the tip of the sheath/guide and the body of the balloon. Do not force the sheath/guide. Coronary balloons are used as anchors to facilitate LV lead placement in one of two ways: **(1)** Anchoring the pacing lead wire in the vein prevents dislodgment of the pacing lead wire as the LV lead is advanced. Two coronary wires were inserted into the target vein via a vein selector or a 5 Fr catheter. The anchor balloon is inserted on one of the wires and is inflated, trapping the second wire in the vein. The pacing lead is advanced over the second wire (Fig. 11.8). If it buckles gentle traction on the pacing lead wire straightens the lead, allowing it to be advanced into the vein. **(2)** Anchoring the wire in the vein allows the guide to be pulled into the vein for subsequent lead placement (Fig. 11.9). Although LV lead placement is facilitated in both cases, using the balloon to get the guide into the vein allows selective contrast injection to locate options in case phrenic pacing or high thresholds are encountered. Furthermore, guide support enables easy repositioning of the lead into the alternative branch if necessary.

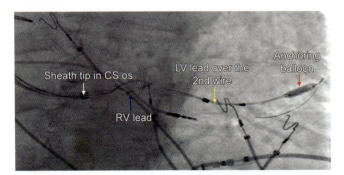

Fig. 11.8 Coronary balloon anchors the pacing lead wire, preventing dislodgment of the pacing wire as the left ventricular lead is advanced

Implantation Technique 241

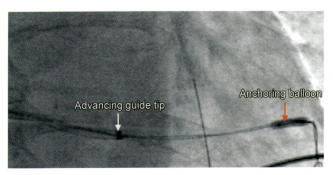

Fig. 11.9 Coronary balloon used as an anchor to "pull" the guide into the target vein for left ventricular lead delivery

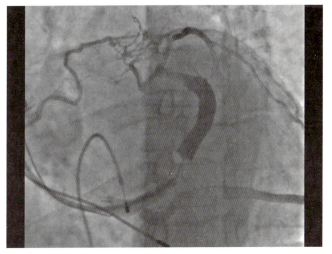

Fig. 11.10 Coronary sinus venogram shows no lateral vein. Posterolateral vein is large caliber vein

Now let us look at another coronary sinus venogram in LAO view (Fig. 11.10).

In this patient postero-lateral vein was not selected for LV lead placement because of its abnormal origin and tortuous course. Also, large caliber of this vein makes it unsuitable for lead placement as lead stability can be an important issue. We planned to position the LV lead on the lateral wall through the antero-lateral vein. But, lead could not be advanced because of the bend despite use of buddy wire (Fig. 11.11). However, we could negotiate a 0.014″ double length coronary wire from the postero-lateral ventricular vein through the collateral into the antero-lateral vein then into the coronary sinus. Finally, we positioned the lead onto the lateral wall **retrogradely over the**

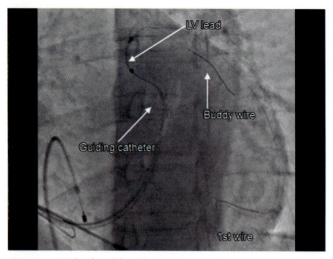

Fig. 11.11 LV lead could not be advanced to the lateral wall through the anterolateral vein despite use of buddy wire

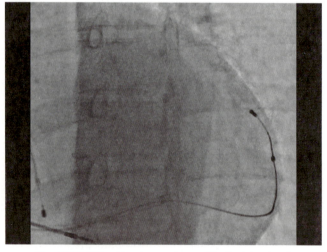

Fig. 11.12 LV lead has been advanced to the lateral wall retrogradely through the posterolateral vein

wire after snaring out the distal end of the wire into the pocket (Fig. 11.12).

ANTEGRADE SNARE TECHNIQUE

In this technique, a floppy hydrophilic wire is advanced into the target vein then into the collaterals of an adjacent vein and finally from the adjacent vein retrogradely into the CS. The distal end of the wire is snared as it reenters CS from the adjacent vein. The distal end of the wire is stabilized either internally (in the CS or in the catheter) or externally (at the hub) depending on the internal diameter of the CS access catheter. The 7F internal diameter of the CS access catheter will not accept the snare catheter and LV lead at the same time. With the distal end of the wire secured by the snare, traction can be placed on the wire as the delivery guide and lead are advanced.

RETROGRADE SNARE TECHNIQUE

When a wire cannot be advanced into the target vein antegradely, it is often possible to enter the target with a wire retrograde by selecting an adjacent vein and directing the wire through the collaterals into the target vein. Through an adjacent vein, a double length (300 cm) coronary wire is directed into the target vein through the collaterals. Once in the target vein, the wire can usually be advanced retrograde out into the CS where it is snared. The distal end of the wire is pulled out of the target vein into the tip of the sheath and out into the pocket. The stiff end of the wire is continuously advanced and the distal (floppy) end is pulled out until 80 cm of wire is on the field. Then the floppy tip of the wire is trimmed of and the lead back loaded onto the distal end of the wire. While holding the proximal (stiff) end of the wire, the lead is advanced into the target vein. If the lead does not advance smoothly, venoplasty of the target vein can be performed.

BALLOON-FACILITATED DELIVERY

In case of very tortuous branch veins which arise at steep angles, advancement of the lead can cause buckling of the guide wire and prolapse of the lead into the CS or great cardiac vein (Figs 11.13A and B). Guide wires with added support may not always allow the advancement of the lead into the lateral vein due to tortuosity and the acute branch angle. In absence of suitable collateral channel between the lateral vein and either the posterior or middle cardiac vein attempt to pull the lead into position with snare technique may not be advisable. After failure of all standard techniques the CS is cannulated with a 6-Fr multipurpose guide catheter, and a large balloon dilatation catheter is positioned in the great cardiac vein, immediately upstream from the ostium of the target vein over a 0.014" coronary wire. The balloon diameter is selected based on visual estimation and is equal to or slightly greater than the diameter of the CS. The balloon was inflated to four atmospheres pressure and held in position with gentle traction (Fig. 11.13C). With the balloon inflated, the LV lead can easily

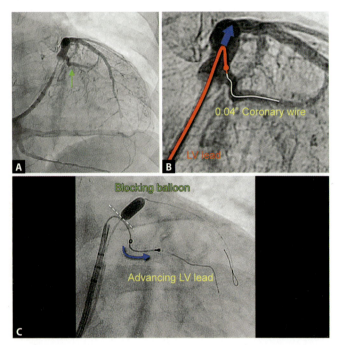

Figs 11.13A to C (A) Occlusive CS venogram in the anteroposterior projection. The target vein (lateral vein) (arrow) is small and tortuous. (B) Attempts to advance the lead result in buckling and prolapse into the great cardiac vein, with dislodgment of the lead tip. (C) Blocking balloon to prevent prolapse. A balloon inflated in the great cardiac vein just above the takeoff of the lateral branch vein provides a barrier (dashed line) that prevents lead prolapse. Forces are redirected toward the lead tip

be advanced through a conventional delivery system. A low-pressure balloon is utilized as a temporary mechanical barrier to prevent prolapse of the guide wire and lead into the great cardiac vein. As an added benefit, the balloon also redirected the force of lead advancement into the long axis of the target vein, helping to overcome resistance associated with vessel tortuosity and small diameter. It is likely that any low-pressure balloon catheter (such as a venography catheter or a wedge angiography catheter typically used to perform CS venogram) would have provided similar results with less expense. Even when using low-pressure balloons, attempts to advance pacing leads around tight bends can lead to CS and branch vein dissections. While dissection of the side branch is usually clinically silent and resolves without any sequel, dissection within the main trunk of CS can be potentially problematic.

In our lab, we put two floppy 0.014" coronary wires through the subselection catheter after selective venography of the target vein and routinely use antegrade buddy wire technique to deliver the LV lead into the target vein. If this technique fails we use balloon anchor technique and venoplasty for severely stenosed or small target vein to deliver the LV lead in the target area. If both the technique fails, we prefer antegrade snare technique if suitable collateral is available. Next, we use retrograde buddy wire followed by retrograde snare technique to deliver the LV lead in the target vein antegradely. In case of prolapse of the lead into the CS during attempt to cross the proximal tortuous segment of the target vein we like to use balloon-facilitated LV lead delivery. If everything fails, we consider advancement of the lead retrogradely over the retrograde wire after gentle balloon dilatation of the collateral. If this also fails, we take help from our surgical colleagues for epicardial LV lead implantation via mini-thoracotomy and tunneling the lead into the pacemaker pocket.

PLACEMENT OF RV LEAD

Conventionally, in a biventricular pacing, initially the RV lead is placed and fixed in the RV apical region, followed by LV lead placement, as determined by the venous anatomy. Transvenous LV lead placement is dependent on the availability of a vein, and due to the variable coronary venous anatomy, there may not always be a suitable 'major' vein in the region of interest. Several reports have indicated that LV lead placement at an optimal anatomic pacing site (usually defined as the lateral and postero-lateral LV wall) is a critical determinant of short- and long-term outcome.[1] Inter-patient variability in the LV electrical activation sequence, inconsistency of the coronary venous anatomy, as well as need for acceptable pacing parameters, may preclude the attainment of an "optimal" LV pacing site in some patients. This may dictate choosing between a sub-optimal LV site or placing the LV by an open surgical procedure. Selecting a RV pacing site complementary to the chosen LV site can potentially expand the range of "optimal" LV site. The concept of "Dialing-in" RV pacing lead coined by Heist and his colleagues entails initial placement of the LV lead at the most suitable available anatomic site (often dictated by the constraints of coronary sinus anatomy and LV pacing parameters) and then RV site selection over the RV endocardial surface of the inter-ventricular septum to maximize electrical separation of the leads by either RV pacing (and sensing electrical delay in the LV lead) or LV pacing with sensing in the RV lead.[2] With the LV viewed as a clock face in fluoroscopic left anterior oblique projection, the RV lead should be dialed-in along the septal surface at a diametrically opposite site (Fig. 11.14).

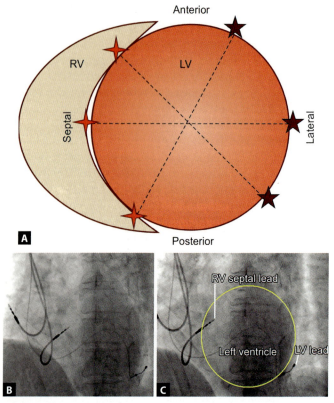

Figs 11.14A and B (A) Cross sectional view of the LV and RV. Red stars present RV pacing sites in relation to diametrically opposite LV lead positions (black stars) along the lateral wall, maximizing the physical distance of the leads in the LV short axis. (B) RV septal lead position in the anterior part of the interventricular septum in a patient with CRT with LV lead positioned in the posterolateral vein in left anterior oblique view

Abbreviations: LV, left ventricle; RV, right ventricle.

Although in some cases maximal physical inter-lead separation may not translate into maximal electrical delay, it is intuitive that physically distant LV and RV sites may have greater electrical separation. This may not hold true in scarred myocardium, and the most electrically distant RV lead position may not be always be diametrically opposite. Lucie R and his colleagues from Czech Republic have shown that septal positioning of the RV lead during cardiac resynchronisation therapy appears to promote reverse LV remodeling (a significant reduction in LVEDD) over 12 months of follow-up. This suggests that additional clinical benefit of cardiac resynchronization therapy can be achieved through the placement of the RV lead in septal location.[2] The SEPTAL-CRT trial (prospective, multicenter, randomized trial) has also demonstrated the non-inferiority of the mid-septal location of the RV lead as compared to the conventional apical location in CRT patients on left ventricular reverse remodeling.[3] However, Khan and his colleagues have shown that the extent of left ventricular reverse remodeling following CRT is not related to the RV lead position, but is significantly higher in patients with a concordant LV lead (LV lead in the latest activated region of the left ventricle).[4]

ANATOMICAL INTER-LEAD DISTANCE

A number of variables including pattern of mechanical dyssynchrony, etiology of heart failure, and site of left ventricle (LV) stimulation[1] have been investigated as predictors of response. With regard to site of LV stimulation, a posterolateral or lateral branch of the coronary venous system generally provides the most optimal pacing site. Maximized physical electrode separation (the distance between LV and RV lead) has been advocated to improve outcomes. Different investigators have evaluated inter-lead distance on postoperative chest X-ray in lateral view and posteroanterior view to find out the relationship between the inter-lead distance and response to CRT. Merchant and co-workers found a positive correlation between inter-lead horizontal distance in lateral view and the inter-lead electrical delay (electrical distance) and acute response to CRT, but not with the vertical distance measured in the posteroanterior view which actually has a negative correlation.[5] Heist and co-workers also described the correlation between horizontal inter-lead distance in the lateral projection with acute response to CRT (Fig. 11.15).[6]

But, none of the above studies have advocated absolute value of inter-lead distance above which there is good response to CRT. However, in lateral view horizontal inter-electrode distance corrected with C/T ratio (cardiothoracic ratio) of more than 9 cm (13.4 ± 5.5 cm) suggests good anatomical separation of the leads.

Echocardiographic projections in parasternal short axis correlates with fluoroscopic left anterior oblique (LAO) view and parasternal long axis view correlates with fluoroscopic right anterior oblique (RAO) view. Neither fluoroscopy nor echocardiography guided measured inter-lead distance correlate with response to CRT. Zoppo and his colleagues showed that the inter-lead anatomical distance measured in either LAO or RAO during implantation do not predict positive reverse remodeling in CRT patients. They have measured the distance with a radiopaque ruler with the centimeter scale positioned over the patient's chest.[7] In my opinion we should look at the interelectrode distance in left lateral (LL) view during implant procedure. The tip to ring distance of the RA or RV lead can be used as reference distance (Fig. 11.16). However, anatomic variations such as rotation of the heart can alter the true intracardiac location of the LV lead compared

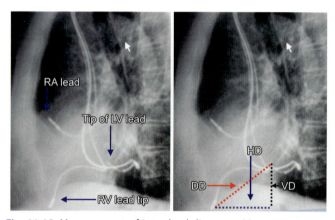

Fig. 11.15 Measurement of inter-lead distances. Measurements are performed on lateral (left) chest radiographs. Inter-lead dimensions are measured as horizontal (HD), vertical (VD), and direct (DD) on radiograph. All inter-lead distances are divided by cardiothoracic ratio obtained from posteroanterior chest radiograph to correct for differences in body habitus

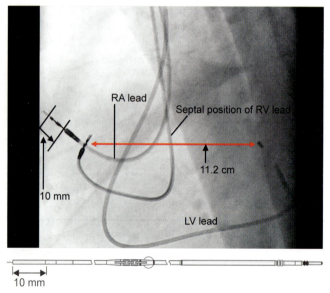

Fig. 11.16 Measurement of inter-lead distance in fluoroscopic left lateral view. The tip to ring distance of a medtronic screw-in lead is 10 mm. keeping it as reference the inter-lead distance in this case is 11.2 cm which seems to be a good anatomical separation

with the perceived location as visualized on chest radiography or fluoroscopy.

ELECTRICAL INTER-LEAD DISTANCE

The first fragmentation or notching of the QRS complex on the 12-lead surface ECG represents the first sign of LV activation. Left ventricular activation time (LVAT) is calculated by subtracting the time until first notch from the total QRS duration. We can measure LV_{sense}-QR_{Send}, using both the surface ECG and LV lead intracardiac electrogram (EGM): LV_{sense}-QR_{Send} represents the duration of LV depolarization starting from local LV depolarization at the site of the LV lead (dominant peak on LV EGM) to the end of the QRS complex. On the other hand, Q-LV_{sense} represents the timing of local LV depolarization on EGM measured from start of the QRS complex, and RV_{sense}-LV_{sense} represents the timing difference between local RV and local LV activation on the ventricular EGMs (Fig. 11.17).

Intraprocedural aspects of lead placement, including anatomic lead position and lead proximity to scar tissue and region of mechanical dyssynchrony play an important role in determining the response to CRT. The electrical activation pattern is different among patients with similar left bundle branch configurations, suggesting that an optimal anatomic site may not be reflective of the site with maximal electrical delay or mechanical dyssynchrony.

A study by Singh and his colleagues indicates that pacing from a site with more delayed electrical activation is associated with a beneficial acute hemodynamic and echocardiographic response in patients with nonischemic cardiomyopathy.[8] They have shown that LV lead electrical delay (Q-LV_{sense}) **greater than half the width of the baseline QRS** is associated with a beneficial long-term outcome in patients receiving CRT. A group of investigators have shown that the **Q-LV_{sense} ≥ 95 msec** predict reverse remodeling in patients receiving CRT.[9]

The presence of complete LBBB and longer Q-LV_{sense} at baseline, and biventricular electrical resynchronization during CRT predicts higher acute hemodynamic response. Singh and his colleagues in a study have shown that the positioning of the LV lead in an area with widest LV_{sense}-QRS predicts most favorable long-term clinical effects.[8] The difference of the RV–LV inter-lead electrical delays measured during RV and LV pacing at the positioned ventricular leads is identified as independent predictor of LV reverse remodeling.[10] RV–LV interval during pacing is a very attractive intraprocedural parameter for optimizing RV–LV lead pacing site configuration and can predict mid-term CRT response. However, changing

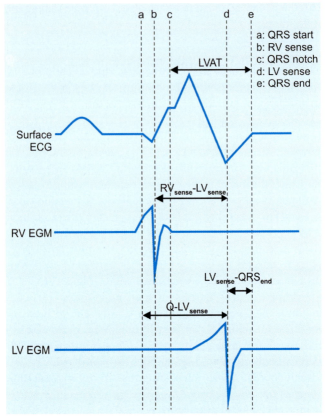

Fig. 11.17 Schematic representation of baseline time interval measurements

Abbreviations: EGM, intracardiac electrogram; LVAT, left ventricular activation time; LV, left ventricular; RV, right ventricular.

LV lead position to different sites during implantation to find site of largest electrical delay is not possible always. So, our practice involves initial placement of the LV lead at the most suitable anatomical site, often dictated by the coronary sinus anatomy and LV pacing parameters, and then subsequent RV site selection based on the obtained LV site. After LV lead placement, the RV endocardial surface of the interventricular septum as well as apex is probed with the RV lead to maximize electrical separation of the leads by RV pacing and sensing the electrical delay in the LV lead. Figure 11.18 shows the measurement of LV electrical delay in a patient during sinus rhythm. Figure 11.19 shows the differences in electrical delay on the LV lead in the same patient after RV pacing from RV apical site and then RV anterior septum. In this case, changing the site of RV pacing altered the activation pattern and extent of delay on the LV lead.

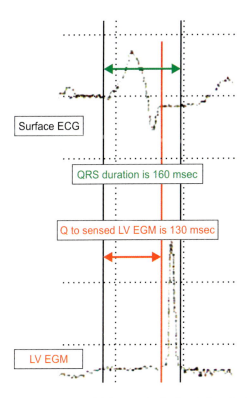

Fig. 11.18 Measurement of left ventricular lead electrical delay = (interval between beginning of surface QRS to sensed LV EGM/QRS duration) × 100%. In this case QRS duration is 160 msec and Q-LV$_{sense}$ is 130 msec. So, the electrical delay is 81% (value of more than 50% is a predictor of favorable outcome)

Pacing the RV apex produced greater delay than pacing the RV anterior septum when measured at a posterolateral region of the LV. Of note, electrical delay can also be different depending on the position of the LV lead (apical vs mid vs basal) in a given coronary sinus branch.

ALTERNATIVE TECHNIQUES

The optimal placement of a LV lead is one of the most challenging technical aspects of CRT device implantation and it is one of the major determinants of response to CRT. The final position of the LV pacing lead depends on the anatomy of the CS, the performance and stability of the pacing lead, and the absence of phrenic nerve stimulation. Despite all of the available technologies and the placement techniques, the rate of failed LV lead implantation into the suitable CS side branch or the risk of late lead dislodgement, phrenic nerve stimulation,

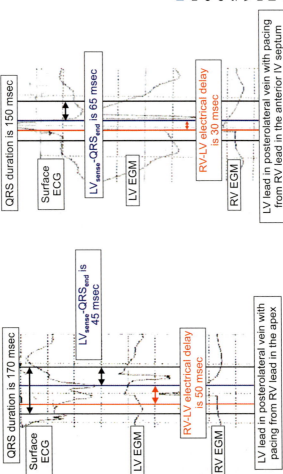

Fig. 11.19 Intracardiac electrocardiograms and measurement of electrical delay. The top row of each electrogram shows surface QRS of the RV paced beat from either the apical region or anterior part of interventricular septum. In this case LV_{sense}-QRS_{end} duration is lesser in patient with RV apical pacing than the RV septal pacing (65 vs 45 msec) and RV-LV inter-lead electrical delay greater with RV apical pacing (50 vs 30 msec respectively) suggesting a greater delay, when paced from the apex

or increasing threshold remains a substantial complication of transvenous CRT. Numerous techniques and technologies have been specifically developed to provide alternatives for the CS LV pacing. The alternative approaches can be epicardial or endocardial LV pacing site, and closed chest/percutaneous or open chest.

Transvenous lead placement in the CS side branch results in epicardial pacing, which is less physiological, reversing the pattern of the normal LV wall activation. Endocardial biventricular pacing results in better LV filling and systolic performance.[11] Epicardial pacing may be more proarrhythmic than endocardial LV pacing, since epicardial activation of the LV wall prolongs QT interval and transmural dispersion of repolarization.[12]

EPICARDIAL PACING TECHNIQUES

Currently, the open chest access epicardial lead placement is most frequently used as a second choice by either thoracotomy or video-assisted thoracoscopy (VAT). The advantage of this approach is the direct visual control with the possibility of choosing the lead-tip position. The risks of lead dislodgement and phrenic nerve stimulation are low and there is no limitation of the CS anatomy. Less fluoroscopy and avoidance of intravenous contrast material are also benefits over conventional CRT.[13] Surgical epicardial LV lead placement has several disadvantages such as the need for general anesthesia, the presence of epicardial fat, adhesions, and it is more invasive than the transvenous approaches. The surgical trauma and the recovery time are appreciably higher than the transvenous LV lead implantation. Finally, surgical implanted epicardial leads have a significantly higher failure rate than those of CS and transvenous right heart leads. There are several surgical approaches to implant the LV pacing lead. Median sternotomy is used at planned coronary artery bypass graft surgery and at valve repair or replacement. The full left thoracotomy offers the widest accessibility of the lateral LV wall; however, at present it is less applied. The minimal thoracotomy (mini-thoracotomy) offers better survival and a lower incidence of mediastinitis or osteomyelitis. Nowadays, the epicardial LV lead is implanted surgically, often through a small left thoracotomy, and two other technologies are increasingly used: VAT techniques and robotic surgery.

Mini-thoracotomy

Under general anesthesia via a lateral mini-thoracotomy LV lead implantation is performed on the beating heart. In the left fourth or fifth intercostal space at mid-axillary level by a 4- to 5-cm incision the access to the pericardium is achieved and the pericardium is opened anterior to the phrenic nerve. The lead is placed on the target area and the proximal end of the lead is tunneled sub-muscular to the provisional pocket after testing and connected to the device. Chest tube drainage is started postoperatively and can be discontinued within 48 hours. This is a safe technique with a very low complication rate.

Video Assisted Thoracoscopy

This offers less postoperative pain and requires smaller incisions without compromising visualization. In the fourth or fifth intercostal space along the anterior and mid-axillary line using two or three incisions (used for ports) under general anesthesia with single-lung ventilation and standard monitoring on the beating heart the procedure is performed. Under visual control, the pericardium is opened laterally to phrenic nerve, the obtuse marginal artery as landmark help to identify the desired site, and an epicardial lead is screwed into the targeted wall region of the LV. After transesophageal echocardiography (TEE) control and the pacing threshold test, the proximal end of the lead passed through the medial incision and is tunneled subcutaneously to the pocket. The VAT approach is a feasible and safe alternative and is well tolerated with minimal postoperative recovery.

Robotically Assisted Surgery

This technique results in more precise LV lead placement on the ventricular wall and significantly reduces postoperative morbidity and the length of hospitalization. This approach also needs general anesthesia, single-lung ventilation, standard monitoring, and TEE control. The robotic camera and instruments are introduced through 5–10-mm port sites. Using the robotic arms, the pericardium is opened posterior to the phrenic nerve to expose the posterolateral wall of the LV. Computer interfacing allows the scaled motion, eliminates tremor, and provides incredibly accurate surgical precision. A screw-in lead is passed into the chest and is secured to the heart using robotic arms. The proximal part is tunneled to the axillary region and is connected to the pacemaker. The minimally invasive robotic approach to epicardial LV lead placement is associated with 98% acute technical success rate and can be performed with a low complication rate.[14] However, the use of robotic surgery is restricted largely by cost implications as the epicardial LV lead fixation on the heart with a robotic arm needs special equipments and the risk of lead dislocation increases without this equipment.

ENDOCARDIAL PACING TECHNIQUES

Transseptal Endocardial LV Lead Implantation

The placement of a transseptal LV endocardial lead requires the puncture of the interatrial septum, to allow the passage of the lead from the right to the left atrium before entering the left ventricle through the mitral valve. Transseptal LV endocardial lead implantation can be accomplished by 3 ways:

Initially the inter-atrial septum is punctured using transfemoral venous approach using Brokenbrough needle. The left atrial end of the guide-wire is snared by a loop advanced from the jugular vein. Then a long sheath is introduced into the left atrium over the guide-wire, and the stimulation lead is advanced through the sheath. Finally, the lead is tunneled over the clavicle. It increases the risk of lead damage and skin erosion and the procedure is little cumbersome. Recently, the implanters are using the steerable introducer catheter sheath (Select Site) to enter from the right atrium to left atrium over a 0.035" wire through the dilated (8F dilator used during PTMC procedure) puncture site. Having gained access to the left atrium, the steerable introducer is advanced from left atrium and across mitral valve orifice into LV. The steerable introducer is orientated towards a pacing location on the posterior high lateral aspect of the LV endocardial wall.[15,16]

Some operators repuncture the IAS from the left axillary vein using a manually shaped transseptal needle using a guide wire placed in the LA through an IAS puncture from the right femoral vein as a fluoroscopic marker. An alternative technique is to pass the guide wire across the IAS puncture through a Judkins right or internal mammary catheter from the left or right subclavian vein. These techniques allow more flexibility for the upper body venous access used for transseptal endocardial LV lead placement. All of these techniques require TEE guidance.

Major advantages are:
- Transvenous access
- More lead placement sites
- Endocardial pacing
- No need to compromise in LV pacing threshold for positional stability or phrenic nerve stimulation.

Major limitations are the lack of reliable long-term safety data and difficulty of the necessary techniques. However, the major concerns are:
- The long-term risk of thromboembolic complication requiring life-long oral anti-coagulation

- Mitral valve endocarditis related to permanent presence of the transmitral LV lead from the RA
- Risk of mitral valve regurgitation due to the presence of the lead across the valve
- Long-term lead integrity (as it is placed in the systemic circulation it is exposed to high shear stress)
- Technical difficulty.

Trans-apical Endocardial LV Lead Implantation

This technique combines the minimal invasive surgical approach and the advantage of endocardial pacing. A small pericardiotomy is performed above the LV apex and a standard active fixation endocardial pacing lead is positioned in the LV cavity through the apex using the Seldinger technique with a peel-way sheath under fluoroscopy guidance under general anesthesia. To reach the target area (optimal pacing site) a "J"-shaped electrode guide-wire is used. Thin commercially available bipolar pacing electrodes are used. The advantage of this minimally invasive technique is the best accessibility of the all LV endocardial segments without the limitations of the anatomy to reach the most delayed segment of the lateral wall.[17] A potential disadvantage is the long-term oral anticoagulation with a target international normalized ratio level of 2–3 to avoid the risk of thromboembolic complication. A recently published study confirms that the trans-apical technique for endocardial CRT is a feasible approach and has potential advantages such as shorter procedure times and a decreased postoperative burden. Lead longevity and long-term outcome requires a lengthy follow-up and large-scale evaluation. The idea of using this method as a second and not as third-line therapy also requires further investigation.

Trans-arterial Endocardial LV Lead Implantation

Access is through the **subclavian or axillary artery** and retrogradely through the aortic valve. However, major concerns are stability of the lead and the need for long-term anticoagulation. Although, the feasibility and safety of deliberately implanting a transaortic LV lead from the right carotid artery has been studied in a pig model.[18] After 6 months of stimulation, and despite the absence of anticoagulation, no thromboembolic complication was observed; aortic insufficiency, when present, remained trivial; and no aortic valve lesion was found on postmortem examination. But, the long-term risk and effects of implanting a lead across the aortic valve have not been ascertained in humans, in whom a subclavian or axillary instead of a carotid approach is probably be the preferred approach.

REFERENCES

1. Ansalone G, Giannantoni P, Ricci R, et al. Doppler myocardial imaging to evaluate the effectiveness of pacing sites in patients receiving biventricular pacing. JACC. 2002;39:489-98.
2. Heist EK, Ruskin JN, et al. "Dialing-in" cardiac resynchronization therapy: overcoming constraints of the coronary venous anatomy. J Interv Card Electrophysiol. 2006;17:51-8.
3. Lucie R, Josef Kautzner, et al. Optimization of right ventricular lead position in cardiac resynchronisation therapy, European Journal of Heart Failure. 2006;8:609-14.
4. Fakhar Z Khan, Pegah Salahshouri, et al. The impact of the right ventricular lead position on response to cardiac resynchronization therapy. PACE. 2011;34:467-74.
5. Merchant FM, Heist EK, Nandigam KV, Mulligan LJ, Blendea D, et al. Inter-lead distance and left ventricular lead electrical delay predicts reverse remodeling during cardiac resynchronization therapy. Pacing Clin Electrophysiol. 2010;33:575-82.
6. Heist EK, Fan D, Mela T, Arzola-Castaner D, Reddy VY, et al. Radiographic left ventricular-right ventricular inter-lead distance predicts the acute hemodynamic response to cardiac resynchronization therapy. Am J Cardiol. 2005;96:685-90.
7. Zoppo F, Berton A, Zerbo F, Frigato N, Michieletto M, et al. Pacing Inter-lead Fluoroscopic RAO and LAO Distance and Cardiac Resynchronization Therapy Response. J Clin Exp Cardiolog. 2014;5:336.
8. Singh JP, Fan D, Heist EK, Alabiad CR, Taub C, Reddy V, Mansour M, et al. Left ventricular lead electrical delay predicts response to cardiac resynchronization therapy. Heart Rhythm. 2006;3:1285-92.
9. Margot D Bogaard, Tim hesselink, Mathias meine, et al. The ECG in cardiac resynchronization therapy: influence of left and right ventricular pre-activation and relation to acute response. J Cardiovasc Electrophysiol. 2012;23:1237-45.
10. Biagio S, Luca G, Luigi P, Barold SS, et al. Value of right ventricular–left ventricular inter-lead electrical delay to predict reverse remodeling in cardiac resynchronization therapy: The INTER-V pilot study. Europace. 2010;12:78-83.
11. Garrigue S, Jais P, Espil G, Labeque JN, Hocini M, Shah DC, Haïssaguerre M, et al. Comparison of chronic biventricular pacing between epicardial and endocardial left ventricular stimulation using Doppler tissue imaging in patients with heart failure. Am J Cardiol. 2001;88:858-62.
12. Fish JM, Di Diego JM, Nesternko V, Antzelevitch C. Epicardial activation of left ventricular wall prolongs QT interval and transmural dispersion of repolarization: Implications for biventricular pacing. Circulation. 2004;109:2136-42.
13. Patwala A, Woods P, Clements R, Albouaini K, Rao A, Goldspink D, Tan LB, et al. A prospective longitudinal evaluation of the benefits

of epicardial lead placement for cardiac resynchronization therapy. Europace. 2009;11:1323-9.
14. DeRose JJ, Ashton RC, Belsley S, Swistel DG, Vloka M, Ehlert F, Shaw R, et al. Robotically assisted left ventricular epicardial lead implantation for biventricular pacing. J Am Coll Cardiol. 2003;41:1414-9.
15. Jais P, Douard H, Shah DC, Barold S, Barat JL, Clementy J. Endocardial biventricular pacing. Pacing Clin Electrophysiol. 1998;21:2128-31.
16. Jais P, Takahashi A, Garrigue S, Yamane T, Hocini M, Shah DC et al. Mid-term follow-up of endocardial biventricular pacing. Pacing Clin Electrophysiol. 2000;23:1744-7.
17. Mihalcz A, Kassai I, Kardos A, Foldesi C, Theuns D, Szili-Torok T. Comparison of the efficacy of two surgical alternatives for cardiac resynchronization therapy: Trans-apical versus epicardial left ventricular pacing. Pacing Clin Electrophysiol. 2012;35:124-30.
18. Reinig M, White M, Levine M, et al. Left ventricular endocardial pacing: a trans-arterial approach. Pacing Clin Electrophysiol. 2007;30:1464-8.

CHAPTER 12

Surface Electrocardiography: CRT Follow up

INTRODUCTION

The 12-lead surface ECG is an indispensable part of device evaluation and troubleshooting in patients with cardiac resynchronization therapy. During follow-up of CRT systems, the 12-lead electrocardiogram (ECG) is essential to ascertain the native QRS, right ventricle (RV) and left ventricle (LV) stimulation configuration, presence of biventricular stimulation with complete capture, presence of fusion between native activation and pacing capture during biventricular stimulation, presence of anodal capture with biventricular stimulation. Ventricular pacing thresholds should ideally be checked independently and in the VVI mode, at a rate exceeding the prevailing ventricular rate, so as to obtain continuous ventricular capture without fusion. Alternatively, thresholds can be performed in the VDD or DDD mode at very short AV delays (e.g. 50% of PR interval), to ensure full ventricular capture without fusion. In general, it is advisable to initiate threshold determinations at maximum output (voltage and pulse duration), because there is often a significant difference in capture thresholds between RV and LV.

ECG OF RIGHT VENTRICULAR PACING IN CRT

Right ventricular apex is located to the right, inferior, and anterior to the left ventricle. So, pacing at RV apex causes positive deflections in I (left lead), aVR, and aVL (superior lead) and negative paced QRS complex in the inferior leads (III is often more negative than II), simply because the activation starts in the inferior part of the heart and travels superiorly, away from the inferior leads. V1 is a right anterior lead and is therefore negative (left bundle-branch block). V5 and V6 (left lateral leads) can be positive in distinctive ways. The mean QRS frontal plane axis is superior either in the left or right superior quadrant. In cases of very apical pacing or a greatly enlarged and deformed right ventricle, and in cases of pacing in a right ventricular outflow tract positioned far to the left, V1 can be positive. Pacing from the RV outflow tract produces a frontal plane axis that is "normal," meaning inferiorly directed (positive QRS in inferior leads) (Fig. 12.1).

A **dominant R wave in V1** (R/S > 1) during right ventricular pacing (often called as right bundle branch block pattern) reflects activation moving from the posterior to the anterior part of the heart and it does not seem related to RV activation delay. The following are possible causes of a dominant R wave in lead V1 (occurs in about 10–20% of cases) during conventional RV pacing:

- Ventricular fusion.
- Inadvertent positioning of the lead into a branch of coronary sinus.
- Lead perforation of the RV or ventricular septum with LV stimulation.
- Uncomplicated RV pacing (lead V1 recorded too high or in the correct place).

A tall R wave extending to V3 and V4 signifies that a pacemaker lead is in all likelihood not in the RV. During RV apical pacing the frontal plane axis points superiorly mostly to the left but it points to the right (superior quadrant) when RV is paced in RVOT mid-septum and thus produces a **negative QRS complex in lead I.** Thus, an ECG of uncomplicated RV pacing with a dominant R wave in lead V1 and a right superior frontal plane axis can closely resemble that from a biventricular pacemaker. A small early r wave (sometimes wide) may occasionally occur in lead V1 during uncomplicated RV apical or outflow tract pacing. There is no evidence that this r wave represents a conduction abnormality at the RV exit site. Furthermore, an initial r wave during biventricular pacing does not predict initial LV activation.

ECG of Left Ventricular Pacing from the Coronary Venous System

LV pacing from a correctly positioned lead in the coronary venous system (lateral or posterolateral veins) invariably produced an RBBB pattern in lead V1 a rightward axis, similar to maximal ventricular pre-excitation over a left-sided accessory pathway (Fig. 12.2). LV pacing from the coronary venous system that generates a positive complex in lead V1 may not necessarily be accompanied by a positive QRS complex in leads V2 and V3. With apical sites, leads V4–V6 are typically negative. With basal locations, leads V4–V6 are usually positive as with the concordant positive R waves during overt pre-excitation in left sided accessory pathway conduction in the Wolff–Parkinson–White syndrome.

RV apical pacing

The frontal plane axis usually left superior. It may also be in the right superior quadrant, where it causes leads I, II and III to be negative and lead aVR to show the largest positive deflection.

Two patterns are possible:

A. A typical LBBB pattern in the left precordial leads may not be present and all leads show a QS pattern

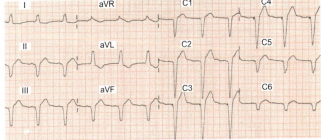

B. The left precordial leads may show a dominant R wave

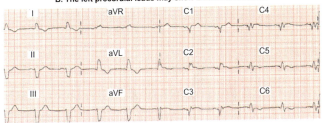

RV outflow tract pacing

The frontal plane axis is normal, i.e. as for normally conducted beats
But as the lead moves towards the pulmonary valve, the axis becomes deviated to the right
A qR pattern can occur only in lead I and aVL
However, true RVOT septal pacing causes dominant negative QRS in aVL

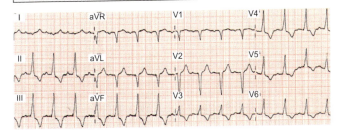

Fig. 12.1 Electrocardiographic QRS patterns during pacing of the right ventricle (RV) from different sites
Abbreviation: LBBB, left bundle branch block

In an occasional patient with uncomplicated LV pacing with a typical RBBB pattern in lead V1, the axis may point to the left inferior or left superior quadrant. The exact reasons for these unusual axis locations are not known. A RBBB pattern may not be seen if leads V1 and V2 are recorded too high, or with unsuspected RV and LV lead reversal when programming only the LV output. The ECGs of a cardiac resynchronization therapy (CRT) patient may sometimes produce two different

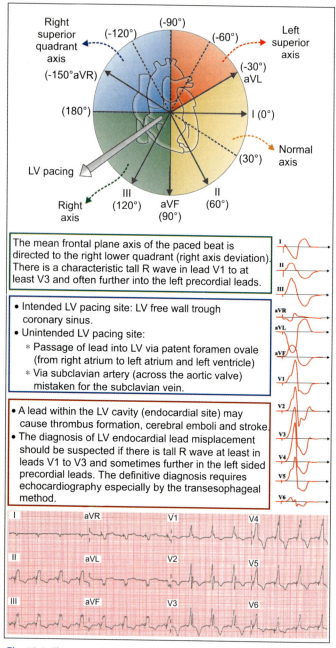

Fig. 12.2 Electrocardiographic QRS patterns during free wall pacing of the left ventricle (LV)

morphologies at two different rates, probably due to delay or the emerging LV impulse in a region of scarring particularly in ischemic cardiomyopathy.[1]

Due to the anatomy of the coronary sinus and its lateral branches, the ECG pattern varies widely depending on the pacing site. Pacing in the area of inferior branches (the middle cardiac vein, which runs parallel to the posterior descending artery (and is also called "posterior" in the old nomenclature) leads to an excitation from inferior to superior and thus to negative deflections in lead II, III, and aVF. Lead I can be isoelectric or negative, depending on whether the pacing is more septal or posteroinferior.

An ECG pattern of LBBB during ventricular pacing from the coronary venous system strongly suggests that the pacing site be either in the great cardiac vein (GCV) or middle cardiac vein (MCV). However, the occurrence of intermittent LBBB and RBBB paced patterns soon after implantation of a lead in the MCV suggests that movement of an unstable lead can produce an RBBB pattern proximally and an LBBB pattern more distally in the MCV. Superior pacing (also called "anterior" in the old nomenclature) or pacing from the great cardiac vein (GCV) (runs parallel to the left anterior descending artery) results in excitation propagation from superior to inferior regions. This can show a RBBB pattern in lead V1 with frontal plane axis deviation to the right inferior quadrant. The inferior limb leads are therefore positive (similar to pacing in the RV outflow tract). The right axis suggests a proximal site as it traverses the basal LV near the septum. In contrast, more distal GCV pacing produced an LBBB pattern possible by the capability of positioning contemporary LV leads more distally in the GCV than in the past.[2] Pacing in the area of the posterior and posteroinferior branches (also called "lateral" and "posterolateral" in the old nomenclature) lead to excitation propagation from left to right. I, aVL, V5 and V6 are therefore negative. While the inferior limb leads are negative during posteroinferior pacing, III can become positive during posterior or posterosuperior. Lead I is negative, especially in the case of pacing in the more postero-superior positioned side branches. Negative deflections in V4–V6 point to more anterior pacing, i.e. pacing close to the apex, and these leads tend to be more positive with pacing close to the base. According to an algorithm by Ploux and his colleagues, the first step is the analysis of the QRS morphology in V1. A positive R wave in V1 suggests lateral or posterior LV free wall stimulation. During biventricular stimulation, most of the anterior LV leads are associated with no positive deflection in V1. Therefore, a QS pattern is specific of an anterior LV lead position. An inferior lead position and a minority of leads in an anterior position are associated with an R wave in V1. Therefore in presence of an R wave in V1, one has to analyze V6 to separate inferior from anterior LV stimulation. Inferior LV leads are never associated with a positive V6. To distinguish a lateral from a posterior position, one has to analyze the QRS in V2. In a majority of patients, lateral wall stimulation is associated with an R wave in V1 and a negative complex in V2. In contrast, posterior wall stimulation was associated with an R wave in both V1 and V2. aVL is usually mostly negative when the lateral LV wall is stimulated, whereas an inferior lead location is exclusively associated with an R wave in this lead (Fig. 12.3).[3]

ECG Patterns and Follow-up of Biventricular Pacemakers

Usually **QRS duration** shortens with biventricular stimulation. There may be little correlation between the degree of QRS shortening after CRT and hemodynamic benefit and/or the clinical response.[4] In some cases, the QRS complex after CRT may actually lengthen or remain unchanged despite substantial improvement in mechanical LV dyssynchrony. Increased QRS duration with CRT does not necessarily reflect the presence of ventricular areas with slow conduction resulting in more heterogeneous myocardial activation. With mono-chamber LV pacing there is an obvious discrepancy between QRS

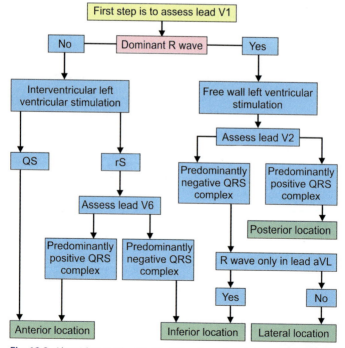

Fig. 12.3 Algorithm to identify the LV lead location. (+) = predominantly positive QRS complex; (−) = predominantly negative QRS complex

duration (compared with baseline) and hemodynamic and clinical improvement. Some patients with mono-chamber LV pacing exhibit an equal or superior degree of mechanical resynchronization compared to biventricular pacing despite a very wide paced QRS complex.[5] Thus, in congestive heart failure patients the paced QRS duration cannot be assumed to reflect a more heterogeneous propagation pattern of LV activation and prolonged duration of mechanical activation. The QRS morphologies during biventricular pacing are highly variable and often deviate significantly from classic bundle branch block. Herweg and his colleagues have classified the QRS morphology in lead V1 as predominantly positive, balanced or negative (Fig. 12.4).[6] A positive R wave (R/S > 1) during simultaneous biventricular pacing almost always indicates successful early LV capture. Also a balanced QRS complex in lead V1 likely indicates both LV and RV activation with sufficient myocardial depolarization via the LV lead stimulation. Patients who exhibit a predominantly negative QRS complex in lead V1 (particularly a QS complex) causes potential problem.

A negative QRS complex in lead V1 may indicate poor LV contribution with predominantly RV activation. The probable reasons are fusion with spontaneous right bundle branch activation, delayed or latent LV activation, poor LV lead position, and LV noncapture. The electrocardiographic diagnosis of these conditions is important because all of them can be associated with a poor clinical response to CRT.

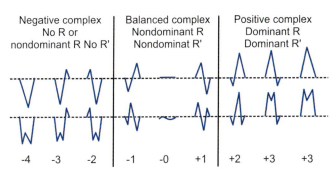

Fig. 12.4 QRS morphology in lead V1 is classified as predominantly negative, balanced, or positive. This schematic shows individual QRS morphologies encountered during CRT. Morphology scores (ranging from −4 to +4) are assigned according to negativity or positivity of the individual QRS complexes. Each QRS complex falls into one of three categories: Predominantly negative (−4, −3, −2), balanced (−1, 0, +1), or positive (+2, +3, +4) QRS complex

Biventricular Pacing with the RV Lead Located at the Apex

The frontal plane QRS axis usually moves superiorly from the left (RV apical pacing) to the right superior quadrant (biventricular pacing) in an anticlockwise fashion if the ventricular mass is predominantly depolarized by the LV pacing lead (Fig. 12.5). The frontal plane axis may occasionally reside in the left superior rather than the right superior quadrant during uncomplicated biventricular pacing.

The QRS complex is often positive in lead V1 during biventricular pacing when the RV is paced from the apex. A

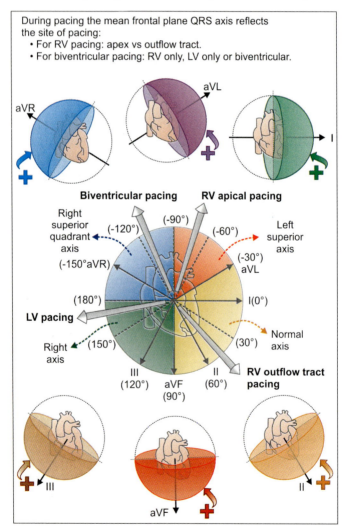

Fig. 12.5 Mean QRS axis in the frontal plane during ventricular pacing. *Abbreviations:* LV, left ventricle; RV, right ventricle. (*Courtesy:* Barold SS, Stroobandt RX, Sinnaeve AF. Cardiac Pacemakers Step by Step. An Illustrated Guide. Malden: Blackwell-Futura, 2004 with permission)

negative paced QRS complex in lead V1 during CRT with RV apical pacing may occur in the following circumstances:
- Incorrect placement of lead V1 (too high on the chest)
- Lack of LV capture
- LV lead displacement, marked LV latency[7]
- Marked delay in the local propagation of LV activation from the stimulation site (with or without abnormal latency)
- Ventricular fusion with the conducted QRS complex
- Coronary venous pacing via the middle cardiac vein (also the anterior cardiac vein)
- Even unintended placement of two leads in the RV.

A negative QRS complex in lead V1 during uncomplicated biventricular pacing probably reflects different activation of a heterogeneous biventricular substrate (ischemia, scar, His-Purkinje participation in view of the varying patterns of LV activation in spontaneous LBBB, etc.) and does not necessarily indicate a poor (electrical or mechanical) contribution from LV stimulation. This is especially important in the presence of a QS complex suggesting that RV pacing depolarizes most, if not all, of the LV. **Q, or q configuration in lead I and lateral leads** is a rule during biventricular pacing using the RV apex (Fig. 12.6). A Q/q wave (followed by positivity) is rare in lead I during uncomplicated mono-chamber RV apical pacing.

Biventricular Pacing with the RV lead in the Outflow Tract

It has been seen that during biventricular pacing with the RV lead in the septal area or outflow tract, the paced QRS in lead V1 is often negative and the frontal plane paced QRS axis is often directed to the right inferior quadrant (right axis deviation). This may create a problem in troubleshooting because the ECG may resemble that of simple mono-chamber RV septal or outflow tract pacing with a LBBB pattern and right inferior frontal axis deviation thereby mimicking loss of LV pacing. Figure 12.7 shows the importance of the frontal plane axis of the paced QRS complex in determining the arrangement of pacing during mono-chamber and biventricular pacemakers. The shift in the frontal plane QRS axis during programming the ventricular output is helpful in determining the site of ventricular stimulation in patients with first-generation devices without separately programmable RV and LV outputs.

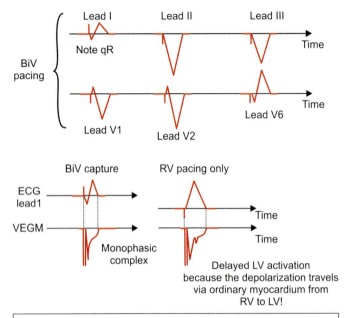

- A change in frontal plane axis may corroborate loss of capture in one ventricle.
- Simultaneous recording of ECG, markers and ventricular electrogram (VEGM) is very helpful.
- Beware of ventricular fusion beats with the conducted spontaneous QRS complex. The absence of fusion is verified by shortening the AV delay whereupon no change in QRS morphology should take place.

- To show ventricular capture in pacemakers with a common output, lower the voltage and/or the pulse width. The left ventricle (LV) will loose capture first in almost all cases because pacing threshold is higher than that of the right ventricle.
- Loss of capture in one ventricle will cause a change in the morphology of the beats in the 12-lead ECG. Examination of a single lead may be misleading.

Fig. 12.6 Analysis of electrocardiographic (ECG) QRS patterns to ascertain right ventricular (RV) and left ventricular (LV) capture in cardiac resynchronization systems without separately programmable ventricular outputs.
Abbreviations: BiV, biventricular; VEGM, ventricular electrogram.
(*Courtesy:* Barold SS, Stroobandt RX, Sinnaeve AF. Cardiac Pacemakers Step by Step. An Illustrated Guide. Malden: Blackwell-Futura, 2004 with permission)

Surface Electrocardiography: CRT Follow up

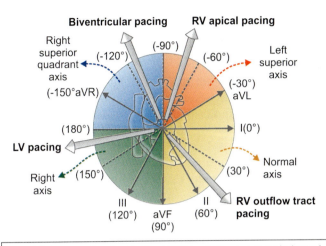

- Establish a template for the best ECG lead showing morphological differences in RV, LV, BiV pacing. Store the pattern and use it for follow-up.
- More than one lead is needed to confirm capture. Lead I and III are often enough. Make sure the leads are properly connected. Consider a 12-lead ECG in all cases.
- Do the thresholds test in DDD mode with a short AV delay or in the VVI mode (if tolerated) at a rate higher than the intrinsic rate.
- When in doubt, start at the maximum output (voltage and pulse width) to ensure pacing of RV and LV.
- Newer devices with separately programmable RV and LV outputs will facilitate ECG interpretation.

Pacing site	QRS in Lead I	QRS in Lead III	Axis shift
BiV→RV	Greater positivity	Greater negativity	Clockwise
BiV→LV	Greater negativity	Greater positivity	Counter clockwise

Fig. 12.7 Diagram showing the usual direction of the mean frontal plane axis during apical right ventricular (RV) pacing, RV outflow tract pacing, left ventricular (LV) pacing from the coronary venous system, biventricular pacing with LV from the coronary venous system + RV from the apex or RV from the outflow tract. Note that the axis during biventricular pacing from the LV from the coronary sinus + RV outflow tract usually points to the right inferior quadrant (right axis) as with mono-chamber LV pacing. The curved arrow indicates that the axis during mono-chamber RVOT pacing can also reside in the right inferior quadrant (*Courtesy:* Barold SS, Stroobandt RX, Sinnaeve AF. Cardiac Pacemakers Step by Step. An Illustrated Guide. Malden: Blackwell-Futura, 2004 with permission)

CASE 1 (FIG. 12.8 TO 12.13)

Combination of pacing from RV apex and posterolateral vein of Coronary Sinus.

The surface ECG will vary in morphology depending on where and how the device is pacing. On Lead I, the QRS morphology will show up positive (upward deflection from baseline) for RV pacing and more or completely negative (downward from baseline) for BV pacing. In fact, on Lead I a BV QRS complex may look almost identical to an inverted RV complex. On Lead III, the LV complex will show up as more positive than the BV, again, sometimes looking like an upside-down version of the same complex. To visualize better why these complexes look the way they do, it is important to review how the electrical energy captured on the ECG is traveling through the heart. BV energy tends to create a more negative morphology on the tracing than either RV pacing alone or LV pacing alone. Because of the way the electrodes are placed, lead I transmit a graphic depiction of what is going on in the right side of the heart, while Lead III shows the same image of the left side.

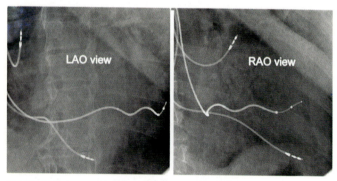

Fig. 12.8 Fluoroscopic left and right anterior oblique view showing RA, RV and LV leads

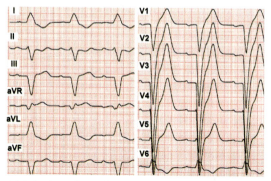

Fig. 12.9 Intrinsic: Sinus rhythm 85/min, PR interval 165 ms, QRS duration 160 ms, left bundle branch block

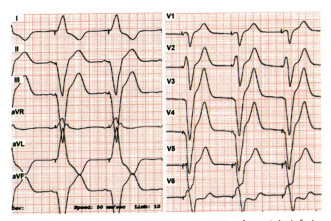

Fig. 12.10 Right ventricular stimulation: Excitation from right inferior
- *Negative:* III, II, aVF (III>II).
- *Positive:* I, aVL, aVR (aVL>aVR).

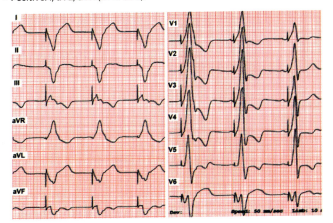

Fig. 12.11 Left ventricular stimulation: Excitation from posterolateral vein
- *Negative:* I, aVL, II (I>aVL).
- *Positive:* III, aVF, aVR, also V1 (III>aVF).

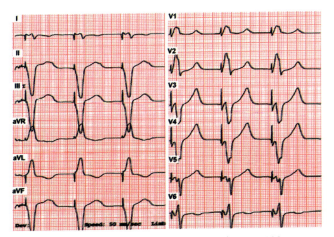

Fig. 12.12 Biventricular stimulation: QRS duration 120 ms:
- LV contribution (*Negative:* I, II. *Positive:* aVR, V1).
- RV contribution (*Negative:* II, III, aVF. *Positive:* aVL, aVR)

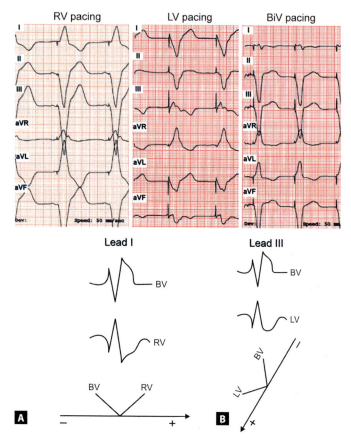

Fig. 12.13 (A) QRS complexes on Lead I. A biventricular (BV) complex shows up as more negative on Lead I than a corresponding right-ventricular (RV) complex. In fact, the BV complex may look like an inverted RV complex. Lead I show mostly right-sided cardiac activity. (B) QRS complexes on Lead III. On Lead III, the waveform depicts what is going on in the left side of the heart. The biventricular (BV) paced QRS complex is more negative than the left-ventricular paced QRS complex. Again, sometimes the BV complex will look like the right ventricular complex upside down

CASE 2 (FIGS 12.14 TO 12.19)

Combination of pacing from RV apex and anterolateral vein of coronary sinus.

ECG during simultaneous biventricular pacing shows fair balanced contribution from both the ventricle. Programming the VV delay to 40 msec (LV followed by RV) causes minimal

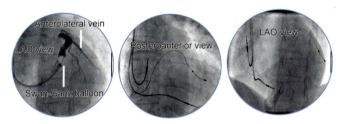

Fig. 12.14 Different fluoroscopic views showing positions of RA, RV, LV leads

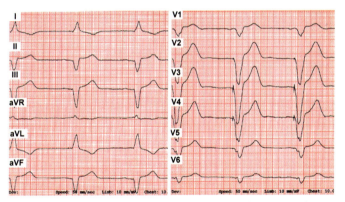

Fig. 12.15 Right ventricular stimulation: Excitation from right inferior
- *Negative:* III, II, aVF (III>II).
- *Positive:* I, aVL, aVR (aVL>aVR).

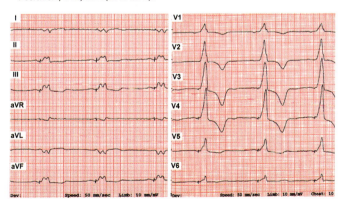

Fig. 12.16 Left ventricular stimulation: Excitation from anterolateral vein
- *Negative:* I, aVL, aVR (I<aVL).
- *Positive:* III, II, aVF, also V1 (II = III).

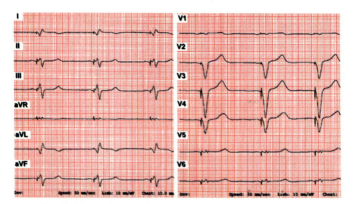

Fig. 12.17 Biventricular stimulation (Simultaneous): QRS duration 125 ms:
- LV contribution (*Negative:* I, aVL, *Positive:* aVR, II, III).
- RV contribution (*Positive:* aVR).

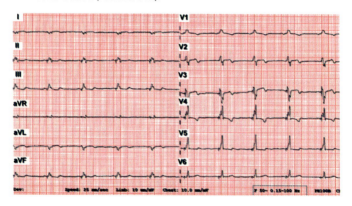

Fig. 12.18 Biventricular stimulation with VV delay of 40 msec (LV followed by RV)

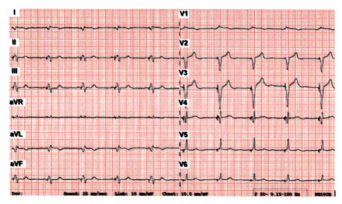

Fig. 12.19 Biventricular delay of 20 msec (LV followed by RV)

contribution from right ventricle and reverse dyssynchrony is evidenced by notching of the QRS complex in the precordial leads. Reducing the delay to 20 msec causes better configuration (QRS width of 115 msec, absence of any notching in the QRS complex and finally little more contribution from the left ventricle as evidenced by prominent R wave in lead V1).

CASE 3 (FIGS 12.20 TO 12.26)

Combination of pacing from RV apex and lateral vein of coronary sinus.

The interval from the pacemaker stimulus to the onset of the earliest paced QRS complex is called **latency.** An isoelectric onset of the QRS complex in one or only a few leads can mimic latency. Consequently, the demonstration of latency requires a 12-lead ECG taken at faster speed for diagnosis. Marked latency is more common with LV than right ventricular (RV) pacing as in LV pacing the activation wave front has to travel from the branch of coronary sinus through the epicardial pad of fat and

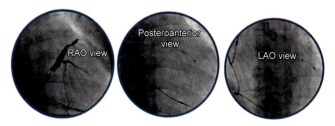

Fig. 12.20 Different fluoroscopic views showing positions of the different leads

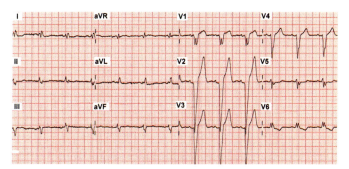

Fig. 12.21 Sinus rhythm ECG shows LBBB with QRS duration of 155 msec with PR interval is 170 msec

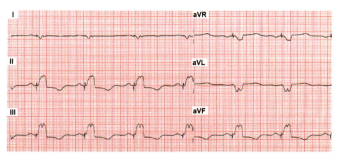

Fig. 12.22 Mono-chamber LV pacing in 6 limb leads show a latency of 40 msec

epicardium to the myocardium. During RV pacing this interval normally measures < 40 msec. At physiologic rates, pronounced latency is uncommon during RV pacing but may be more prevalent during LV pacing because of LV pathology including scars, ischemic myocardium, nonischemic cardiomyopathy, hyperkalemia, and antiarrhythmic drugs. Prolonged LV latency delays LV depolarization during simultaneous biventricular pacing producing an ECG pattern dominated by the pattern of RV pacing with left bundle branch block (LBBB) configuration. In a patient with CRT, we want a balanced contribution from both ventricles towards the cardiac contraction in a timely fashion (Fig. 12.24). Simultaneous biventricular stimulation in an uncomplicated CRT causes undisturbed impulse

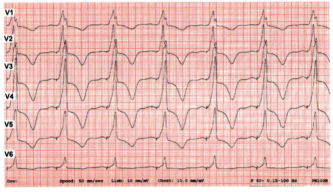

Fig. 12.23 6 precordial leads show lowest latency period of 40 msec

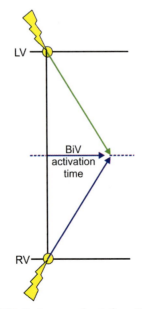

Fig. 12.24 Pacing wave fronts from RV and LV

propagation from both the pacing sites leading to balanced fusion of left and right ventricular wave front and a short biventricular activation time.

Prolonged LV latency intervals during stimulation from within epicardial cardiac veins may be owing to interposed venous tissue and epicardial fat and/or electrode proximity to a scar preventing direct contact between electrode and healthy LV myocardium. Latency may be related to nonhomogeneous impulse propagation from the paced site, conduction block in proximity to the electrode, or prolonged refractoriness. The conventional surface ECG cannot differentiate failure of excitation from delayed propagation in the myocardium around the electrode. The deleterious effects of LV latency can be treated with V-V programming by advancing LV stimulation ahead of RV stimulation.

An increase in the **pacing rate** may prolong the abnormal stimulus to QRS interval during RV and LV stimulation while a prolonged latency interval may be shorten by slowing the pacing rate. An increase in **stimulus amplitude** may shorten the stimulus-QRS interval and a decrease accentuates the latency interval. In this respect, some investigators have shown that increasing the LV stimulus output decreases interventricular conduction time.

Investigations with temporary unipolar LV pacing (anode in the inferior vena cava) have shown that patients with an LV scar or infarction near the pacing site may exhibit a change in paced QRS configuration, a decreased latency interval, shorter QRS duration and conduction time to the RV when the LV output is increased.[9]

Increasing the LV output strength probably works by decreasing the latency interval and/or enlarging the area of myocardial capture beyond a site of conduction block, creating a larger virtual electrode. In patients with implanted CRT devices (unipolar LV lead and anode in the RV proximal electrode), increasing the LV output may also reduce the paced QRS duration, the conduction time from LV to RV and may alter QRS configuration by a combination of RV anodal pacing and a larger virtual electrode effect. A larger virtual electrode may be of particular importance during pacing of diseased myocardium but may be complicated by phrenic nerve stimulation, rapid battery depletion, and RV anodal capture. Bipolar LV leads are needed to show the true impact of increasing the LV output because they are not associated with RV anodal capture.

Prolonged LV latency intervals with delayed LV activation can result in a suboptimal hemodynamic CRT response that is potentially correctable by advancing LV stimulation (before RV stimulation) via a **programmable interventricular (V-V)**

delay. The hemodynamic consequences depend on the difference (delta latency) between right- and left-sided latency intervals during biventricular pacing rather than absolute values. RV anodal stimulation during BiV pacing interferes with a programmed V-V delay (often programmed with the LV preceding the RV) aimed at optimizing CRT because RV anodal capture causes simultaneous RV and LV activation (the V-V interval becomes zero). In patients with a biventricular system using the RV apex and abnormal LV latency, programming of incremental left to right ventricular (V-V) delays can unmask a dominant R wave in lead V1. When the largest offset is insufficient, the RV channel should be turned off to provide better hemodynamics. When attempting to provide better electrocardiographic electrical synchrony by programming the V-V interval, it is important to appreciate that the relationship between the presence and/or amplitude of the paced R wave in lead V1 has not yet been correlated with the best mechanical or hemodynamic response in individual patients.

However, simultaneous biventricular pacing (V-V delay is 0 msec) in this patient results in profound right ventricular contribution with low left ventricular contribution as evidenced by identical QRS morphology in lead V1 with right ventricular pacing. This can happen because either of **profound left ventricular latency or slow left ventricular conduction at the proximity to the stimulation site or combination of both.**

In presence of prolonged left ventricular latency, left ventricular activation occurs late and more myocardium is depolarized by the right ventricular wave front leading to a prolonged biventricular activation time and reduced left ventricular contribution towards cardiac contraction (Fig. 12.25). Slow conduction in the proximity to the LV pacing site due to myocardial fibrosis or scar tissue has similar effect (Fig. 12.25). Both the slow conduction and prolonged left ventricular latency can coexist in some patients. In that case, major portions of the left ventricle are depolarized by the right ventricular wave front with minimal fusion from two pacing sites and further prolongation of the biventricular activation time (Fig. 12.25). Prolonged left ventricular latency can be compensated by pre-exciting the left ventricle with a VV delay (equal to latency period) resulting in a synchronous biventricular activation and a shorter biventricular activation time. The problem of slow conduction can be partially managed by increasing left ventricular pacing output. In case of severe delay, pacing only the left ventricle and allowing fusion with the intrinsic right bundle branch conduction can results in satisfactory result.

In this patient, left ventricular latency is 50 msec (shortest) in lead III and V2. In programming, the V-V delay to 40 msec results in balanced contribution by both the ventricle (Fig. 12.26).

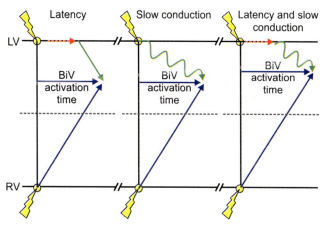

Fig. 12.25 Various patterns of pacing wave front fusion in presence of LV latency and slowed LV conduction

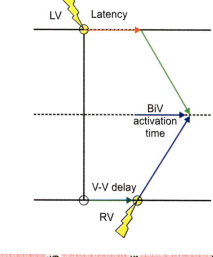

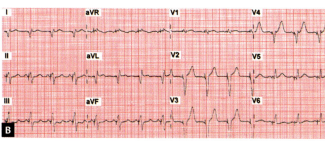

Figs 12.26A and B (A) Fusion of both LV and RV pacing wave front; (B) Biventricular stimulation of VV delay programmed at 40 msec

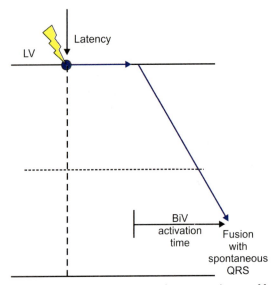

Fig. 12.27 Pacing the LV only may results in some degree of fusion with native conduction

In case of markedly prolonged LV latency interval, pacing the LV only may results in some degree of fusion with native conduction on the right side depending on the programmed atrioventricular delay and may yield satisfactory hemodynamic results (Fig. 12.27). Dual chamber pacemaker with the ventricular lead placed in the suitable CS branch and atrial lead in its proper position and pacing in VDD mode can be also an acceptable alternative in this situation.

CASE 4 (FIGS 12.28 TO 12.30)

A 42-year-old, nondiabetic, normotensive lady presented with idiopathic dilated cardiomyopathy with severe LV systolic dysfunction. Her sinus rhythm ECG shows LBBB.

Characterization of ventricular activation during LBBB: Typical LBBB with dominant R in I and aVL, indicates R → L activation; rS or QS in II, III, aVF, and rS or QS in V1–V3, indicates anterior → posterior activation. In some patients, RS and Rs emerge in V4–V6. Left superior axis is caused by QS in leads II, III, aVF.

Generation of ventricular activation fusion after CRT: Note the reversal of activation by regions which yields a global pattern of ventricular activation fusion [R wave emergence where there were previously S waves; Q, QS, or S wave emergence where

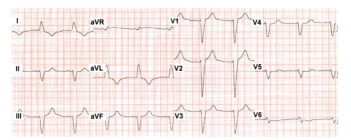

Fig. 12.28 Sinus rhythm ECG

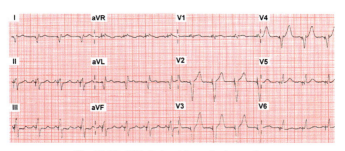

Fig. 12.29 ECG during biventricular pacing

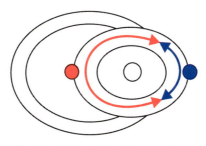

Fig. 12.30 Wavefront fusion during biventricular stimulation

there were previously R waves. R waves in leads I and aVL have been replaced by QS and qR complexes; indicating reversal of activation in the frontal plane (L→R). QS waves in V1 and V2 have been replaced by R waves, indicating reversal of activation in the horizontal plane (P→A)]. This patient had QRS score = 2 (inferior scar: R/S ≤ 0.5), LVATmax = 130 msec, and robust evidence of fusion postCRT. Predicted probability of ≥10% reduction in ESV at 6 months was 80%, actual ESV reduction was 20%. LV activation plot (upper right) indicates fusion (red arrows, RV pacing wave front; blue arrows, LV pacing wave front).

CASE 5 (FIGS 12.31 TO 12.34)

Combination of pacing from RV anterior septum and posterolateral vein of coronary sinus.

This is a case of ischemic cardiomyopathy with severe left ventricular systolic dysfunction with complete LBBB in sinus rhythm with QRS duration of 160 msec. The left ventricular lead was placed in the lateral vein, tributary of coronary sinus. The right ventricular active fixation lead was placed in the interventricular septum in a place, diametrically opposite to the position of the LV lead. The parameters of both the leads during implantation were satisfactory without any phrenic stimulation. However, in the 2nd postoperative day, she developed phrenic stimulation. Adjustment of the LV output was not effective in avoidance of phrenic stimulation.

Sometimes, phrenic stimulation can be difficult to demonstrate during implantation when the patient is supine and sedated but may be immediately evident when the patient is later active and changes body positions, even in the absence of lead dislodgment. Once phrenic nerve stimulation is observed acutely (during implantation), it is mandatory to seek

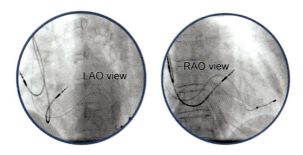

Fig. 12.31 Fluoroscopic left and right anterior oblique projections showing RV and LV lead positions

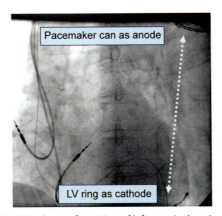

Fig. 12.32 Unipolar configuration of left ventricular stimulation

an alternative site for LV pacing. However, phrenic stimulation in post-implantation period can be managed by:
- If there is a significant differential in the capture thresholds for phrenic nerve stimulation versus LV capture, this can be overcome by manipulation of LV voltage output in devices that permit separate RV and LV outputs.
- Algorithms for automatic adjustment of LV output voltage based on periodic threshold testing. LV output voltage can be automatically "capped" beneath the phrenic nerve capture voltage without compromising LV capture.
- Some LV leads have two or more electrodes that permit selection of specific LV sites for dual cathodal biventricular stimulation, BiV stimulation with true bipolar LV stimulation, or true bipolar LV—only univentricular stimulation. Selecting alternate LV electrodes for dual cathodal BiV stimulation may occasionally overcome phrenic stimulation by altering the LV-RV pacing vector. This can be achieved noninvasively using some pulse generators and is referred to as **"electronic repositioning."**

In any case, the problem of phrenic nerve stimulation is more reliably addressed by LV lead repositioning at implant. If phrenic stimulation during attempted transvenous LV pacing cannot be overcome by any means, surgical placement of LV leads should be considered. Phrenic stimulation can occur with surgically placed epicardial leads if careful visualization of the course of the nerve sheath is not performed prior to fixation.

The interelectrode distance in bipolar left ventricular leads varies from 8 to 21 mm. The advantages of bipolar leads are two-fold. **First,** there is the option of programming between multiple different pacing electrode permutations, including true bipolar and extended bipolar configurations, with the option of selecting whether to use the LV tip or the LV ring electrode as the pacing cathode. These programming options may be invaluable in the patient with posterolateral LV fibrosis or a large field of phrenic nerve capture, where an alternate pacing polarity may obviate the need for lead revision. **Second,** true bipolar LV pacing also eliminates the problem of simultaneous right ventricular (RV) anodal capture, which can be seen in the setting of unipolar LV lead use and can sometimes partially undermine the benefit of LV pacing. There are possible 6 programmable permutations of electrodes:
- Using LV lead tip as cathode and
  - LV ring as anode (conventional).
  - Can as anode.
  - RV ring as anode (common anode for both LV and RV stimulation).

- Using LV lead ring as cathode and:
  - LV lead tip as anode (reverse of conventional).
  - Can as anode.
  - RV ring as anode.

In this patient, we used the LV ring as cathode and the can as anode and achieved good electrical resynchronization (biventricular paced QRS duration is 118 msec) (Fig. 12.32).

In case of LV stimulation using RV ring as anode and LV ring as cathode, there is possibility of RV **anodal capture**. In case of a true unipolar LV pacing, the pacemaker can is utilized for left ventricular pacing as anode. In case of BiV pacing system which utilizes a unipolar lead for LV pacing and a bipolar RV lead; sometimes with high output LV pacing, the pacing is achieved with the tip electrode of the LV lead as the cathode and the proximal electrode of the bipolar RV as the anode. This arrangement leads to myocardial capture at the RV anode in a dual cathodal arrangement. This could theoretically occur in isolation with the LV cathode, but most often occurs with both RV and LV cathodes, and is referred to as "capture at three sites during biventricular pacing." Anodal capture is more common at high-voltage outputs and with true bipolar RV leads because of the small surface area and higher current density of the ring electrode, as opposed to the larger surface area and lower current density of the coil electrode in integrated bipolar leads.[11,12] Although anodal capture may occur with high output traditional bipolar RV pacing, this phenomenon is almost always indiscernible electrocardiographically.

Anodal capture involving the proximal electrode of the bipolar RV lead can occur with BiV pacemakers with separately programmable ventricular outputs. During mono-chamber LV pacing at a relatively high output (with the RV output programmed off), RV anodal capture produces a paced QRS complex identical to that registered with BiV pacing (Fig. 12.33 and 12.34). With the proper electrode arrangement as described above this form of anodal stimulation can occur in almost 80% of systems programmed to a high LV output. The threshold for RV anodal pacing is almost always above the LV pacing threshold. This means that during LV testing, and gradual reduction of the LV output anodal capture will disappear before LV pacing is lost. Theoretically, this type of anodal capture could prevent electrocardiographic documentation of pure LV pacing if the LV pacing threshold is higher than that of RV anodal stimulation. Such anodal stimulation may complicate LV threshold testing and should not be misinterpreted as pacemaker malfunction. Furthermore if loss of anodal capture is misinterpreted as loss of capture, it may lead to an inappropriately high LV output above the anodal threshold

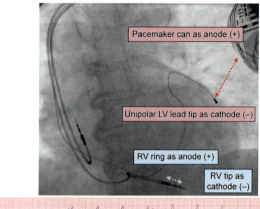

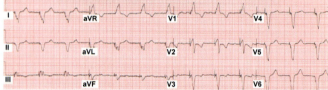

Fig. 12.33 Pacing arrangement with a unipolar LV lead and bipolar RV lead: 12 lead ECG shows biventricular pacing with simultaneous LV and RV stimulation with LV output at 2.0 V. No anodal capture

precluding the programming of an effective V-V interval. A high current density (from two sources) at the common anode during BiV pacing may cause anodal capture manifested as a paced QRS complex with a somewhat different configuration from that derived from standard BiV pacing. RV anodal capture can be recognized on the ECG during BiV pacing but in only about 40% of cases where the phenomenon is documented during LV mono-chamber pacing. Thus, anodal stimulation is present but concealed. When apparent in the ECG, it has been called "triple stimulation" with one LV electrode and two RV electrodes. The electrocardiographic manifestations during BiV pacing are usually slight, minimal or even subtle.

Although anodal capture is generally benign, it should be avoided as recent reports described patients with worsening LV dysfunction. If the LV threshold is not too high, appropriate programming of the LV output should eliminate anodal stimulation in most cases. It is important to understand that in the presence of anodal capture because it is impossible to advance LV activation by V-V interval programming because the effective V-V interval remains at zero. The use of true (dedicated) bipolar LV leads eliminates all forms of RV anodal stimulation. If due to anatomical constraint or some other reason, the use of an unipolar LV lead is inevitable; programming the RV lead also to unipolar configuration may also solve the problem.

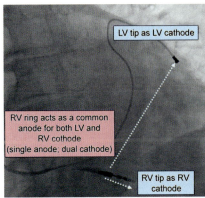
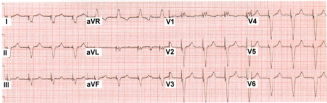

Fig. 12.34 Effect of anodal capture on ventricular activation sequence during simultaneous biventricular (BiV) pacing: RV apex and LV posterior wall capture thresholds are less than 1 V. Simultaneous, BiV pacing when LV output is 5 V (5 times > threshold) resulting in anodal capture. Simultaneous BiV pacing when LV output is 2 V and no anodal capture. Note change in activation sequence. During high-LV-output BiV pacing, anodal capture is indicated by attenuation of monophasic R wave in V1 and loss of R (QS) in V2 (horizontal plane) and attenuation of QS in lead I and aVL (frontal plane). QRS duration is shorter. During lower-output BiV pacing, loss of anodal capture is indicated by dominant QS in I, aVL, and dominant R (V1) and RS (V2). QRS duration is longer

CASE 6 (FIGS 12.35 TO 12.41)

Combination of pacing from RV apex and anterolateral vein of coronary sinus.

This is a patient of idiopathic dilated cardiomyopathy with LBBB (QRS duration of 165 msec) with severe left ventricular systolic dysfunction (LVEF = 30%) received CRT-D device from St Jude Medical (Quadra Assura) with a quadripolar LV lead.

The RV lead was paced in the interventricular septum. Pacing from the mid-superior RV septum also generates right to left activation in the frontal plane and anterior to posterior activation in the horizontal plane, but the mean QRS frontal plane axis is typically left inferior. Mono-chamber LV pacing produces a variety of activation sequences depending on stimulation site and conduction blocks.

A quadripolar LV lead has at least two distinct advantages over unipolar and bipolar LV lead:
1. Avoids phrenic stimulation by LV stimulation from the proximal poles.

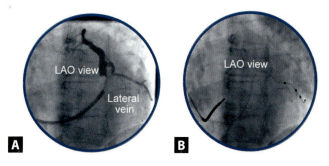

Fig. 12.35 (A) CS ventricular in LAO view showing the target vein; (B) Fluoroscopic LAO projection showing positions of RV and LV lead

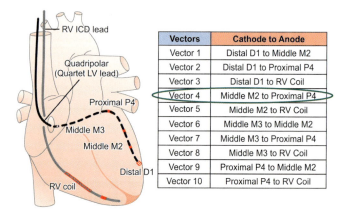

Vectors	Cathode to Anode
Vector 1	Distal D1 to Middle M2
Vector 2	Distal D1 to Proximal P4
Vector 3	Distal D1 to RV Coil
Vector 4	Middle M2 to Proximal P4
Vector 5	Middle M2 to RV Coil
Vector 6	Middle M3 to Middle M2
Vector 7	Middle M3 to Proximal P4
Vector 8	Middle M3 to RV Coil
Vector 9	Proximal P4 to Middle M2
Vector 10	Proximal P4 to RV Coil

Fig. 12.36 Different programmable vectors in ST. Jude CRT-D device with quadripolar LV lead.

2. Pacing from various vectors (programmable) gives different QRS morphology and gives option for choosing the narrowest QRS complex during LV stimulation and thereby gives the best electrical resynchronization.

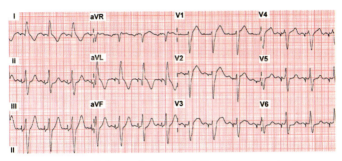

Fig. 12.37 Left ventricular stimulation through vector-1

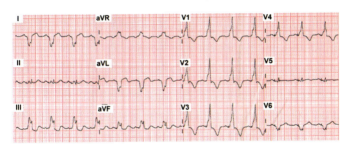

Fig. 12.38 Left ventricular stimulation through vector-6

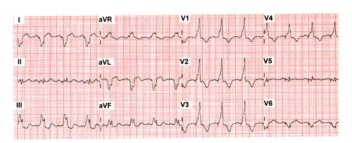

Fig. 12.39 Left ventricular stimulation through vector-7

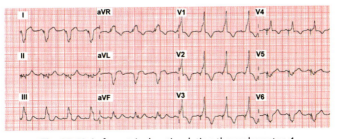

Fig. 12.40 Left ventricular stimulation through vector-4

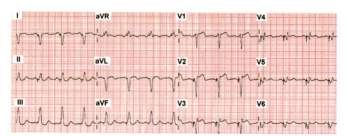

Fig. 12.41 Biventricular stimulation with left ventricular stimulation through vector-4

Quadripolar LV lead from St Jude Medical (Quartet) allows us to program 10 vectors.

Conventional LV stimulation (vector 1) (Fig. 12.36) in this patient results in diaphragmatic stimulation (Fig. 12.37). LV stimulation by vector 6 and 7 gives different QRS morphology with a narrower QRS complex (Figs 12.38 and 12.39). In an effort to recruit more myocardium, we programmed LV stimulation by vector 4 which gives narrowest QRS complex (QRS duration is 125 msec) during simultaneous biventricular stimulation (Figs 12.40 and 12.41).

Stimulation from vector 1 involves stimulation of part of the anterior wall in addition to lateral wall as the lead is placed little distally in the branch. So its morphology is different from other vectors.

Simultaneous biventricular stimulation with LV stimulation from vector 4 and RV stimulation from mid IVS.

FUSION

The underlying spontaneous ECG should be exposed periodically to confirm the continuing presence of a LBBB type of intraventricular conduction abnormality where reverse electrical remodeling may slightly shorten the QRS complex. In this respect, turning off the pacemaker could potentially improve LV function and heart failure in the rare patients who have lost their intraventricular conduction delay or block through electrical reverse ventricular remodeling.[9] In other words, a spontaneous narrow QRS is better than biventricular pacing. In patients with sinus rhythm and a relatively short PR interval, **ventricular fusion** (defined as involving spontaneous conduction) with competing native conduction during biventricular pacing may cause misinterpretation of the ECG, and is a common pitfall in device follow-up (Fig. 12.42). Substantial QRS shortening mandates exclusion of ventricular fusion with the spontaneous QRS complex and rather than

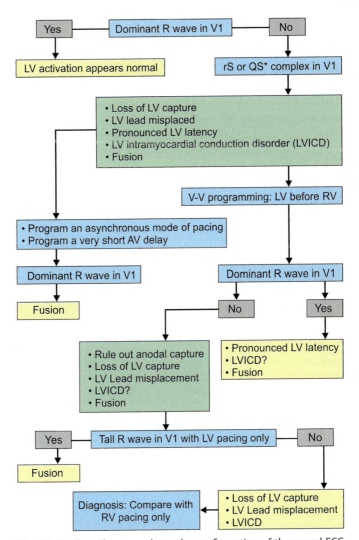

Fig. 12.42 Algorithm to evaluate the configuration of the paced ECG in lead V1 during simultaneous biventricular pacing. Ventricular fusion with the intrinsic rhythm is the great ECG imitator and appears at several levels. A misplaced left ventricular (LV) lead means location in the anterior or the middle cardiac vein; LVICD — LV intramyocardial conduction delay. Little is known about this entity and precisely where it fits in the algorithm. It should always be a diagnosis of exclusion. A QS complex (barring fusion with the intrinsic rhythm) is not diagnostic of any problem but cause for concern (*) as it often represents an unfavorable situation with right ventricular (RV) preponderance when LV activation is delayed (or absent) and being overshadowed by RV activation. Note that fusion appears at many sites in this algorithm to emphasize the ubiquity of fusion in cardiac resynchronization therapy. The operator can evaluate the presence or absence of fusion by using only the first step of the protocol. For more precise LV lead location another algorithm can be consulted (*Courtesy:* Ploux S, Bordachar P, Deplagne A, et al. Electrocardiogram-based algorithm to predict the left ventricular lead position in recipients of cardiac resynchronization systems. Pacing Clin Electrophysiol. 2009;32 (Suppl 1):S2–S7).

attributing the pattern to near-perfect electrical ventricular resynchronization.

Fusion and pseudofusion are the cause of much confusion in any paced ECG, and these phenomena can occur in CRT pacing as well as conventional pacing. A fused beat occurs when an electrical stimulus 'collides' with an intrinsic event in such a way that the stimulus contributes to the beat but does not entirely cause it. A fusion beat has distinct 'hybrid' morphology, in that it is neither entirely paced nor entirely sensed. When fusion occurs, the electrical stimulus contributes to the paced beat but it is 'wasted energy' in that the heart was starting to beat on its own anyway. **Pseudofusion** occurs when an electrical stimulus falls exactly on top of a sensed event. The result is that the output pulse is delivered once the heart was already beating; the output spike appears on top of the paced beat. The morphology of the pseudofusion beat is similar to the morphology of a true sensed event; the pacemaker spike is gratuitous. The spike contributes nothing to the beat and also represents a waste of energy.

So, fusion actually confirms capture, because the hybrid fused morphology shows that the electrical energy is depolarizing the heart, even though the heart is trying to beat on its own anyway. Pseudofusion neither confirms nor disproves capture. Fusion and pseudofusion are primarily timing problems that the output pulse is delivered once the heart was already beating; the output spike appears on top of the paced beat. The morphology of the pseudofusion beat is similar to the morphology of a true sensed event; the pacemaker spike is gratuitous. The spike contributes nothing to the beat and also represents a waste of energy.

The presence of ventricular fusion should be ruled out by observing the paced QRS morphology during progressive shortening of the atrial sensing-ventricular pacing (AS-VP) interval in the VDD mode or the atrial pacing-ventricular pacing (AP-VP) interval in the DDD mode. Alternatively, BiV pacing in the VVI mode at a rate faster than the spontaneous rate can also be used to evaluate the presence of fusion. The absence of first-degree AV block is associated with a better response to CRT. Patients with first-degree AV block have a poorer outcome than patients with a normal PR interval. Enhanced hemodynamic response in patients with normal AV conduction may have occurred by concealed resynchronization or fusion from the right bundle branch with the impulse initiated by the LV electrode together with the avoidance of RV apical stimulation. As present, it is best to first program the AV delay to avoid all forms of ventricular fusion because fusion may sometimes be associated with a suboptimal CRT response in some patients.

Configuration of the P wave

Interatrial conduction delay causes late left atrial activation and systole; the latter may even occur during LV systole.[13] The diagnosis is important because it is a cause of a potentially correctible suboptimal CRT response. Interatrial conduction delay in CRT patients is not rare but its true incidence is unknown. **Interatrial conduction delay** is characterized electrocardiographically by a wide and notched P wave (> 120 ms) traditionally in ECG lead II, associated with a wide terminal negativity in lead V1. When the ECG suggests interatrial conduction delay, and it is confirmed at implantation, the atrial lead should be placed in the interatrial septum where pacing produces a more homogeneous activation of both atria and abbreviates total atrial conduction time.

In the presence of established CRT with an atrial lead already in the right atrial appendage, restoration of optimal mechanical left-sided AV synchrony occasionally requires simultaneous biatrial pacing performed by the addition of a second atrial lead near or into the proximal coronary sinus. Difficult cases of interatrial conduction delay can be managed by AV nodal ablation, whereby the AV delay can then be extended with impunity, though some biventricular ICDs may limit the maximum programmable AV delay.

To summarize, the ECG evidences of resynchronization of LV and RV activation wave fronts during biventricular pacing is assessed by 3 observations: **First,** rightward frontal plane axis shift: baseline QRS axis is left, intermediate or undefined, and changes to a right inferior or right superior axis during biventricular pacing. **Second,** activation wave front reversal in leads I, aVL, V1, and V2. Evidence for electrical resynchronization is considered present if leftward forces changed into right ward forces or if anterior forces emerged where initially posterior forces are present. This is reflected by a change from dominant positive QRS complex to dominant negative in leads I and aVL, and a change from dominant negative QRS complex to dominant positive in leads V1 and V2, respectively. **Third,** change in R-wave amplitude in the expected direction in lateral (I, aVL) and anterior (V1-V2) leads by CRT.

REFERENCES

1. Grimley SR, Suffoletto MS, Gorcsan J 3rd, Schwartzman D. Electrocardiographically concealed variation in left ventricular capture: A case with implications for resynchronization therapy in ischemic cardiomyopathy. Heart Rhythm. 2006;3: 739-42.

2. Giudici MC. Tigrett DW, et al. Electrocardiographic patterns during: Pacing the Great Cardiac and Middle Cardiac Veins. PACE. 2007;30:1376-80.
3. Ploux S, Bordachar P, Deplagne A, et al. Electrocardiogram-based algorithm to predict the left ventricular lead position in recipients of cardiac resynchronization systems. Pacing Clin Electrophysiol. 2009;32(Suppl 1):S2–S7.
4. Lecoq G, Leclercq C, Leray E, et al. Clinical and electro-cardiographic predictors of a positive response to cardiac resynchronization therapy in advanced heart failure. Eur Heart J. 2005;26:1094-100.
5. Leclercq C, Faris O, Tunin R, et al. Systolic improvement and mechanical resynchronization does not require electrical synchrony in the dilated failing heart with left bundle-branch block. Circulation. 2002;106:1760-3.
6. Herweg B, Barold SS. Three-Step Electrocardiographic Evaluation of Cardiac Resynchronization. PACE. 2012;35:249-52.
7. Herweg B, Ilercil A, Madramootoo C, et al. Latency during left ventricular pacing from the lateral cardiac veins: A cause of ineffectual biventricular pacing. Pacing Clin Electrophysiol. 2006;29:574-81.
8. Herweg B, Ali R, Ilercil A, et al. Site-specific differences in latency intervals during biventricular pacing: Impact on paced QRS morphology and echo-optimized V-V interval. Pacing Clin Electrophysiol. 2010;33:1382-91.
9. Tedrow UB, Stevenson WG, Wood MA, et al. Activation sequence modification during cardiac resynchronization by manipulation of left ventricular epicardial pacing stimulus strength. Pacing Clin Electrophysiol. 2007;30:65-9.
10. Dendy KF, Powell BD, Cha YM, et al. Anodal stimulation: An under recognized cause of nonresponders to cardiac resynchronization therapy. Indian Pacing Electrophysiol J. 2011;11:64-72.
11. Barold SS, Herweg B. Usefulness of the 12-lead electrocardiogram in the follow-up of patients with cardiac resynchronization devices. Part II. Cardiol J. 2011;18(6):610-24.
12. Dizon J, Horn E, Neglia J, Medina N, Garan H. Loss of left bundle branch block following biventricular pacing therapy for heart failure: evidence for electrical remodeling? J Interv Card Electrophysiol. 2004;10:47-50.
13. Daubert JC, Pavin D, Jauvert G, Mabo P. Intra- and interatrial conduction delay. Implications for cardiac pacing. Pacing Clin Electrophysiol. 2004;27:507-25.

CHAPTER 13

Optimizing Response

DEFINITION OF RESPONSE

There is no clear consensus or standardized definition of what is considered to be an adequate response to cardiac resynchronization therapy (CRT) or when a patient should be considered as a non-responder. However, interpretation of the response to CRT can be done in respect of the following parameters, 6 months post CRT implantation:

Clinical

- Reduction of symptoms by at least one New York Heart Association (NYHA) class or symptomatic status post-CRT of class I or II.
- Improvement in 6 minutes walking by > 25% or > 50 meters.
- Improvement in quality of life (QOL) scores by > 15 points.

Echocardiographic

- The patients with an increase in left ventricular end-diastolic volume (LVESV) are considered as **negative responders**; patients with a decrease in LVESV ranging from 0% to 14% are known as **non-responders**; patients with a decrease in LVESV ranging from 15% to 29% are defined as **responders**; and patients with a decrease in LVESV ≥ 30% are known as **super-responders**.[1]
- Increase in LVEF by at least 25% from baseline level.
- Increase in stroke volume by 15%.

Although successful CRT implantation causes significant narrowing of QRS width and considered useful marker of electrical resynchronization during and after implantation, it is not used to define responders to CRT as, QRS duration does not always reflect degree of left ventricular dyssynchrony or resynchronization.[2]

RESPONDERS AND SUPER-RESPONDERS

The response to CRT is not uniform and varies significantly among individuals; some patients exhibit a significant improvement in clinical status with extensive LV reverse remodeling and almost normalization of LV function, whereas other patients show deterioration of both clinical and functional parameters. Importantly, reversal of LV remodeling in heart failure patients by either pharmacological or interventional therapies is proposed as a surrogate for improved outcome.[3] The extent of reverse LV remodeling varies significantly among patients undergoing CRT. More extensive LV reverse remodeling is related to greater clinical and functional improvement after 6 months of CRT and more LV reverse remodeling results in better survival and less hospitalization for decompensated heart failure after 6 months of CRT.[4] Immediately after a successful CRT implantation, assuming adequate LV lead position and thresholds, systolic blood pressure, cardiac output, and stroke work usually increase, whereas end systolic volumes and pulmonary capillary wedge pressure decrease as a result of immediate correction of ventricular dyssynchrony which leads to direct improvement of LV systolic function.[5,6] Some patients may feel the effects as early as one month after implant though others may require a longer period of time for symptom relief.[7] After 12 months of CRT, super-responders exhibit normalization in LVEF ($\geq$ 50%) with $\geq$ 30% decrease in LVESV associated with clinical improvement to NYHA functional class I to II. The super-responders more frequently have nonischemic etiology of heart failure, longer QRS duration, more often LBBB configuration, less severe mitral regurgitation, and more extensive LV dyssynchrony.[4] The exact mechanism of this super-response is not known. In patients with chronic heart failure (CHF) subjected to CRT, RV apical pacing increases the LV activation time and changes the location of the latest LV endocardial activation area (in 80% of cases to more anterior positions). Programming the CRT device to allow partial or complete intrinsic depolarization of the interventricular septum (fusion pacing), creates three activation fronts (intrinsic wave front, right ventricular pacing wave front and left ventricular pacing wave front) instead of two during pure biventricular pacing (Fig. 13.1). Acute invasive hemodynamic data proved that in patients with normal AV conduction, CRT with fusion is superior to any optimized biventricular (Biv) configuration in improving LV as well as RV systolic performance.[8] The mechanism of this improved performance is a shorter LV activation time, which probably produces superior resynchronization. However, due

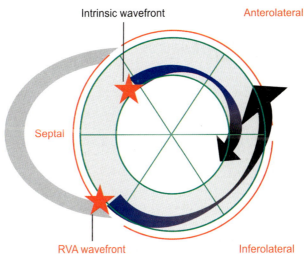

Fig. 13.1 Schematic of the mechanism by which the fusion between RV apical pacing and partial intrinsic LV endocardial depolarization shortens LV activation time. The most delayed area during sinus rhythm (intrinsic LV endocardial depolarization) was posterolateral or lateral in > 80% of patients. During RV apical pacing, the most delayed area shifted to anterior or anterolateral in ~ 90% of patients. Thus, fusion between these two wavefronts takes less time to depolarize the LV. Adding a third wavefront from the epicardial LV further diminishes the total duration of the LV activation time (*Courtesy:* Radu Vatasescu, Antonio Berruezo, Lluis Mont, et al. Midterm 'super-response' to cardiac resynchronization therapy by biventricular pacing with fusion: insights from electro-anatomical mapping. Europace (2009) 11, 1675–1682)

to presumed variability in AV conduction and lack of data on chronic effects of fusion, the majority of authors try to avoid it and prefer biventricular (Biv) pacing with the shortest possible AV delay, as determined by echocardiography. A recent long-term prospective study used a non-invasive algorithm to obtain CRT with optimal fusion, observing high rate of structural response, with a very high level of reverse remodeling at 6 months.[9]

Non-responders

With optimal background medical therapy for HF, about 70% of patients respond to CRT and about 30% don't respond adequately. This non-responder rate is derived from several clinical trials in which 30% to 35% of patients show either no improvement or worsening symptoms after six months of CRT.[7,10] Table 13.1 demonstrates different responsible factors for CRT non-responders.

Based on current CRT data, re-evaluation of a CRT patient should be considered if there is no improvement in

Table 13.1 Causes of non-responders		
Inappropriate patient selection	*Inappropriate lead position*	*Inappropriate device programming*
Absence of mechanical dyssynchrony despite wide QRS complex. Very advanced end stage cardiomyopathy. Severe right ventricular failure. Presence of significant ischemia. Advanced renal failure. Presence of atrial fibrillation.	Lead should be positioned in the latest activated region of LV. Target area of LV should be viable without any significant scar. Lead should have stable position with acceptable threshold without diaphragmatic stimulation.	AV optimization: • Prolonged AV delay causing AV asynchrony may compromise cardiac performance. • Individual optimization of AV delay should be performed in all CRT patients. • Minimum AV delay without truncated A wave in transmitral flow with maximum LVOT VTI and filling time considered as optimum delay. VV optimization

symptoms after 6 months of CRT or there is worsening heart failure with increased ventricular remodeling within the first several months after initiation of CRT. Figure 13.2 represents an algorithm of strategy to manage HF patients who are not responding to CRT.

Atrial Fibrillation

The prevalence of atrial fibrillation (AF) in patients with heart failure is 10-25% for patients in NYHA class II-III and approximately 50% in NYHA class IV. Rapid AF results in conducted beats, diminishing biventricular capture. Effective suppression of rapid intrinsic AV conduction in patients with AF is mandatory to achieve consistent biventricular capture and prevent inhibition of resynchronization. In patients with paroxysmal AF or persistent AF of short duration, pharmacological treatment to control ventricular rate may be sufficient to maintain high ventricular pacing percentages. In patients with permanent AF, guideline favors AV node ablation for eliminating native AV conduction in order to achieve 100% biventricular pacing. However, AV node ablation should be considered in patients with any form of AF, if the biventricular pacing percentage is $\leq 80\%$.

Myocardial Ischemia

The implantation of an LV lead at an area with transmural myocardial scar reduces the beneficial effects of CRT on clinical outcome and cardiac performance. Hence, results in ineffective CRT. Myocardial ischemia is also responsible for suboptimal response to CRT. So, all attempts at complete revascularization should be done in a patient with ischemic cardiomyopathy prior to considering CRT. A non-responder patient to CRT should be reevaluated for provokable myocardial ischemia with either of the non-invasive modalities. If the test becomes positive, one should go for coronary angiography followed by revascularization to get an optimal response to CRT.

Medical Treatment

Cardiac resynchronization therapy is not a replacement for standard pharmacologic therapy, but it may offer the opportunity to augment the medical therapy. The combination of device therapy and optimal medical management may provide synergistic effects on reverse LV remodeling, improved systolic and diastolic function, and increased long-term survival. If a HF patient with near optimal filling pressures receives CRT and has adequate diuresis, failure to reduce diuretics will result in pre-renal azotemia which may mask or delay the beneficial effects of CRT. On the contrary patients after CRT implantation with hypervolemic state should receive increased dose of diuretics. Cardiac resynchronization therapy improves HF symptoms and blood pressure while restoring synchrony by pacing both ventricles.[5,7,11] Therefore, some of the clinical problems for which beta-blocker therapy is abandoned or not aggressively pursued are stabilized with CRT. The COMPANION trial demonstrated that systolic blood pressure increases with CRT and that outcome of hospitalization and mortality are better with CRT or CRT and defibrillator with concomitant beta-blocker therapy.[11] So, all patients after CRT implantation should receive enhanced dose of beta-blockers. In addition all patients should receive ACE-Inhibitors.

Evaluation and Interrogation of the CRT Device

In absence of pre-renal azotemia, atrial fibrillation, or cardiac ischemia a CRT non-responder should undergo evaluation and interrogation of the CRT device. Comparison of a current chest X-ray (deep penetrating PA and left lateral) with a chest X-ray from the time of implant is a simple screening procedure to look for lead dislodgement of either LV or RV lead. 12 lead surface ECG analysis is very essential in a non-responder patient to

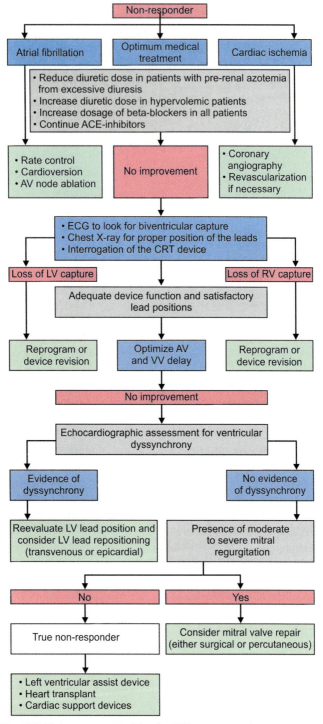

Fig. 13.2 Management algorithm for CRT non-responders
Abbreviations: AV, atrioventricular; CXR, chest X-ray; ECG, electrocardiogram; LV, left ventricular; RV, right ventricular; VV, interventricular

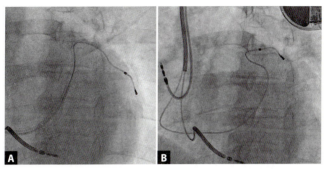

Figs 13.3A and B (A) Fluoroscopic LAO view during CRT implantation; (B) Same view after 6 months. During follow up the patient developed loss of LV capture. Quite evidently the LV lead displaced proximally. Because of the larger caliber of the proximal vein the anode of the LV does not have good contact to the venous wall. Changing the conventional bipolar pacing vector from conventional to unipolar configuration (LV tip to can) solved the problem

CRT to ascertain proper biventricular capture. Comparing a current electrocardiogram with a baseline electrocardiogram from the time of implant gives a definite clue towards detection of loss of RV or LV capture. The ECG signs of biventricular electrical resynchronization which have been linked to LV reverse remodeling are **(1)** rightward axis shift; **(2)** activation wave front reversal to dominant negative in leads I, aVL and dominant positive in leads V1, V2; **(3)** significant R-wave amplitude decrease in leads I, aVL and increase in leads V1, V2.[12] Increment of R-wave and diminution of S-wave amplitude in lead II and/or no change in bundle branch morphology in V1 was associated with loss of RV capture (positive predictive value 93%, negative predictive value 93%). Deepening of S-wave in lead II and/or no change in bundle branch morphology in V1 was associated with loss of LV capture (positive predictive value 71%, negative predictive value 89%).[13] Thus, it may be useful to have a baseline electrocardiogram from the time of implant readily available for comparison with future electrocardiograms to evaluate right and left ventricular capture. This can be confirmed with interrogation of the device. Loss of LV capture due to minor lead dislodgement of LV lead in a case of bipolar LV lead can be managed by changing the pacing vector (using LV ring as cathode) (Fig. 13.3). Loss of capture of either can be tackled sometimes with increasing the output. However, gross dislodgement of either LV lead or RV lead warrants device revision. But, if these investigations indicate satisfactory lead positions with adequate device function one should look for proper AV and VV delay optimization.

Atrioventricular (AV)/Interventricular (VV) Delay Optimization

Adequate device function in a CRT patient with persistent or worsening symptoms should lead to evaluation of AV and VV delay (if available).

The optimal AV delay has been defined as that which allows completion of the end-diastolic filling flow prior to ventricular contraction, thereby providing the longest diastolic filling time.[14] When programmed optimally, the mitral valve closes immediately after completion of the A wave. If the AV delay is too long, time available for transmitral flow is reduced, with fusion of the E and A waves and a reduction in the total duration of diastolic transmitral flow. Because the LV pressure can exceed the LA pressure during late diastole, diastolic mitral regurgitation may occurs further reducing left ventricular end diastolic pressure and volume. If the AV delay is too short, active filling cannot be completed before the onset of LV contraction and the A wave is either absent or is truncated by abrupt closure of the mitral valve during the rise in LV systolic pressure. So, the optimum AV delay provides maximized LV preload and maximized diastolic filling time. No single method of AV resynchronization has demonstrated convincing clinical superiority, such as reduction in heart failure hospitalization or reductions in LV end-systolic volume (ESV) (reverse remodeling). The available methods of AV interval optimization are discussed below:

Left Ventricular Inflow Analysis

The method described by Ritter requires programming the AV delay to a short and a long interval while testing each setting for its impact on end diastolic filling with Doppler echocardiography.[15] According to this method, optimal pacemaker AV interval during atrial sensing (SAVI) can be stated algebraically as: $SAVI_{optimal} = SAVI_{short} + d$, where $d = (SAVI_{long} + QA_{long}) - (SAVI_{short} + QAI_{short})$, Q = ventricular pacing stimulus, and A = termination of A wave.

- $SAVI_{long}$ and QA_{long} are determined by programming a "long" sensed AVI ($SAVI_{long}$). $SAVI_{long}$ is the longest AVI that results in (a) ventricular capture without fusion of native conduction and (b) spontaneous closure of the mitral valve before LV ejection (Fig. 13.4). QA_{long} is then measured as the time from the ventricular pacing stimulus to the end of the A wave.
- $SAVI_{short}$ and QA_{short} are determined by programming a "short" sensed AVI ($SAVI_{short}$). $SAVI_{short}$ is the longest AVI that results in A-wave truncation (Fig. 13.5). QAshort is then

Optimizing Response 303

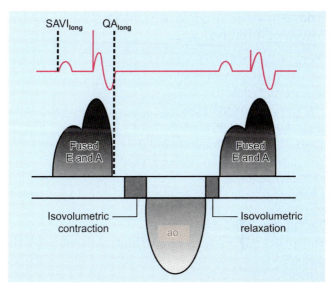

Fig. 13.4 Ritter method for atrioventricular resynchronization: step 1. Determination of optimal pacemaker atrioventricular interval during atrial sensing: $SAVI_{long}$ and QA_{long}. The longest AV interval that yields full ventricular capture without A-wave truncation is $SAVI_{long}$. The time from the ventricular pacing stimulus to the end of the A wave is QA_{long}.

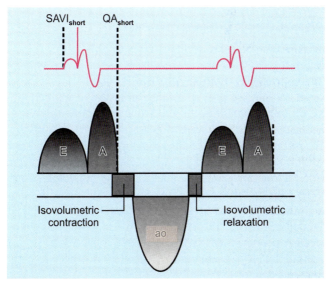

Fig. 13.5 Ritter method for AV resynchronization: step 2. Determination of $SAVI_{short}$ and QA_{short}. The SAVI is shortened until A-wave truncation is observed. This is $SAVI_{short}$. The time from the ventricular pacing stimulus to the end of the A wave is QA_{short}

measured as the time from the ventricular pacing stimulus to the end of the A wave.
- The SAVIoptimal is then calculated from these values. AV optimization is confirmed by noting the return of normal E- and A-wave separation indicating improved diastolic filling time and optimized AV timing relationship.

In an another "simplified" two-step approach, firstly a "long" sensed AVI that results in (a) ventricular capture without fusion of native conduction and (b) spontaneous closure of the mitral valve before LV ejection is selected. The time between the end of the A wave (representing the end of the diastolic filling period) to the time of onset of high-velocity systolic mitral regurgitation (representing the onset of ventricular contraction) is recorded. Then, the time from the end of the A wave to the onset of low-velocity diastolic mitral regurgitation is denoted as t1. The optimal AVI is then calculated as the "long" AVI-t1.[16] The Ritter method is a very cumbersome process. As with all methods for AV synchronization using visual analysis of LV inflow patterns, subjective error is common because the terminal portion of the A wave is often difficult to discern. The Ritter method was developed for AV resynchronization in complete AV block and during mono-chamber RV pacing. Ventricular conduction is entirely different during biventricular pacing.

Left ventricular Outflow Analysis

Measurement of the continuous-wave Doppler aortic velocity time integral (VTI) provides an estimate of stroke volume. This approach is often applied during manipulation of the paced AV interval (pAVI). A range of pAVIs is scanned, and the optimal interval is the pAVI that generates the largest increase in aortic VTI (stroke volume). The aortic VTI method is simple to perform, assuming an adequate echocardiographic window can be obtained. Data acquisition is generally rapid, which allows for screening a broad range of pacing control parameters in abbreviated time. However, VTI measurements are influenced by extraneous factors (e.g., respiratory phase, sympathetic tone). The accuracy of the method is degraded because of at least 10% variation between measurements, and it cannot reliably discriminate changes in VTI smaller than this inherent error.

Electrogram Analysis

The sensed AV-delay is programmed to approximately 75% of the PR interval to ensure complete ventricular pacing. Pulsed-wave Doppler is performed at the tips of the mitral leaflets in the apical four-chamber view to obtain transmitral flow. E and A waves are recorded and the AV delay is shortened by 20 msec until the A-wave is truncated. The truncated A-wave represents early mitral valve closure during ventricular systole. The AV delay is then lengthened by 10 msec until the A-wave is no longer truncated. At this point ventricular contraction should begin just at the end of atrial contraction.

The aortic VTI method is superior to mitral inflow method.[17] The optimal AV interval predicted by the mitral inflow method is significantly shorter than the VTI method. It is argued that the aortic VTI method performs better than the mitral inflow method because it titrates a measure of LV ejection, whereas the mitral inflow method titrates a measure of LV filling.

During normal electrical activation in patients with normal QRS durations, the delay between RV and LV contraction is about 6 msec.[18] To optimize the LV-RV interval, the AV delay is first optimized. Once the best RA-LV interval is determined, an apical 5-chamber echocardiographic view with sampling from aortic root is used to obtain time velocity integral (VTI). The VV delay which gives maximal aortic VTI is considered to be the optimum VV delay. The optimized VV delay results in short-term improvement in hemodynamic measurements of ejection fraction, cardiac output, and increased LV filling times as compared to simultaneous ventricular pacing.[19, 20] There are little data on long-term clinical outcomes after VV optimization. The optimal VV interval may vary according to etiology of heart failure. Patients with ischemic cardiomyopathy may require longer VV intervals necessitating more pre-excitation of the left ventricle due to the presence of scar tissue resulting in a slower conduction velocity.[21] The VV delay usually can be programmed between 80 or 100 msec left ventricular (LV) pre-activation and 80 or 100 msec right ventricular (RV) pre-activation, and a VV delay of 0 denotes simultaneous biventricular pacing. During individual optimization of the VV delay, various degrees of LV and RV pre-activation are applied while measuring hemodynamic or echocardiographic changes. However, in case of LV pre-activation of 40 msec or more, the effective VV delay may become shorter than programmed VV delay.[22]

Echocardiographic Assessment

In case of persistent symptoms after device optimization, noninvasive echocardiographic dyssynchrony studies should be considered. Specifically, septal to posterior wall motion delay of ≥ 130 msec as measured by M-mode echocardiography at the level of papillary muscle, interventricular mechanical delay of ≥ 40 msec defined as the time difference between LV and RV pre-ejection intervals, and interventricular dyssynchrony of ≥ 65 msec as detected by tissue Doppler imaging are significant measurements of dyssynchrony and predict response to CRT.[23-25] After successful CRT there should be minimal interventricular or intraventricular dyssynchrony. If significant interventricular or intraventricular dyssynchrony is still present in a CRT non-responder, then proper LV lead position should be considered through transvenous or epicardial approach. Proper LV lead positioning essentially means putting the lead in the latest activating, viable left ventricular region usually through lateral or postero-lateral branch with late intra-cardiac LV sensed signal (at the end of QRS complex in surface ECG). The LV lead should be kept in a stable wedged position (secondary curves provides more stability) with satisfactory lead parameters (R wave amplitude of ≥ 5 mV with pacing threshold of ≤ 2.0 V without diaphragmatic stimulation at high output) with good anatomical and electrical separation of RV and LV lead.

Persistent symptoms in absence ventricular dyssynchrony or after correction of ventricular dyssynchrony should be followed by evaluation for significant mitral regurgitation. Causes of functional mitral regurgitation (MR) in dilated cardiomyopathy range from ventricular dilation with increasing distance between papillary muscles and the enlarged mitral annulus restricting leaflet motion, to delayed activation of the posteromedial papillary muscle resulting from ventricular dyssynchrony. Functional MR is reduced by CRT.[26] Persistent MR despite correction of ventricular dyssynchrony may mask the effects of CRT. Studies have shown that mitral valve surgery offers symptomatic improvement to MR patients with poor LV function.[27, 28] In selected patients, mitral valve surgery should be considered to correct persistent significant MR in a CRT non-responder.

CARDIAC ASSIST DEVICES

HF patients with CRT whose symptoms persist despite adequate device function and absence of dyssynchrony or significant mitral regurgitation should be considered as a true non-responder. In selected non-responder patients who progress to NYHA functional class IV heart failure, the use of LV assist devices or cardiac transplantation should be considered seriously.

REFERENCES

1. Ypenburg C, van Bommel RJ, Willem Borleffs CJ, et al. Long-term prognosis after cardiac resynchronization therapy is related to the

extent of left ventricular reverse remodeling at midterm follow-up. J Am Coll Cardiol. 2009; 53:483-90.
2. Bleeker GB, Schalij MJ, Molhoek SG, Verwey HF, Holman ER, Boersma E, Steendijk P, van der Wall EE, Bax JJ. Relationship between QRS duration and left ventricular dyssynchrony in patients with end-stage heart failure. J Cardiovasc Electrophysiol 2004;15:544-9.
3. Cohn JN, Ferrari R, Sharpe N. Cardiac remodeling—concepts and clinical implications: a consensus paper from an international forum on cardiac remodeling. J Am Coll Cardiol. 2000;35:569-82.
4. Yu CM, Bleeker GB, Fung JW, Schalij MJ, Zhang Q, van der Wall EE, et al. Left ventricular reverse remodeling but not clinical improvement predicts long-term survival after cardiac resynchronization therapy. Circulation. 2005;112:1580-6.
5. Kass DA. Chen CH, Curry C, et al. Improved left ventricular mechanics from acute VDD pacing in patients with dilated cardiomyopathy and ventricular conduction delay. Circulation. 1999;99:1567-73.
6. Leclercq C, Cazeau S, Le Breton H, et al. Acute hemodynamic effects of biventricular DDD pacing in patients with end-stage heart failure. J Am Coll Cardiol. 1998;32:1825-31.
7. Abraham WT, Fisher WG, Smith AL, Delurigic DB, et al. Cardiac resynchronization in chronic heart failure. N Engl J Med. 2002;346:1845-53.
8. Castellant P, Fatemi M, Bertault-Valls V, et al. Cardiac resynchronization therapy: "nonresponders" and "hyperresponders." Heart Rhythm. 2008;5:193-7.
9. Radu Vatasescu†, Antonio Berruezo, Lluis Mont, et al. Midterm 'super-response' to cardiac resynchronization therapy by biventricular pacing with fusion: insights from electro-anatomical mapping. Europace. 2009;11:1675-82.
10. Young JB, Abraham WT, Smith AL, et al. Combined cardiac resynchronization and implantable cardioversion defibrillation in advanced chronic heart failure. JAMA. 2003;289:2685-94.
11. Bristow MR, Saxon LA, Boehmer J, et al. Cardiac-resynchronization therapy with or without an implantable defibrillator in advanced heart failure. N Engl J Med. 2004;350:2140-50.
12. Sweeney MO, van Bommel RJ, Schalij MJ, Borleffs CJ, Hellkamp AS, Bax JJ. Analysis of ventricular activation using surface electrocardiography to predict left ventricular reverse volumetric remodeling during cardiac resynchronization therapy. Circulation. 2010;121:626-34.
13. Hart DT, Petre L, Arshad R, King M, Herwes B, Steinberg J. Assessment of ventricular capture in patients with cardiac resynchronization devices: a simple surface electrocardiographic algorithm (abstr). Pacing Clin Electrophysiology. 2003;26:618.
14. Ronaszeki A. Hemodynamic consequences of the timing of atrial contraction during complete AV block. Acta Biomedica Lovaniensia. 1989:15.
15. Ritter P, Padeletti L, Gillio-Meina L, et al. Determination of the optimal atrioventricular delay in DDD pacing: comparison between echo and peak endocardial acceleration measurements. Europace. 1999;1:126-130.

16. Meluzin J, Novak M, Mullerova J, et al. A fast and simple echocardiographic determination of the optimal atrioventricular delay in patients after biventricular stimulation. Pacing Clin Electrophysiol. 2004;27:58-64.
17. Kerlan JE, Sawhney NS, Waggoner AD, et al. Prospective comparison of echocardiographic atrioventricular delay optimization methods for cardiac resynchronization therapy. Heart Rhythm. 2006;3:148-154.
18. Grines CL, Bashore TM, Boudoulas H, Olson S, Shafer P, Wooley CF. Functional abnormalities in isolated left bundle branch block. The effect of interventricular asynchrony. Circulation. 1989;79:845-53.
19. Sogaard P, Egeblad H, Pederson AK, et al. Sequential versus simultaneous biventricular resynchronization for severe heart failure: evaluation by tissue Doppler imaging. Circulation. 2002;106:2078-84.
20. Bordachar P, Lafitte S, Reuter S, et al. Echocardiographic parameters of ventricular dyssynchrony validation in patients with heart failure using sequential biventricular pacing. J Am Coll Cardiol. 2004;44:2157-65.
21. Van Gelder BM, Bracke FA, Meijer A, Lakerveld LJ, Pijls NH. Effect of optimizing the VV interval on left ventricular contractility in cardiac resynchronization therapy. Am J Cardiol. 2004; 93:1500-03.
22. Margot D. Bogaard, Mathias Meine, Pieter A. Doevendans, et al. Programmed versus Effective VV delay during CRT Optimization: When what you see is not what you get. PACE. 2013;36:403-9.
23. Pitzalis MV, Iacoviello M, Romito R, et al. Cardiac resynchronization therapy tailored by echocardiographic evaluation of ventricular asynchrony. J Am Coll Cardiol. 2002; 40:1615-22.
24. Rouleau F, Merheb M, Geffroy S, et al. Echocardiographic assessment of the interventricular delay of activation and correlation to the QRS width in dilated cardiomyopathy. Pacing Clin Electrophysiol. 2001;24:1500-6.
25. Bax JJ, Bleeker GB, Marwick TH, et al. Left ventricular dyssynchrony predicts response and prognosis after cardiac resynchronization therapy. J Am Coll Cardiol. 2004;44:1834-40.
26. Breithardt OA, Sinha AM, Schwammenthal E, et al. Acute effects of cardiac resynchronization therapy on functional mitral regurgitation in advanced systolic heart failure. J Am Coll Cardiol. 2003;41:765-70.
27. Haan CK, Cabral CI, Conetta DA, Coombs LP, Edwards FH. Selecting patients with mitral regurgitation and left ventricular dysfunction for isolated mitral valve surgery. Ann Thorac Surg. 2004;78:820-5.
28. Bishay ES, McCarthy PM, Cosgrove DM, et al. Mitral valve surgery in patients with severe left ventricular dysfunction. Eur J Cardiothorac Surg. 2000;17:213-21.

CHAPTER 14

Newer Advances

MULTISITE AND MULTIPOINT LV PACING

Simultaneous (or near simultaneous) stimulation of the left ventricular free wall and interventricular septum is thought to improve the mechanical synchrony in patients with left bundle branch block by enhancing myocardial recruitment in the regions of late activation. However, the conduction properties of the myocardium affect both the progression of the depolarizing wave front and the hemodynamic response to biventricular (BiV) pacing. About 30-40% of patients receiving cardiac resynchronization therapy (CRT) do not experience symptomatic improvement and up to 50% may not show echocardiographic evidence of positive remodeling.[1] Failure of response is probably due to a combination of factors including the presence of scar in the left ventricular wall, placement of the pacing lead over a zone of slow conduction, variable electrical response of the diseased ventricle to pacing, or suboptimal positioning of the pacing leads with regard to the area of latest contraction.[2,3]

The assessment of therapy efficacy in a patient with CRT is little complex. Echo evaluation and quality of life assessment may reveal that some measurements improved while others remained the same or stabilized.

Therefore, the goal of CRT technology innovation is to address not only the 30-40% of patients who are classified as non-responders, but to also further enhance the hemodynamic results of the responders.

Both the extent and position of myocardial scar influence the response to pacing either because there is an inadequate volume of healthy myocardium to recruit and improve hemodynamics, or because regions of scar prevent progression of the activation wave front and the synchronized engagement of viable tissue. So, pacing from multiple sites (multisite) in the left ventricle (two coronary sinus branches) may offer a more effective and reliable means of depolarizing the left ventricle by either directly recruiting more myocardial tissue simultaneously or ensuring the depolarizing wave front bypasses regions of scar to reach the other viable sites.

In multisite left ventricular (LV) pacing, two LV leads and one right ventricular (RV) lead are inserted. One LV lead is inserted into a lateral or posterolateral branch of the CS and the second LV lead is implanted into another lateral or anterolateral branch of the CS or into the middle cardiac vein, aiming for maximal orthogonal separation between the pacing sites of the three ventricular leads. Two left ventricular leads are paired together using a twin bipolar-to-bipolar connector. The paired leads are connected to the LV port and the unpaired right ventricular lead is connected to the RV port (Fig. 14.1).

Lenarczyk et al. have done a retrospective analysis of clinical and procedural data on 27 patients receiving three ventricular leads and found improved exercise capacity and left ventricular ejection fraction (LVEF) compared with a group with a conventional biventricular (BiV) system.[4] Rogers and his colleagues in a randomized double-blind cross-over trial have shown better outcome in patients with triple-site ventricular pacing (two LV leads and one RV lead or one LV lead and two RV leads where second LV lead implantation was not possible) in comparison to conventional biventricular pacing in term of 6 minutes walk test, reduction in LV end systolic volume and increased LVEF.[5]

However, Shetty and his colleagues have shown that multisite pacing in the heart from three, four, or five sites simultaneously does not appear to confer an advantage over conventional DDD biventricular (BiV) pacing with an optimal LV coronary

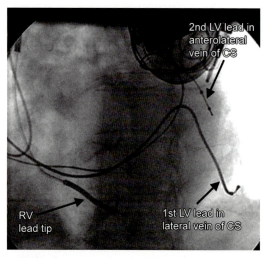

Fig. 14.1 Triple site ventricular pacing: Left anterior oblique (LAO) Fluoroscopic view: RV ICD lead in RV apex, 1st LV lead in lateral vein of coronary sinus and 2nd LV lead in anterolateral vein of coronary sinus

sinus (CS) site.[6] DDD LV endocardial pacing appears to confer a similar benefit to optimal CS site pacing. Pacing the heart from more than two sites simultaneously does, however, appear to be safe acutely and multi-site pacing using a Quartet lead appears to give rise to a similar acute hemodynamic response to pacing from two separate LV CS sites.

Triple-site ventricular pacing is technically difficult and the favorable coronary sinus anatomy is very essential for successful multisite ventricular pacing. With the development of multipolar pacing leads, improved delivery systems, and increasingly sophisticated programming capabilities of CRT devices, it is possible that multisite pacing can be done from the quadripolar lead from the single coronary sinus branch. The advantages of a quadripolar leads are:
- Avoidance of phrenic stimulation (LV stimulation can be done from the proximal poles).
- Pacing from various vectors (programmable) gives different QRS morphology. We have to obtain the vector which gives narrowest QRS complex during LV stimulation and thereby gives the best electrical resynchronization.
- Multisite LV pacing with the lead in a single coronary sinus branch can be done by simultaneous LV stimulation from two vectors.

The quadripolar LV lead provides pace/sense capability from 4 electrodes (tip and 3 rings):
- Distal tip (D1),
- Mid 2 (M2),
- Mid 3 (M3),
- Proximal 4 (P4)

Figure 14.2 shows the sequence of 4 poles at lead tip and arrangement of their connection sites at the proximal end of the lead. Figure 14.3 demonstrates quadripolar leads from various pacemaker companies.

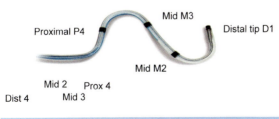
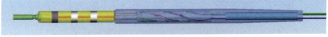

Fig. 14.2 Quadripolar LV lead: Sequence of pacing poles and their connection slot

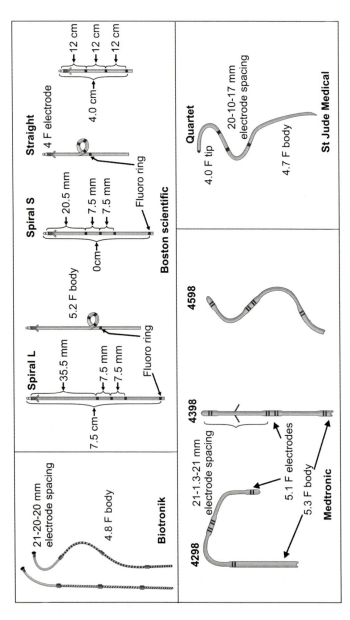

Fig. 14.3 Quadripolar LV lead from different companies

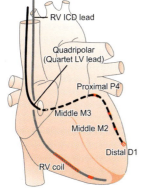

Vectors	Cathode to Anode
Vector 1	Distal D1 to Middle M2
Vector 2	Distal D1 to Proximal P4
Vector 3	Distal D1 to RV Coil
Vector 4	Middle M2 to Proximal P4
Vector 5	Middle M2 to RV Coil
Vector 6	Middle M3 to Middle M2
Vector 7	Middle M3 to Proximal P4
Vector 8	Middle M3 to RV Coil
Vector 9	Proximal P4 to Middle M2
Vector 10	Proximal P4 to RV Coil

Fig. 14.4 Programmable vectors in a St Jude quadripolar CRT-D system

With quadripolar LV lead from St. Jude Medical (Quartet) allow us to program 10 vectors (Fig. 14.4).

Quadripolar LV lead in a CRT-D system from Medtronic has 16 programmable vectors (Fig. 14.5). It has an interpolar distance of 21 mm between distal 1 and mid 2, 1.3 mm between mid 2 and mid 3, and 21 mm between mid 3 and proximal 4. Short bipolar spacing between mid 2 and mid 3 helps in less phrenic nerve stimulation occurrence (Figs 14.6A to C). Shorter electrode spacing results in significantly higher phrenic nerve thresholds and lower phrenic nerve stimulation occurrence and maximize phrenic nerve stimulation management, both at implantation and at follow-up, while allowing individual targeting of the LV pacing site.[7]

Steroid on every electrode improves pacing thresholds by reducing pacing energy significantly and increased pacemaker longevity. Programmable vectors maximizes flexibility and reverse polarity benefits. Decreased pacing energy means increased margin between LV pacing threshold and phrenic nerve capture.

MultiPoint Pacing (MPP) is a new innovation from St Jude Medical in heart failure treatment. This new type of heart failure therapy delivers two LV pulses from the Quartet (quadripolar) LV lead per pacing cycle resulting in a more uniform ventricular contraction shown to improve therapy response (Fig. 14.7).[7,8] The benefits of uniform ventricular contraction are:
- Augmented contractility
- Improved transventricular activation time
- Reduced LV dyssynchrony.

Multipoint pacing involves pacing the left ventricle (LV) from 2 vectors (LV1 and LV2) with a programmable delay (Delay 1) of 5 to 40 msec followed by pacing the right ventricle (RV) with

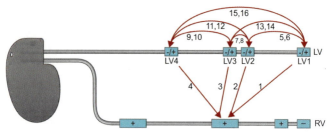

Fig. 14.5 Programmable 16 vectors in a Medtronic CRT-D system

another programmable delay of 5 to 40 msec (Delay 2). Two LV vectors can be defined on anatomical basis as **Apical** (LV1) and **Basal** (LV2) or based on electrical delay from RV pacing to LV sensing and termed as **Early** (LV1) or **Late** (LV2). This ultimately results in triple site ventricular stimulation with programmable delays. In order to allow the MPP feature to be turned **on**, a patient needs to have **at least 2 vectors from different groups** (with different cathodes) that fulfills the following conditions with the capture threshold of less than 4.5 V at 0.5 ms pulse width without any phrenic nerve stimulation (PNS) at 1 Volt above the pacing capture threshold.

Multipoint pacing improves hemodynamics by:
- Improves acute systolic function over single-site pacing in 80% of patients in a study assessing hemodynamics with dP/dt max.[9]
- Reduces mechanical dyssynchrony as assessed by echo tissue Doppler imaging in 12-segment LV contraction time in more patients than single-site pacing alone.[10]
- May improve CRT responders rate: After 3 months, 22% more patients are classified as responders than with traditional Bi-V single-site pacing (73% vs 89%).[11]

So, multipoint pacing may be beneficial to further improve CRT patients' hemodynamics and increase the number of CRT responders. However, it is questionable that whether multipoint pacing can induce multiple reentry mechanism in future.

Adaptive CRT Algorithm

In patients with sinus rhythm and normal atrioventricular (AV) conduction, pacing only the left ventricle with appropriate AV intervals in comparison to conventional biventricular (BiV) pacing can result in similar and sometimes superior improvement of left ventricular (LV) function and right ventricular (RV) function.[12,13] Optimization of the AV and VV intervals during BiV pacing is an option to maximize the

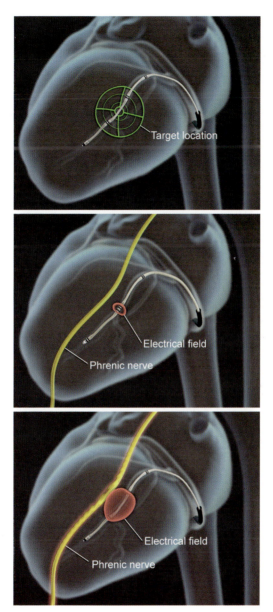

Figs 14.6A to C Mechanism of avoidance of phrenic stimulation. (A) Target location of LV stimulation; (B) Wide spacing between 2nd and 3rd pole increases chance of phrenic stimulation; (C) Short inter-electrode distance decreases electrical field and reduces chance of phrenic nerve capture

positive effects of CRT. Adaptive CRT is an algorithm introduced by Medtronic Co. has been developed to further increase in the CRT response. This algorithm provides RV-synchronized LV pacing when AV conduction is normal, or BiV pacing

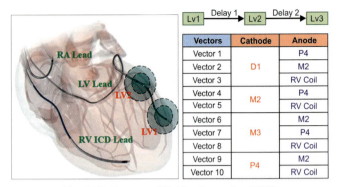

Fig. 14.7 Concept of Multi-point pacing (MPP)

otherwise.[14] The main two logics behind this algorithm are: 1) avoidance of RV pacing and greater recruitment of intrinsic conduction in patients with normal conduction into the right ventricle and 2) dynamic adjustment of AV and VV delays based on the electrical conduction intervals. Among patients with intact AV conduction, LV dysfunction, and a narrow QRS, it is well accepted that RV pacing is to be avoided as it results in a higher incidence of HF, presumably due to iatrogenic ventricular dyssynchrony caused by RV pacing.[15] So, speculatively substituting intrinsic RV activation with RV-paced activation may also be unnecessary in patients with left bundle branch block and LV dysfunction. RV pacing can have deleterious effects on RV function. RV pacing, whether alone or as part of BiV pacing, produced RV activation delays, which are avoided with LV only pacing. The algorithm also adjusts AV and VV delays on the basis of periodic automatic evaluation of intrinsic conduction intervals. The algorithm is intended to provide ambulatory CRT optimization and allow more physiologic ventricular activation and greater device longevity in patients with normal AV conduction by reducing unnecessary RV pacing.

If a patient has LBBB with normal conduction to the RV, LV pacing is sufficient for cardiac resynchronization. Device AV delay would be adjusted based on resynchronization with the RV activation. On the other hand if a patient has first or advanced degree AV block in addition to LBBB, bi-ventricular pacing would be used to restore both atrioventricular and interventricular synchrony (Fig. 14.8). AV delay would be chosen based on considerations of LV filling. Specifically, it would be adjusted to pace after the end of the P-wave. Since conduction can change with time, the algorithm would periodically re-evaluate it and adjust the pacing settings.

Newer Advances

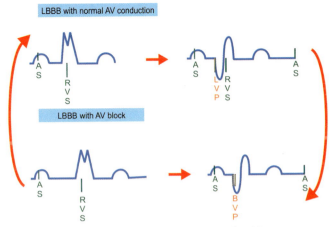

Fig. 14.8 The concept of AdaptivCRT algorithm

The algorithm first assesses intrinsic conduction every minute and determines if a patient's AV interval is normal or prolonged. Based on that assessment it determines the pacing method to be either Adaptive LV, for normal AV intervals or Adaptive BiV, for prolonged AV intervals (Fig. 14.9). Then it optimizes timing. For Adaptive LV pacing, the algorithm will determine when to pre-pace the LV to synchronize with the intrinsic RV activation. For Adaptive BiV pacing, it will optimize AV/VV delays based on AV interval, P wave and QRS waveform width measurements.

Adaptive LV pacing leverages intrinsic RV conduction by pre-pacing the LV to synchronize with intrinsic RV activation. It promotes physiologic pacing for patients with normal AV intervals, increases longevity, and improves in clinical outcomes for patients with normal AV intervals. It assesses automatically and continuously AV and VV delays. Automatically adapts as needed to changes in conduction status and provides optimal CRT settings and maximizes CRT benefit by optimizing ventricular filling and ejection. There is no need for time consuming manual echo optimization.

The Adaptive BiV setting provides biventricular pacing with automatically optimized CRT parameters based on the patient's activity level and conduction status. The optimized CRT parameters are the AV delays, VV delays, and ventricular pacing configuration (meaning which chamber is paced first). This CRT pacing method is programmed by selecting the 'Adaptive BiV' CRT setting. Adaptive BiV will also operate within the 'Adaptive BiV and LV' setting when the patient's heart rate rises, when LV capture loss is suspected, or most commonly when the patient's AV conduction lengthens (Figs 14.10 and 14.11). Adaptive BiV maximizes CRT benefit

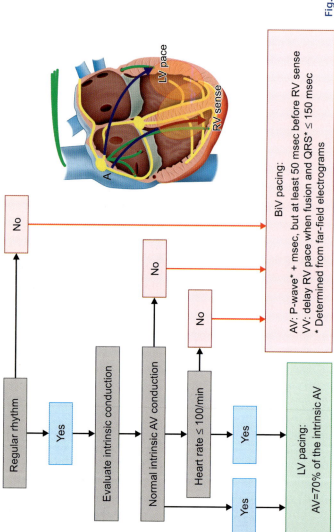

Fig. 14.9 The mechanism of AdaptivCRT algorithm

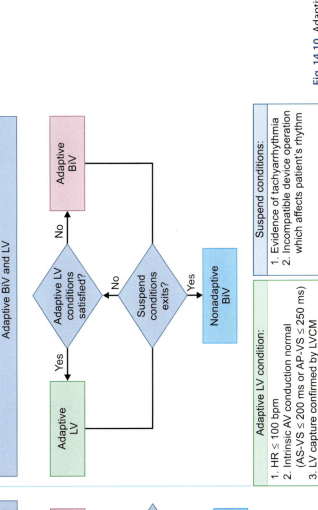

Fig. 14.10 AdaptivCRT programmable settings

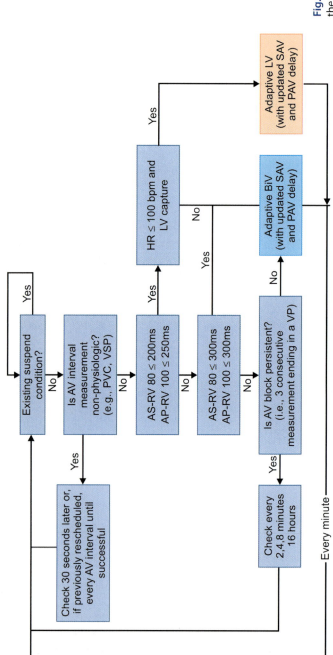

Fig. 14.11 Calculation of the SAV and PAV interval

by optimizing the programmed parameters between device checks.

Adaptive CRT measures the **AV interval once per minute**. For one beat, the sensed AV and paced **AV delays are extended to 300 msec** to allow time for an RV sense to occur after either an atrial pace or an atrial sensed event. During this beat, the device measures the duration from the atrial sensed or paced event to the following right ventricular sensed event. The AV interval measurement is defined as:

- **Normal,** if the sensed AV interval is **80 ms to ≤ 200 msec** or the paced AV interval is **100 to ≤ 250 msec.**
- **Prolonged,** if the SAV interval is **> 200 to ≤ 300 msec** or the paced AV interval **> 250 to ≤ 300 msec.**
- **Non-physiologic**, if the sensed AV interval is **< 80 msec**, the paced AV interval is **< 100 msec** or if the measured AV interval contains a PVC, PAC, NCAP, VSP.

The AV delays for Adaptive LV operation are calculated as approximately 70% of the intrinsic AV interval with the minimum pre-excitation of the LV with respect to the RV sensing by 40 msec. The aim is to pace ~30 msec after the end of the P-wave but at least 50 msec before onset of the intrinsic QRS, as ~50% of intrinsic AV delay, but at least 30 msec before the intrinsic QRS and to pace 40 msec before the onset of the intrinsic QRS. The interval from VS to QRSend of 90 msec would correspond to the surface ECG QRS duration of 90 + 40 =130 msec. V sense - to- QRS is set to the default value of 110 ms if VS-QRS measurement is outside of the 50-180 msec range.

Operating values for Adaptive LV vs Adaptive BiV		
AdaptivCRT operation	Parameter	Operating value range (msec)
Adaptive LV	Sensed AV Delay	80–140
	Paced AV Delay	100–170
Adaptive BiV	Sensed AV Delay	80–140
	Paced AV Delay	100–180
	V-V Pace Delay	RV → LV 20 to LV → RV 40

Adaptive CRT automatically optimizes every patient with no negative impact to battery longevity. In addition the reduction of RV pacing when operating in Adaptive LV, results in increased longevity - up to one year. Viva-XT CRT-D device by Medtronic has incorporated this algorithm.

The Adaptive CRT trial showed that this algorithm results in 44% absolute reduction in the percentage of RV pacing and optimization provided by the this algorithm is safe and non-inferior to echocardiographic optimization with respect to clinical, structural, and functional improvement at 6-month follow up post-procedure.[16] However, further investigation of clinical outcomes over longer follow-up is needed to support the benefit of synchronized LV pacing.

REFERENCES

1. Bleeker GB, Bax JJ, Fung JW, van der Wall EE, Zhang Q, Schalij MJ, et al. Clinical versus echocardiographic parameters to assess response to cardiac resynchronization therapy. Am J Cardiol. 2006;97:260-3.
2. Bleeker GB, Kaandorp TA, Lamb HJ, Boersma E, Steendijk P, de RA, et al. Effect of posterolateral scar tissue on clinical and echocardiographic improvement after cardiac resynchronization therapy. Circulation. 2006; 113:969-76.
3. Auricchio A, Fantoni C, Regoli F, Carbucicchio C, Goette A, Geller C, et al. Characterization of left ventricular activation in patients with heart failure and left bundle-branch block. Circulation. 2004;109:1133-9.
4. Lenarczyk R, Kowalski O, Kukulski T, Pruszkowska-Skrzep P, Sokal A, Szulik M, et al. Mid-term outcomes of triple-site vs. conventional cardiac resynchronization therapy: a preliminary study. Int J Cardiol. 2009;133:87-94.
5. Dominic PS Rogers, Pier D Lambiase, Martin D Lowe, Anthony WC Chow. A randomized double-blind crossover trial of tri-ventricular versus biventricular pacing in heart failure European Journal of Heart Failure. 2012;14:495-505.
6. Shetty AK, Sohal M, Chen Z, Ginks MR, Bostock J, Amraoui S, et al. A comparison of left ventricular endocardial, multisite, and multipolar epicardial cardiac resynchronization: an acute haemodynamic and electroanatomical study. Europace. 2014;16:873-9.
7. Forleo, G et al. Left ventricular pacing with a new quadripolar transvenous lead for CRT: early results of a prospective comparison with conventional implantation outcomes. Heart Rhythm. 2011;8:31-7.
8. Ryu K, Ghanem RN, Khrestian CM, et al. Comparative effects of single- and linear triple-site rapid bipolar pacing on atrial activation in canine models. Am J Physiol Heart Circ Physiol. 2005;289(1):H374-84.
9. Fagagnini A, Martino A, Minati M, et al. Quadripolar left ventricular pacing for cardiac resynchronization therapy: Acute echocardiographic evaluation. Heart Rhythm. 2012; 9(5):S373; Abstract PO05-24.
10. Thibault B, Dubuc M, Khairy P, Guerra PG, Macle L, Rivard L, et al. Acute hemodynamic comparison of multisite and biventricular pacing with a quadripolar left ventricular lead. Europace. 2013; 15(7):984-91.
11. Pappone C, et al. Improvement in 3-month echocardiographic response with multisite left ventricular pacing in cardiac resynchronization therapy patients. HRS 2013 Poster session PO02. May 9, 2013.
12. Kass DA, Chen CH, Curry C, et al. Improved left ventricular mechanics from acute VDD pacing in patients with dilated

cardiomyopathy and ventricular conduction delay. Circulation. 1999;99:1567-73.
13. Lee KL, Burnes JE, Mullen TJ, Hettrick DA, Tse HF, Lau CP. Avoidance of right ventricular pacing in cardiac resynchronization therapy improves right ventricular hemodynamics in heart failure patients. J Cardiovasc Electrophysiol. 2007;18:497-504.
14. Krum H, Lemke B, Birnie D, et al. A novel algorithm for individualized cardiac resynchronization therapy: rationale and design of the adaptive CRT trial. Am Heart J. 2012;163:747-52.e.1.
15. Wilkoff BL, Cook JR, Epstein AE, et al. Dual-chamber pacing or ventricular backup pacing in patients with an implantable defibrillator: the Dual Chamber and VVI Implantable Defibrillator (DAVID) trial. JAMA. 2002;288:3115-23.
16. David OM, Bernd L, David B, Henry K, et al. Investigation of a novel algorithm for synchronized left ventricular pacing and ambulatory optimization of cardiac resynchronization therapy: Results of the adaptive CRT trial. Heart Rhythm. 2012; 9:1807-14.

Index

Page numbers followed by *f* refer to figure

A

Albert Hyman's artificial pacemaker 2*f*
Anchor balloon technique 240
Angiotensin converting-enzyme inhibitors 164
Angiotensin receptor blockers 164
Anisotropic conduction 21
Annular dilatation 35
Anodal capture 285
Antegrade snare technique 242
Anterior interventricular vein 216, 218*f*
Anti-tachycardia pacing 56
Aorta 62
Artificial pacemaker 2
Atrial auto-decremental ramp 57
Atrial based pacing 37
Atrial burst 57
Atrial fibrillation 35, 52, 58, 298
Atrial myocardium 220
Atrial pacing algorithms 55*f*
Atrial preference pacing 53
Atrial ramp 57
Atrial rate stabilization 53
Atrial tachyarrhythmias 172
Atrioventricular block 167
Atrioventricular conduction 37
Atrioventricular dyssynchrony 184
   measurement of 185*f*
Atrioventricular node 16
Atrioventricular resynchronization 303*f*
Axillary artery 256

B

Bachmann's bundle 56, 151
   pacing 134, 134*f*, 136
Bakken's pacemaker 4
Balloon anchor technique 239
Balloon facilitated delivery 243
Berenstein angiography catheters 236
Biventricular pacing 13, 96, 167, 170, 266, 267, 281*f*
Biventricular stimulation 271*f*, 274*f*, 290*f*
B-natriuretic peptide 163
Buddy wire technique 236, 237*f*
Bundle of His 18

C

Cardiac assist devices 306
Cardiac desynchronization 170
Cardiac memory 31
Cardiac resynchronization 33, 166, 171
   therapy 163, 165, 194, 195*f*, 215, 230, 261, 295, 309
Cardiotoxic triad 164
Cardioverter-defibrillator, implantation of 71
Central fibrous body 92
Conduction delay, types of 202
Congestive heart failure 164
Contact electroanatomical mapping system 19*f*
Contrast-enhanced magnetic resonance 227
Conventional biventricular system 310
Coronary angiogram 221
Coronary balloon anchors pacing lead wire 240*f*
Coronary catheter 232*f*
Coronary sinus 215, 216, 217*f*, 221
   anatomy of 215
   cannulation 231, 232*f*, 233*f*
   diverticulae 221
   ostium 221
   principal tributaries of 216*f*
   venogram 241*f*
Coronary venous system 260
Crista supraventricularis 61

D

Diastolic mitral regurgitation 34
Dual chamber cardiac pacing 41
Dynamic atrial overdrive algorithm 53
Dynamic atrial refractory period 43

E

Echocardiography guided cardiac resynchronization therapy 169
Electrical activation sequence 63, 172
Electrical delay, measurement of 252*f*
Electrical dyssynchrony 23, 28, 138
  mechanism of 22*f*
Electrical inter-lead distance 249
Electrocardiogram 259, 300
Electrogram analysis 304
Endocardial catheter 203
Endocardial pacing 255
  techniques 255
Endocardial sclerosis 23
End-systolic volume 302
Epicardial pacing techniques 253
European Society of Cardiology 170

F

Fat infiltration 23
Fibrosis, chronic 204
Frank-Starling mechanism 29
Frank-Starling relation 28
Functional mitral regurgitation 32
  causes of 306

G

Great cardiac vein 216, 263

H

Heart failure 13, 35, 36, 58, 163, 166, 167
  ambulatory 168
  chronic 296
  dyssynchronous 169
  Society of America 170
Heart Rhythm Society 170
His bundle 16, 17, 90-92, 95, 97, 100
  block 157
  capture 93, 157
  pacing 90, 92, 93, 95, 96
  stimulation, types of 92
His-Purkinje system 22, 23, 93, 174
His-Purkinje tissue 93, 96

I

Implantable defibrillators 36
Implantable pacemaker 6
Incomplete mitral leaflet closure 32
Inferior vena cava 18
Infranodal conduction system 18*f*
Interatrial conduction delay 293
Inter-lead distances, measurement of 248*f*
Internal mammary artery catheter 236
Interpapillary muscle activation delay 33
Interstitial fibrosis 23
Interventricular conduction delay 165
Interventricular dyssynchrony 27, 185
  measurement of 186*f*, 187
Interventricular septum 21*f*, 63, 63*f*, 252*f*
Interventricular synchrony 36
Intracardiac electrocardiograms 252*f*
Intracardiac electrogram 250
Intracardiac noncontact electrograms 175*f*
Intracardiac therapy 1
Intraventricular dyssynchrony 28, 186
Ischemic cardiomyopathy 212, 262
Isovolumic contraction time 187
  prolongation of 33
Isovolumic relaxation time 187

L

Large caliber vein 241*f*
Lateral cardiac veins 218
Lead implantation order 231
Lead stability 97
Left anterior descending artery 62
Left atrium, oblique vein of 21
Left bundle branch 18, 92
  block 20, 95, 138, 165, 179, 202, 203, 210, 212, 231, 261, 276
Left ventricular activation time 202, 250

Left ventricular ejection fraction 169, 196, 310
Left ventricular end-diastolic volume 295
Left ventricular inflow analysis 302
Left ventricular outflow analysis 304
Left ventricular stimulation 271*f*, 273, 289*f*
Left ventricular systolic dysfunction 159
Left ventricular systolic function 159
Left ventricular transmural conduction 173
Lengthened diastolic filling time 194
Lidwell's efforts 1

M

Masquerading bundle branch block 154
Maximum left ventricular activation time, measurement of 208
Middle cardiac vein 216, 219, 263
Mini-thoracotomy 253
Mitral regurgitation 32, 194
Mode selection trial 36, 41
Multipoint pacing 313, 314
 concept of 316*f*
Multi-slice computed tomography 224
Myocardial capture 95
Myocardial contrast echocardiography 227
Myocardial ischemia 299
Myocardial muscular tissue 18
Myocardial performance index 187
 evaluation of 188*f*
Myocardial scar burden 204, 210, 225
Myocardium 95
Myofiber hypertrophy 23

N

National Health and Nutrition Examination Survey Criteria 163
National Research Council of Canada 2
New York Heart Association 166, 295

Nonischemic cardiomyopathy, magnetic resonance imaging of 206*f*

O

Optimal physiological pacing 159, 162

P

Para-Hisian pacing 92, 93, 97, 157
Percutaneous coronary intervention 234
Phrenic stimulation 311
Physiological pacing, Canadian trial of 36
Positron emission tomography 193
Posterior anterior fluoroscopic images 238*f*
Posterior ventricular vein 219
Posterolateral vein 241*f*, 242*f*
Postpaced electron microscopy 24
Premature atrial complex 52
Pulmonary valve 61*f*
Purkinje system 18, 20, 22
Purkinje-myocardial junction 18, 151, 165

Q

QRS score 210, 212

R

Reducing atrial fibrillation burden, strategies of 52
Resynchronization therapy 162
Retrograde buddy wire technique 237
Retrograde snare technique 243
Reverse mode switch 50
Right bundle branch 18, 20, 92
 block 202
Right ventricle contraction 20
Right ventricular apex 17, 41, 92
Right ventricular outflow tract 19, 62
Right ventricular septal pacing 60
Right ventricular stimulation 271*f*, 273*f*
Ritter method 303*f*
Robotically assisted surgery 254
Rotational coronary venous angiography 224

S

Screening techniques, evaluation of 169
Septal hypertrophy, asymmetric 23
Septal hypoperfusion 23
Septal pacing 159
Septal ventricular pacing 93
Septomarginal trabeculation 61
Septoparietal trabeculation 61, 63, 63*f*
Severe functional mitral regurgitation 182
Severe left ventricular systolic dysfunction 212
Severe sinus node disease 157
Single chamber ventricular pacing 36
Single photon emission computed tomography 193, 227
Sinus node dysfunction 36
Small cardiac vein 216
Speckle tracking echocardiography 65
Subclavian artery 256
Superior vena cava 18
Swan-Ganz catheter 72
Systolic heart failure 138
Systolic left ventricular dysfunction 166

T

Tei-index 187
Thebesian veins 215
Tissue Doppler imaging 65, 183, 189

Transesophageal echocardiography 254
Transitional zone index 76, 77*f*
Transseptal conduction 173
Transvenous access 255
Tricuspid annulus 98
Tricuspid valve, anterior papillary muscle of 61
Triple site ventricular pacing 210*f*
Triple stimulation 286

V

Valvular insufficiency 64
Vasodilator therapy 163
Vena contracta 182
Venography 221
Ventricular activation time 207
Ventricular asynchrony 37
Ventricular dilatation 23
Ventricular electrogram 268*f*
Ventricular fusion 260, 290
Ventricular intrinsic preference 47, 48*f*
Ventricular synchrony 36
Video assisted thoracoscopy 254

W

Wolff-Parkinson-White syndrome 260